ROGRESS IN CLINICAL AND BIOLOGICAL RESEARCH

RECENT TITLES

Vol 231: **Detection of Bacterial Endotoxins With the Limulus Amebocyte Lysate Test,** Stanley W. Watson, Jack Levin, Thomas J. Novitsky, *Editors*

Vol 232: **Enzymology and Molecular Biology of Carbonyl Metabolism: Aldehyde Dehydrogenase, Aldo-Keto Reductase, and Alcohol Dehydrogenase**, Henry Weiner, T. Geoffrey Flynn, *Editors*

Vol 233: **Developmental and Comparative Immunology,** Edwin L. Cooper, Claude Langlet, Jacques Bierne, *Editors*

Vol 234: **The Hepatitis Delta Virus and Its Infection**, Mario Rizzetto, John L. Gerin, Robert H. Purcell, *Editors*

Vol 235: **Preclinical Safety of Biotechnology Products Intended for Human Use,** Charles E. Graham, *Editor*

ol 236: **First Vienna Shock Forum,** Günther chlag, Heinz Redl, *Editors*. Published in two lumes: Part A: *Pathophysiological Role of ediators and Mediator Inhibitors in Shock.* rt B: *Monitoring and Treatment of Shock.*

l 237: **The Use of Transrectal Ultrasound in e Diagnosis and Management of Prostate ancer,** Fred Lee, Richard McLeary, *Editors*

l 238: **Avian Immunology,** W.T. Weber, .L. Ewert, *Editors*

l 239: **Current Concepts and Approaches to e Study of Prostate Cancer,** Donald S. offey, Nicholas Bruchovsky, William A. ardner, Jr., Martin I. Resnick, James P. Karr, *ditors*

ol 240: **Pathophysiological Aspects of Sickle ell Vaso-Occlusion,** Ronald L. Nagel, *Editor*

ol 241: **Genetics and Alcoholism,** H. Werner oedde, Dharam P. Agarwal, *Editors*

Vol 242: **Prostaglandins in Clinical Research,** Helmut Sinzinger, Karsten Schrör, *Editors*

Vol 243: **Prostate Cancer,** Gerald P. Murphy, Saad Khoury, Réne Küss, Christian Chatelain, Louis Denis, *Editors*. Published in two volumes: Part A: *Research, Endocrine Treatment, and Histopathology.* Part B: *Imaging Techniques, Radiotherapy, Chemotherapy, and Management Issues*

Vol 244: **Cellular Immunotherapy of Cancer,** Robert L. Truitt, Robert P. Gale, Mortimer M. Bortin, *Editors*

Vol 245: **Regulation and Contraction of Smooth Muscle,** Marion J. Siegman, Andrew P. Somlyo, Newman L. Stephens, *Editors*

Vol 246: **Oncology and Immunology of Down Syndrome,** Ernest E. McCoy, Charles J. Epstein, *Editors*

Vol 247: **Degenerative Retinal Disorders: Clinical and Laboratory Investigations,** Joe G. Hollyfield, Robert E. Anderson, Matthew M.LaVail, *Editors*

Vol 248: **Advances in Cancer Control: The War on Cancer—15 Years of Progress,** Paul F. Engstrom, Lee E. Mortenson, Paul N. Anderson, *Editors*

Vol 249: **Mechanisms of Signal Transduction by Hormones and Growth Factors,** Myles C. Cabot, Wallace L. McKeehan, *Editors*

Vol 250: **Kawasaki Disease,** Stanford T. Shulman, *Editor*

Vol 251: **Developmental Control of Globin Gene Expression,** George Stamatoyannopoulos, Arthur W. Nienhuis, *Editors*

Vol 252: **Cellular Calcium and Phosphate Transport in Health and Disease,** Felix Bronner, Meinrad Peterlik, *Editors*

Vol 253: **Model Systems in Neurotoxicology: Alternative Approaches to Animal Testing,** Abraham Shahar, Alan M. Goldberg, *Editors*

Vol 254: **Genetics and Epithelial Cell Dysfunction in Cystic Fibrosis,** John R. Riordan, Manuel Buchwald, *Editors*

Vol 255: **Recent Aspects of Diagnosis and Treatment of Lipoprotein Disorders: Impact on Prevention of Atherosclerotic Diseases,** Kurt Widhalm, Herbert K. Naito, *Editors*

Vol 256: **Advances in Pigment Cell Research,** Joseph T. Bagnara, *Editor*

Vol 257: **Electromagnetic Fields and Neurobehavioral Function,** Mary Ellen O'Connor, Richard H. Lovely, *Editors*

Vol 258: **Membrane Biophysics III: Biological Transport,** Mumtaz A. Dinno, William McD. Armstrong, *Editors*

Vol 259: **Nutrition, Growth, and Cancer,** George P. Tryfiates, Kedar N. Prasad, *Editors*

Vol 260: **EORTC Genitourinary Group Monograph 4: Management of Advanced Cancer of Prostate and Bladder,** Philip H. Smith, Michele Pavone-Macaluso, *Editors*

Vol 261: **Nicotine Replacement: A Critical Evaluation,** Ovide F. Pomerleau, Cynthia S. Pomerleau, *Editors*

Vol 262: **Hormones, Cell Biology, and Cancer: Perspectives and Potentials,** W. David Hankins, David Puett, *Editors*

Vol 263: **Mechanisms in Asthma: Pharmacology, Physiology, and Management,** Carol L. Armour, Judith L. Black, *Editors*

Vol 264: **Perspectives in Shock Research,** Robert F. Bond, *Editor*

Vol 265: **Pathogenesis and New Approaches to the Study of Noninsulin-Dependent Diabetes Mellitus,** Albert Y. Chang, Arthur R. Diani, *Editors*

Vol 266: **Growth Factors and Other Aspects of Wound Healing: Biological and Clinical Implications,** Adrian Barbul, Eli Pines, Michael Caldwell, Thomas K. Hunt, *Editors*

Vol 267: **Meiotic Inhibition: Molecular Control of Meiosis,** Florence P. Haseltine, *Editor*

Vol 268: **The Na^+,K^+-Pump,** Jens C. Skou, Jens G. Nørby, Arvid B. Maunsbach, Mikael Esmann, *Editors*. Published in two volumes: Part A: *Molecular Aspects*. Part B: *Cellular Aspects*.

Vol 269: **EORTC Genitourinary Group Monograph 5: Progress and Controversies in Oncological Urology II,** Fritz H. Schröder, Jan G.M. Klijn, Karl H. Kurth, Herbert M. Pinedo, Ted A.W. Splinter, Herman J. de Voogt, *Editors*

Vol 270: **Cell-Free Analysis of Membrane Traffic,** D. James Morré, Kathryn E. Howell, Geoffrey M.W. Cook, W. Howard Evans, *Editors*

Vol 271: **Advances in Neuroblastoma Research 2,** Audrey E. Evans, Giulio J. D'Angio, Alfred G. Knudson, Robert C. Seeger, *Editors*

Vol 272: **Bacterial Endotoxins: Pathophysiological Effects, Clinical Significance, and Pharmacological Control,** Jack Levin, Harry R. Büller, Jan W. ten Cate, Sander J.H. van Deventer, Augueste Sturk, *Editors*

Vol 273: **The Ion Pumps: Structure, Function, and Regulation,** Wilfred D. Stein, *Editor*

Vol 274: **Oxidases and Related Redox Systems,** Tsoo E. King, Howard S. Mason, Martin Morrison, *Editors*

Vol 275: **Electrophysiology of the Sinoatrial and Atrioventricular Nodes,** Todor N. Mazgalev, Leonard S. Dreifus, Eric L. Michelson, *Editors*

Vol 276: **Prediction of Response to Cancer Therapy,** Thomas C. Hall, *Editor*

Vol 277: **Advances in Urologic Oncology,** Nasser Javadpour, Gerald P. Murphy, *Editors*

Vol 278: **Advances in Cancer Control: Cancer Control Research and the Emergence of the Oncology Product Line,** Paul F. Engstrom, Paul N. Anderson, Lee E. Mortenson, *Editors*

Vol 279: **Basic and Clinical Perspectives of Colorectal Polyps and Cancer,** Glenn Steele, Jr., Randall W. Burt, Sidney J. Winawer, James P. Karr, *Editors*

Vol 280: **Plant Flavonoids in Biology and Medicine II: Biochemical, Cellular, and Medicinal Properties,** Vivian Cody, Elliott Middleton, Jr., Jeffrey B. Harborne, Alain Beretz, *Editors*

Vol 281: **Transplacental Effects on Fetal Health,** Dante G. Scarpelli, George Migaki, *Editors*

Please contact the publisher for information about previous titles in this series.

Transplacental Effects on Fetal Health

Transplacental Effects on Fetal Health

Proceedings of a Symposium Held in Bethesda, Maryland, November 5–6, 1987

Editors

Dante G. Scarpelli
Department of Pathology
Northwestern University Medical School
Chicago, Illinois

George Migaki
The Registry of Comparative Pathology
Armed Forces Institute of Pathology
Washington, D.C.
and
Universities Associated for Research and Education in Pathology, Inc.
Bethesda, Maryland

ALAN R. LISS, INC. • NEW YORK

Address all Inquiries to the Publisher
Alan R. Liss, Inc., 41 East 11th Street, New York, NY 10003

Printed in the United States of America

Library of Congress Cataloging-in-Publication Data

Main entry under title:

Transplacental Effects on Fetal Health

ISBN 0-8451-5131-2 LC 88-12956

Contents

Contributors

Charles A. Anderson, Department of Pathology, University of California, Davis, Davis, CA 95616; present address: Department of Safety Assessment, Merck, Sharp, and Dohme Research Laboratories, West Point, PA 19486 **[59]**

S. Bolin, Virology Group, National Animal Disease Center, Ames, IA 50010 **[49]**

J.P. Dubey, Animal Parasitology Institute, Agricultural Research Service, Protozoan Diseases Laboratory, U.S. Department of Agriculture, Beltsville, MD 20705 **[153]**

Ronald Fayer, Animal Parasitology Institute, Agricultural Research Service, U.S. Department of Agriculture, Beltsville, MD 20705 **[153]**

Ronnie Guillet, Department of Psychology, University of Rochester, Rochester, NY 14627 **[265]**

James E. Haddow, Research Center for Perinatal and Child Health, Foundation for Blood Research, Scarborough, ME 04074 **[289]**

Paula K. Haddow, Research Center for Perinatal and Child Health, Foundation for Blood Research, Scarborough, ME 04074 **[289]**

James W. Hanson, Department of Pediatrics, University of Iowa, Iowa City, IA 52242 **[327]**

Robert J. Higgins, Department of Pathology, University of California, Davis, Davis, CA 95616 **[59]**

Lewis B. Holmes, Embryology-Teratology Unit, Children's Service, Massachusetts General Hospital, and Department of Pediatrics, Harvard Medical School, Boston, MA 02114 **[177]**

David M. Judge, Pathology Department, Baylor College of Medicine, Houston, TX 77030 **[87]**

Carol K. Kellogg, Department of Psychology, University of Rochester, Rochester, NY 14627 **[265]**

George J. Knight, Radioimmunoassay Laboratory, Research Center for Perinatal and Child Health, Foundation for Blood Research, Scarborough, ME 04074 **[289]**

Edward J. Lammer, California Birth Defects Monitoring Program, Berkeley, CA 94703 **[193]**

Harvey L. Levy, Department of Neurology and Joseph P. Kennedy Jr. Laboratories, Harvard Medical School and Massachusetts General Hospital, Boston, MA 02114 **[227]**

The numbers in brackets are the opening page numbers of the contributors' articles.

N. James MacLachlan, Departments of Microbiology, Pathology, and Parasitology, School of Veterinary Medicine, North Carolina State University, Raleigh, NC 27606 **[33]**

Neil J. MacLusky, Department of Obstetrics and Gynecology, Yale University Medical School, New Haven, CT 06510 **[243]**

V. Moennig, Institute for Virology, Tierärztliche Hochschule Hannover, Hannover, D-3000, Federal Republic of Germany **[49]**

Hugo W. Moser, Kennedy Institute, Baltimore, MD 21205 **[339]**

Richard L. Naeye, Department of Pathology, Milton S. Hershey Medical Center, Pennsylvania State University, Hershey, PA 17033 **[73,165]**

Herbert L. Needleman, Department of Psychiatry, School of Medicine, University of Pittsburgh, Pittsburgh, PA 15213 **[279]**

Bennie I. Osburn, Department of Pathology, School of Veterinary Medicine, University of California, Davis, Davis, CA 95616 **[15,33,59]**

Mary Lou Oster-Granite, Departments of Physiology and Neuroscience, Developmental Genetics Laboratory, The Johns Hopkins University School of Medicine, Baltimore, MD 21205 **[203]**

Glenn E. Palomaki, Research Center for Perinatal and Child Health, Foundation for Blood Research, Scarborough, ME 04074 **[289]**

J.F.L. Pohlenz, Institute for Pathology, Tierärztliche Hochschule Hannover, Hannover, D-3000, Federal Republic of Germany **[49]**

Patricia A. Quinn, Department of Bacteriology, The Hospital for Sick Children, Toronto, Ontario, Canada, M5G 1X8 **[107]**

George H. Sack, Jr., Departments of Medicine, Biological Chemistry, and Pediatrics, The Johns Hopkins University School of Medicine and the John F. Kennedy Institute, Baltimore, MD 21205 **[303]**

Mary M. Sawyer, Department of Pathology, University of California, Davis, Davis, CA 95616 **[59]**

Dante G. Scarpelli, Department of Pathology, Northwestern University Medical School, Chicago, IL 60611 **[xi,xiii]**

John L. Sever, Infectious Diseases Branch, National Institute of Neurological and Communicative Disorders and Stroke, National Institutes of Health, Bethesda, MD 20892 **[3]**

Marion E. Smith, Department of Neurology, Veterans Administration Medical Center, Palo Alto, CA 94304 **[59]**

Elizabeth J. Thomson, Department of Pediatrics, University of Iowa, Iowa City, IA 52242 **[327]**

G. Trautwein, Institute for Pathology, Tierärztliche Hochschule Hannover, Hannover, D-3000, Federal Republic of Germany **[49]**

Preface

This volume contains contributions presented at the Symposium on Transplacental Effects on Fetal Health, held at the National Institutes of Health, Bethesda, Maryland, November 5–6, 1987. The growing numbers of natural and manmade hazards that can impinge on the developing fetus and cause damage demand not only efforts toward their elimination or control but also a fuller understanding of processes involved in the numerous calamitous developmental effects that result.

The precise cellular and molecular mechanisms responsible for most developmental defects remain to be elucidated, but considerable details of their nature and pathogenesis are in hand. It is hoped this book will serve to enhance communication with a larger audience of basic and clinical scientists engaged in the study, treatment, and prevention of fetal diseases and defects induced by exogenous and endogenous factors during pregnancy.

Dante G. Scarpelli, M.D., Ph.D.

Acknowledgments

The Registry of Comparative Pathology is supported in part by Public Health Service grant RR00301 from the Division of Research Resources, National Institutes of Health, United States Department of Health and Human Services under the auspices of Universities Associated for Research and Education in Pathology, Inc.

Introduction

Our preoccupation with fetal health continues to intensify as it becomes increasingly apparent that the developing embryo and fetus are exquisitely sensitive to the myriad adverse natural and synthetic substances and infectious agents in the external environment, as well as endogenous hazards such as the metabolic disturbance associated with maternal diseases such as diabetes, and more rarely, inborn errors. Recent studies suggest that even the preimplantation embryo, once considered to be relatively immune, may be at risk of damage from exposure to mutagenic chemicals. While the serious consequences for the fetus of maternal exposure to noxious elements have taught us some very important lessons, catastrophes similar to those resulting from maternal infection by rubella, or exposure to thalidomide or diethylstilbestrol will continue to occur. The current tragedy of infant AIDS is a case in point. Because developing tissue systems respond so readily to even relatively minor perturbations, they serve as sensitive monitors of their *milieu*.

It was a pleasure to welcome such a diverse group of active researchers and clinicians to this symposium on "Transplacental Effects on Fetal Health." The goal met by this symposium was the elucidation of new and emerging studies on the deleterious actions of infectious agents, inappropriate metabolites, and various drugs and chemicals on the developing fetus of the human and other mammalian species. This meeting was conceived several years ago by the Scientific Advisory Committee of the Registry of Comparative Pathology of the Armed Forces Institute of Pathology, Drs. Charles C. Capen, Linda C. Cork, Jacob K. Frenkel, T. Carlyle Jones, Robert M. Lewis, John M. Pletcher, Dante G. Scarpelli (Chairman), and Robert W. Wissler, with the assistance of outstanding consultants chosen for their special expertise in this area: Drs. Kurt Benirschke, Richard L. Naeye, Hugo W. Moser, and Bennie I. Osburn.

Special thanks are due Dr. George Migaki, Chief Pathologist for the Registry, for his tireless efforts, especially in compiling this volume, and to his assistants, Mrs. Charmaine Goetz and Rebecca Warner, for attending to the many details that are required to ensure a successful meeting; to my secretary, Nancy Starks, for helping with the task of organizing this meeting, and to Drs. Leo A. Whitehair and William I. Gay from the National Institutes of Health for arranging conference space.

Finally, I wish to express the gratitude of the entire committee to the following benefactors for their generous financial support which made this symposium a reality: The Armed Forces Institute of Pathology; the U.S. Food and Drug Administration; Universities Associated for Research and Education in Pathology, Inc.; Burroughs Wellcome Company, The Coca-Cola Company; Hoffmann-La Roche, Inc.; McNeil Pharmaceutical; Merrell Dow Research Institute; Ortho Pharmaceutical Corporation; Sandoz Research Institute; Smith Kline and French Laboratories; and The Upjohn Company.

Dante G. Scarpelli, M.D., Ph.D.

I. CONGENITAL VIRAL INFECTIONS

Transplacental Effects on Fetal Health, pages 3–13
Published 1988 by Alan R. Liss, Inc.

PERINATAL INFECTIONS AND IMMUNITY

John L. Sever, M.D., Ph.D.
Chief, Infectious Diseases Branch
National Institute of Neurological and
Communicative Disorders and Stroke
National Institutes of Health,
Bethesda, Maryland 20892

INTRODUCTION

A large number of infectious agents can infect the human fetus during the perinatal period and cause significant disease and damage. Some of these agents produce malformations while others may result in severe, sometimes fatal illness in the child. In each case the infectious agent is transmitted from the mother to the fetus, usually by the hematogenous route. The damage is caused by the agent multiplying in the fetal tissues. Both the mother and the fetus produce immunological responses but in many cases the fetus remains chronically infected. Prevention of the perinatal infection is best accomplished by preventing infection of the mother. In some cases, early treatment of the mother or child prevents or reduces the severity of the disease.

Perinatal Infections

A listing of the perinatal infections that are of major importance is given in Table I. Among the viral infections, rubella early in pregnancy results in chronic infection of the child and malformations of the heart, deafness, cataracts, mental retardation and other defects. The HIV virus of AIDS is transmitted to the child in 30 to 50% of the pregnancies of infected mothers. Quite frequently the infected child becomes symptomatic with AIDS while the mother is still completely well and unaware of her infection. The parvovirus B-19 is now recognized to cause abortions and hydrops fetalis. Varicella can cause malformations when the infection occurs early in pregnancy

Table I

Perinatal Infections

Viral	Parasitic
Rubella	Toxoplasmosis
AIDS	Malaria
Parvovirus B-19	
Varicella	**Bacterial**
Cytomegalovirus	
Herpes Simplex	Syphilis
Western equine encephalitis	Group B Streptococci
Venezuelan equine encephalitis	Tuberculosis
Echovirus	Listeriosis
Poliovirus	Leprosy
Smallpox	

and severe, fatal disease in the child when the mother has varicella at term. Primary cytomegalovirus infections occur in about 2% of pregnant women, and 10% of congenitally infected children have impaired hearing and/or mental retardation. Herpes simplex early in pregnancy is now recognized to cause *in utero* infection and damage, and herpes acquired by the child at delivery can result in severe or fatal disease in the newborn. Western equine encephalitis virus can produce encephalitis in newborns. Venezuelan equine encephalitis can result in severe brain damage and death. Echovirus infections can transmit to the fetus and cause fatal liver disease. Polioviruses can be transmitted to the fetus and cause paralytic disease. Smallpox is no longer seen but the virus was shown to infect the fetus and produce disease.

Parasitic infections of importance include toxoplasmosis and malaria. Primary toxoplasmosis infection of the mother can cause severe disease or death of the fetus or newborn. Malaria can also be transmitted to the child.

Bacterial infections with *Tryponema pallidum* have been known to be important causes of fetal damage and special efforts are made to identify and treat infected women. Group B streptococci are now recognized to cause meningitis and sepsis in the newborn. Tuberculosis, listeriosis and leprosy can all be transmitted from infected mothers to their children during pregnancy.

Pathogenesis

Perinatal infections are transmitted from the infected mother to the child. The severity of fetal damage is usually influenced by the time of the maternal infection and the immune status of the mother.

Transmission of Infection To The Fetus. The perinatal infections which are recognized to be important causes of morbidity or mortality in the child all involve transmission of the infection from the mother to the child. This transmission usually occurs across the placenta by the hematogenous route; however, in some cases the infection ascends from the infected vagina or the child is exposed at the time of delivery. Certain infections also can be acquired through infected breast milk.

Time of the Maternal Infection. Examples of the importance of the time of maternal infection are provided by rubella and toxoplasmosis. Rubella in the first trimester results in placental infection in almost all cases; however, only about 60% of the fetuses are infected (Monif et al., 1965). In some cases the virus is present in almost all tissues of the fetus while in other instances only a few organs are infected (Table II). Fetal damage is associated with the time of maternal infection (Figure 1) (South et al., 1985). Cardiac and eye defects occur primarily with rubella in the first two months of pregnancy while hearing loss is associated with infection throughout the first 5 months of gestation. The presence of rubella virus in certain tissues appears to interfere with cell growth at key points in morphogenesis, thus causing the defects of the "Congenital Rubella Syndrome" (CRS). Generalized fetal infection can also cause systemic disease including hepatosplenomegaly, encephalitis, pneumonia and death. Maternal infection in the last trimester of pregnancy may be transmitted to the fetus but there is no evidence of fetal damage with these infections. Recent studies have shown that there are also delayed manifestations of the CRS including the development of diabetes in approximately 20% of children during the second decade of life (Sever et al., 1985).

Table II. Recovery of rubella virus from individual organs

Organs	*Patients*							
	M. E.	*M. T.*	*B. C.*	*B. K.*	*E. H.*	*J. L.*	*L. K.*	*O. G.*
Brain	+*	–†	–	+	–	–	–	–
Eye	+	–	–	+	–	–	–	–
Inner ear	+	–	–	+	–	–	–	–
Thymus	+	–	–	+	–	–	–	–
Heart	+	–	–	+	–	–	+	–
Lungs	+	–	–	+	–	–	–	–
Liver	–	–	–	–	–	–	–	–
Spleen	+	–	–	+	–	–	–	–
Kidney	+	–	–	+	–	–	–	–
Gastrointestinal tract	+	–	–	+	–	–	–	–
Adrenal gland	+	–	–	N.T.‡	–	–	–	–
Gonads	+	–	–	N.T.	–	–	–	–
Urine	+	U.A.§	U.A.	U.A.	–	U.A.	U.A.	U.A.
Amniotic fluid	+	U.A.	U.A.	U.A.	–	U.A.	U.A.	U.A.
Placenta	+	+	+	+	+	+	+	+
Maternal blood	–	–	–	–	–	–	–	–
Gestational age at the time of rash	15 Days	27 Days	46 Days	55 Days	63 Days	78 Days	92 Days	128 Days
Interval between clinical onset of rubella and therapeutic abortion	77 Days	64 Days	53 Days	48 Days	27 Days	12 Days	38 Days	61 Days

*+, Rubella virus recovered.

†–, Rubella virus not recovered.

‡N.T., not tested.

§U.A., Unavailable.

Monif G, Sever J, Schiff G, Traub R (1965). Am J Obstet Gynecol 91(8):1143-1146.

Toxoplasmosis results in varying degrees of fetal damage, depending on the time of maternal infection (Table III). Data from Desmonts and Couvieur showed that toxoplasmosis early in pregnancy is less likely to infect the fetus, but if infection occurs, severe damage frequently takes place (Desmonts et al., 1974). Maternal infection late in pregnancy is usually transmitted to the fetus, but in most instances the infection is asymptomatic.

Immune Status Of The Mother

With some infections, such as rubella, prior infection or immunization results in immunity of the mother. If the immune mother is reexposed to the virus during pregnancy she is protected and the fetus is not at risk. With other infections however,

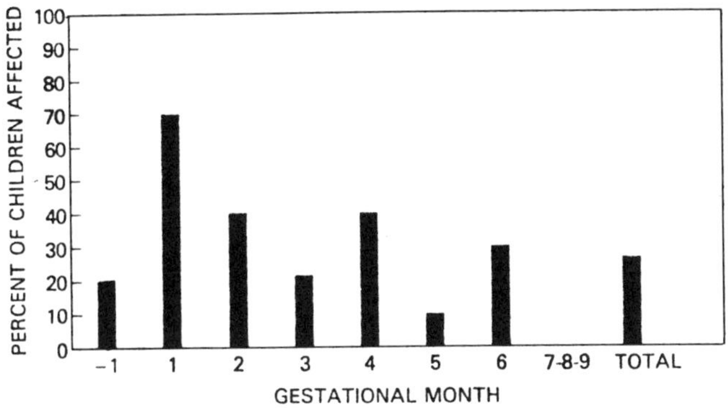

Children in the Collaborative Study, 1964 rubella epidemic, analyzed for frequency of rubella associated defects by gestational month of maternal rubella.

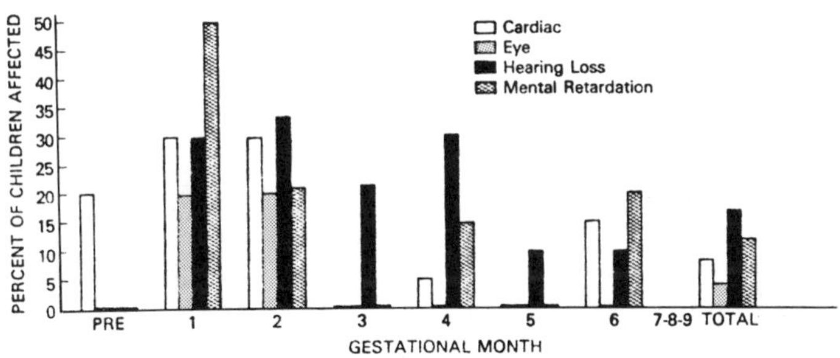

Children in the Collaborative Study, 1964 rubella epidemic, analyzed for the four major rubella associated defects by gestational month of maternal rubella.

Figure 1
South M, Sever J (1985). Teratology 31:297-307

maternal infection does not result in complete immunity and the mother may have recurrences of the infection resulting in some risk to the fetus.

Infections with herpes simplex and cytomegalovirus (CMV) are examples of recurring infections with reduced risk to the fetus associated with the recurrence. Primary herpes simplex infection at term is transmitted to the fetus in about 50% of vaginal deliveries. Recurrent infection, however, carries risk of <8% Prober et al., 1987). It appears that the reduced severity of the recurrent infection and the antibody provided to the fetus by the

Table III

Incidence Of Congenital Toxoplasmosis

Related To Time Of Maternal Infection

Time of Maternal Infection (Trimester)	No. of Women (%)	Congenital Toxoplasmosis			
		No. Cases (%)	Severe	Mild	Asymptomatic
1	29 (20)	5 (17)	3	1	1
2	79 (54)	20 (25)	6	5	9
3	37 (26)	24 (65)	0	2	22

Desmonts, G. and Couvier, J. Bulletin N.Y. Acad. Med. 50:146-159, 1974.

mother contribute to the low frequency of fetal infection and damage. Primary CMV infection is transmitted to the fetus in about 30% of pregnancies and 10% of these children have damage. Recurrent infection is also transmitted to the fetus but damage is rare.

Immune Responses of the Child

The fetus infected *in utero* receives maternal antibody (IgG) across the placenta. With some perinatal infections, antibody (IgM) produced by the fetus becomes detectable at about 20-22 weeks gestation and persists for 6 to 12 months after birth. The presence of this antibody can be used to identify the child congenitally infected with rubella, toxoplasmosis and certain other perinatal infections. Newer techniques for sampling blood *in utero* have provided an opportunity for intrauterine diagnosis of fetal infection using IgM specific antibody determinations. It is likely that the humoral and cellular responses of the older fetuses provide some protection from severe disease with agents such as rubella virus and toxplasma.

Prevention and Treatment of Perinatal Infections

Mother. The most effective approach to the prevention of perinatal infections is to prevent the infection in the mother. This has been accomplished for rubella in the United States by the widespread use of rubella vaccine. In 1964-1965, for example, there were 20,000 damaged children with CRS. In recent years there have been less than 10 cases of CRS each year.

With other infections, education of the mother is used to help reduce exposure of the child. For example, with AIDS, efforts are now being made to inform infected and high risk women of the possibility of transmission of infection to the fetus. It is recommended that these women delay becoming pregnant.

Child. If the woman is infected, it is sometimes possible to avoid exposing the child to the agent by the use of cesarean section. This approach is used when herpes simplex virus is present in the vagina at the time of delivery. With some infections the newborn may receive some benefit from the use of specific gamma globulin or chemotherapy. For example, when a woman experiences varicella at term, varicella-zoster immunoglobulin is given to the child shortly after birth. Most children are protected from severe or fatal varicella with the use of this special gamma globulin. In a similar approach, women with vaginal Group B streptococci are treated with penicillin near the time of delivery to protect the child from this infection, and the child may also be treated. Chemotherapy is also available for children with perinatal herpes infection.

SUMMARY AND CONCLUSIONS

An increasing number of infectious agents are now recognized to be important causes of perinatal morbidity and mortality. Most of these agents produce asymptomatic or mild infections in the mother; however, some can cause severe or fatal disease in the fetus. In each case, the infectious agent is transmitted from the mother to the child, usually by the transplacental, hematogenous route.

The time of maternal infection during gestation frequently influences the chance of fetal infection and severity of fetal disease. The pathogenesis of these infections involves direct infection of the developing fetal tissues. In some cases this infection can interfere with morphogenesis or cause severe tissue destruction. Very late effects are now recognized with some perinatal infection, thus it is important to conduct longitudinal studies of infected children.

Fetal disease can be prevented or reduced if prior exposure of the mother has resulted in complete or partial immunity. Immune responses in the fetus, which become detectable at about 20 to 22 weeks gestation, can be used for diagnostic purposes. They also appear to provide some degree of protection of the fetus from severe or fatal disease with certain agents when infection occurs late in gestation.

The prevention of fetal damage by perinatal infections can be accomplished by protection of the mother through the appropriate use of vaccines, avoidance of exposure, treatment with immunoglobulins or the use of chemotherapy. Treatment of the child also involves the use of immunoglobulins and chemotherapy.

REFERENCES

Desmonts G, Couvreur J (1974). Toxoplasmosis in pregnancy and its transmission to the fetus. Bull NY Acad Med 50:146-159.

Monif G, Sever J, Schiff G, Traub R (1965). Isolation of rubella virus from products of conception. Am J Obstet Gynecol 91(8):1143-1146.

Prober G, Sullender W, Yasukawa B, Au D, Yeager A, Arvin A (1987). Low risk of herpes simplex virus infections in neonates exposed to the virus at the time of vaginal delivery to mothers with recurrent genital herpes simplex virus infections. N Engl J Med 316:240-244.

Sever J, South M, Shaver K (1985). Delayed manifestations of congenital rubella. Rev Infect Dis 7 Suppl 1:S164-169.

South M, Sever J (1985). Teratogen update: the congenital rubella syndrome. Teratology 31:297-307.

DISCUSSION

DR. HOLMES: The observation that infection with rubella virus in the third trimester of pregnancy has no effect on the fetus is in contrast to the data on the effects of cytomegalovirus and toxoplasmosis during the third trimester. Are you satisfied with the quality of the information on rubella infection in the third trimester?

DR. SEVER: I am confident with the data through the 7-year follow-up. In those studies, the children were followed through 7 years of age and they had IQ tests, hearing tests, and a battery of psychological tests, as well as complete physical examinations. I am not sure of the possible occurrence of diabetes, hyperparathyroidism, hypoparathyroidism and some of the other late defects because we did not follow the children in the second decade of life, when those defects appear.

DR. QUINN: You mentioned the sampling of fetal blood in the analysis of IgM antibodies to toxoplasmosis. Could you comment on the validity or potential of this testing?

DR. SEVER: Several studies have been reported by Daffos in France. We also have tested a small number of patients for IgM antibodies using fetal blood samples. The data for rubella from France look quite good. The children who were sampled *in utero* also were studied in the newborn period.

The study of toxoplasmosis by Desmonts and by Daffos *et al* included fetal blood and amniotic fluid which were tested for *Toxoplasma* in mice, IgM antibody, and several "laboratory measurements" at 20-24 weeks. These investigators tested 278 women who had serological evidence of toxoplasmosis and were receiving spiramycin. From the fetal blood, *Toxoplasma* organisms were isolated in 9 cases and IgM antibody was positive in 4 of these cases. There were abnormal "laboratory tests" in 7 of the 9 cases (eosinophilia, thrombocytopenia, elevated total IgM, etc.). From the amniotic fluid, *Toxoplasma* was isolated from 7 of the 9 cases and none had specific IgM antibody in this fluid. The 9 pregnancies were terminated and 8 were studied. In all 8 cases *Toxoplasma* was found in the placenta and there was a necrotic encephalitis in the fetuses. Ultrasonography had shown an increased ventricle/hemisphere ratio in 6 cases. Studies performed at delivery of the remaining children showed *Toxoplasma* in 3 of 157 placentas and CNS toxoplasmosis in 1 of 199 infants. Based on this data, the combined studies of umbilical cord blood and amniotic fluid identified 9 infected babies and missed 1 infected child. All of the mothers had received spiramycin. Isolation of the organism by mouse inoculation, specific IgM tests, and other laboratory tests were necessary to identify the infected children.

There just has been a recent report on finding the HIV in amniotic fluid and those approaches as well as IgM should certainly be worthy of further study.

DR. QUINN: In situations where you have a background colonization with a potentially infectious agent or where the presence of the organism is asymptomatic in the mother, one cannot differentiate who is at risk. The key relates to what is happening in the fetus. Fetal sampling has tremendous potential, for example, in the mycoplasma investigations, where you cannot tell which fetus is infected.

DR. SEVER: I think the combination of IgM antibody plus detection of the agent or the antigen has opened many opportunities for the diagnosis of perinatal infections.

DR. MOSER: I remember a comment you made about 20 years ago or more, that IgM levels in fetal blood were frequently high, but that in only a relatively small percentage of these fetuses could the viral agent be identified. This would suggest that viral infections were a more frequent cause of later deficit than we recognized. Has that percentage of the unknown been diminished or are we still in a situation where there may be viral infections in fetal life that cause brain damage of which we are unaware?

DR. SEVER: The list of infectious agents which cause perinatal damage keeps expanding. We now have to add human immunodeficiency viruses (HIV) and parvoviruses to our list. In the case of rubella which I was probably including about 20 years ago, we now know about late-appearing defects which expand the spectrum of the damage which is associated with the illness. We have maintained the serum bank from the Collaborative Study which was conducted in the 1960's. We have serial collections of sera from 60,000 pregnant women and cord blood from about 30,000 of those children. From this collection, we have been able to retrieve sets of sera to answer questions about perinatal infections and other diseases. For example, just recently, we were able to study paroviruses. We asked the questions: how often does parovirus infection occur in pregnant women and how often is it transmitted to the child? I would recommend that each of you save sera from mothers and children and amniotic fluid so that you can go back and ask these types of questions using those specimens. Also, since the technique of fetal blood sampling is now done by ultrasonography instead of fetoscopy, more samples are becoming available. The foregoing offer an additional way to study the fetus at various times in gestation.

Transplacental Effects on Fetal Health, pages 15–32

ONTOGENY OF HOST DEFENSE SYSTEMS AND CONGENITAL INFECTIONS

B. I. OSBURN

University of California, Davis
1018 Haring Hall, Davis, CA 95616

Competent host defense systems are critical for existence during extrauterine life. These systems consist of innate immune and accessory immune systems. The importance of these systems became very apparent after the recognition of a variety of immune deficiency diseases. Without competent immune systems, microbial agents overwhelm the individual, resulting in death. Most domestic animal species differ from primates and laboratory rodents in the respect that passive transfer of immunity from maternal circulation to the fetus does not occur during pregnancy. Instead, the newborn animal must obtain colostrum immediately after birth in order to benefit from the maternal immune experience with microbes and toxins. As a result of the absence of placental transfer of immunity in domestic animals such as the ruminants, there is an inordinately high incidence of reproductive failure caused by a number of infectious disease agents. Observations on congenital infections in domestic animals have led to the appreciation of a number of factors which play important roles in deficient/immature host defense responses that permit an inordinately high prevalence of microbial-induced congenital diseases in domestic ruminants. In this review an attempt will be made to discuss some of the factors which appear to play a role in permitting these infections. In addition, the immunodeficient fetuses permit a better understanding of the role of host-virus and maternal-fetal-microbial relationships which occur in congenital infections.

IMMUNE STATUS IN THE UNGULATE FETUS

Innate Immunity

Very little is known about innate immunity in the fetus. The embryo/fetus is sheltered from most microbial agents by an intact maternal immune system and by its own innate immunity. The principal barriers that can be associated with innate immunity once the maternal-fetal barrier is broached are the placental membranes. Once infectious agents pass this barrier they have direct access to the fetal blood vascular system. The only known report on innate immunity in the fetus is the report of bacteriocidal activity in serum of 75 day fetal calves (Barta et al., 1972). It is not known how effective this bacteriocidal activity is *in vivo.*

Immune System

There is a slow progressive maturation of the immune system during fetal and early neonatal life. Appearance of lymphoid cells and the subsequent seeding of lymphoid organs occurs sequentially (Tables 1 and 2). Stem cells are located in the yolk sac in early embryonic life and later these cells are found in the liver. Around the time of birth, the stem cells migrate to the bone marrow. Lymphocytes appear initially in blood in the early fetal period. This is followed by a seeding of the thymus gland, lymph nodes, spleen and finally the intestinal tract (Table 1). The appearance of lymphocytes in the intestine occurs later than lymphocytes in peripheral lymph nodes and spleen. This suggests that the local immune system is somewhat delayed in development when compared to the systemic immune system.

Development of immune responses in the ungulate fetus occurs in a sequential manner. Although considerable information in recent years has greatly enhanced our understanding of the genetic reassorting which takes place in the genome of lymphoid cells to create specific immune responses, the ungulate fetus immune system matures at a leisurely and predictable pace. In the fetal lamb, antibody responses to a bacteriophage appear by 41 days gestation. This is

TABLE 1.
MORPHOLOGIC AND PHYSIOLOGIC ONTOGENY OF LYMPHOID AND LEUCOCYTE SYSTEMS IN THE FETAL LAMB

Day of Gestation	Development of Lymphoid and Accessory Systems	Sequential Maturation of Immune Response
32	Lymphocytes in blood	ϕX174
39	C_1 in fetal plasma	
41	Lymphocytes in thymus	
44-45	Lymphocytes in lymph nodes	
56	Lymphocytes in spleen IgG in serum	Ferritin
58	Ig bearing cells in blood monocytes	Flagellin, Chicken RBC's
60	Neutrophils	
63	IgM in serum	
68	Thymocytes respond to Lectin	Akabane
70	Antigen binding-B-cells	
75	Lymphocytes in gut	IgM antibodies to *Salmonella flagellin* Graft rejection
80		Hemocyanin

(Continued)

TABLE 1.
MORPHOLOGIC AND PHYSIOLOGIC ONTOGENY OF LYMPHOID AND LEUCOCYTE SYSTEMS IN THE FETAL LAMB

Day of Gestation	Development of Lymphoid and Accessory Systems	Sequential Maturation of Immune Response
91		*Brucella ovis*
93	γm Gobulin produced by spleen cells *in vitro*	
95		Bluetongue virus
99		Cell mediated immunity to PPD
112	Eosinophils	Functional T-helper for ovalbumin
114		Antibodies to PPD
120	C_3 receptors on lymphocytes	Antibody to ovalbumin
123	Hemolytic complement activity	
135	Esterase positive neutrophils	
Birth 150	Fc receptors on lymphocytes	*Brucella abortus* Chlamydia, Chuzan virus
10	Lipase positive macrophages	
6-8 weeks		Antibody to BCG, *Sal. typhosa*, Diptheria toxoid

(Osburn, 1977; Osburn, 1981)

TABLE 2.
MATURATION OF THE BOVINE IMMUNE SYSTEM DURING ONTOGENY

Sequential Maturation of Lymphoid and Accessory Systems	Gestation Day	Defined Immune Responses
Thymus	42	...
Lymphocytes in blood	45	...
Spleen	55	...
IgM-bearing lymphocytes	59	...
Peripheral lymph nodes	60	...
Bacteriocidal activity in serum	75	...
Phytohemagglutinin lymphocyte blastogenesis	78	...
Hemolytic complement activity measurable C3 in serum	90	...
Mesenteric lymph node	100	...
...	120	Antibody to parainfluenza-3 virus
IgM in serum	130	Interferon to bluetongue
Neutrophils	130	Neutralizing antibody to parvovirus
...	137	IgM and IgG to bluetongue
...	140	Neutralizing antibody to parvovirus
...	141	Antibody to _Anaplasma marginale_
IgG-bearing lymphocytes	145	Agar-gel precipitating antibody to bluetongue virus

(Continued)

TABLE 2.
MATURATION OF THE BOVINE IMMUNE SYSTEM DURING ONTOGENY

Sequential Maturation of Lymphoid and Accessory Systems	Gestation Day	Defined Immune Responses
IgG in serum	145	Increased IgM to parvovirus Interferon produced to bovine viral diarrhea virus
...	155	Antimaternal RBC antibody
...	162	Antibody to *Leptospira saxkoebing*
...	165	Anti-infectious bovine rhinotracheitis antibody
...	170	Antibody to inactivated infectious bovine rhinotracheitis virus
Lymphoid tissue--gastrointestinal tract	175	...
...	190	Neutralizing antibody to bovine viral diarrhea virus
...	210	Cytotoxic antibody to mouse cells
...	243	Complement-fixing antibodies to Chlamydia Neutralizing antibody Chuzan virus, epizootic hemorrhagic disease virus. Ibaraki virus, Akabane virus.
IgA plasma cells in intestine	Newborn	Agglutinins to *Brucella abortus*, cell-mediated response to *Mycobacterium bovis*, tetanus toxoid, and *B. abortus*

(MacLachlan et al., 1984; Osburn et al., 1982)

before lymphoid cells populate lymph nodes or the spleen. Antibody activity to ferritin occurs at 56 days, flagellin and chicken red blood cells at 58 days, graft rejection at 75 days and cell mediated immunity to PPD at 99 days gestation (Silverstein, Uhr, Kraner, and Lukes, 1963). Antibody to BCG, _Salmonella_ _typhosa_ and diphtheria toxoid is not present until 6 weeks after birth (Table 1). The reason for the progressive development of the immune response is not known. Factors which play a role include maturation of antigen presenting cells, the maturation of T-lymphocytes as well as B-lymphocytes. The appearance of Class II antigens on cells involved in the immune response is also important. A successful immune response requires the maturation of each of these cellular components before immune response to any one antigen occurs.

ACCESSORY IMMUNE SYSTEM

The accessory immune system consists of cells and humoral factors which complement and extend the capabilities of the immune system. The cellular components of this system include neutrophils, monocytes, eosinophils and basophils. Monocytes are present in peripheral blood relatively early in fetal life. Neutrophils are usually found by midway through fetal development whereas basophils and eosinophils are not found in peripheral blood of unstimulated fetuses until the last one third of pregnancy. Although monocytes and neutrophils can be found during much of gestation, these cells are not fully differentiated as they lack lysosomal enzymes for lipase and esterase (Sawyer et al., 1978). Neutrophils in normal lambs do not have demonstrable esterase activity until 2 weeks before birth and lipase activity is not evident in monocytes until after birth. Neutrophils and monocytes in lambs infected with Brucella will acquire these 2 lysosomal enzymes shortly after infection (Gorham et al., 1986).

An important humoral component of the accessory immune system is complement. The multifactorial components of the hemolytic complement system are present in the fetal calf as early as 90 days gestation (Culbertson, 1976) and fetal lamb serum by 123 days gestation (Rice and Silverstein, 1964). However, activity gradually increases from very modest measurable activity by the end of the first one-third of gestation to less than 50% of the adult activity by the time of birth (Culbertson, 1976). Even though very low levels of complement are present, the inoculation of endotoxin into fetuses did not result in complement consumption (Sawyer et al., 1978). The marginal complement activity and relatively small amounts of C_3 may be responsible for the modest or nonexistent neutrophil response in fetal calf as early as 90 days gestation (Culbertson, 1976) and in fetal lamb serum by 123 days gestation (Rice and Silverstein, 1964).

FETAL RESPONSE TO INJURY AND/OR MICROBIAL AGENTS

The response of the fetus to microbial agents or irritants depends on the maturation of the immune and accessory immune systems during the time that the irritants are present. Fetal inflammatory responses to specific irritants or microbes differ considerably from those observed in postnatal life. The response to injury in the fetus may be 1) no response, 2) mononuclear/ /macrophage responses without lymphocytes, 3) mixed population mononuclear response, and 4) neutrophil response (Table 3) (Schwartz and Osburn, 1974). In the early fetal period, the responses are nonexistent or minimal consisting of collections of mononuclear cells. The responses are slow developing and if cellular damage occurs, the chemoattractant appears to be a cellular or tissue derived cytokine (Enright and Osburn, 1979). Once maturation of cellular immune system to the inciting irritant occurs, lymphocytes become a part of the inflammatory response. In most fetal inflammatory responses, neutrophils are not found until shortly before birth. If present in mid to late fetal ages, the neutrophils are large and immature. For example, killed staphylococcal organisms when injected intradermally into fetal rhesus at 90 and 120 days gestation cause a mononuclear response at 24 hours. In contrast, the same preparation injected intradermally in newborn causes a mixed mononuclear and neutrophil response whereas in the juvenile and adult rhesus the preparation causes a vigorous neutrophil response leading to an abscess (Schwartz and Osburn, 1974). The response with neutrophils was apparent at 24 hours in 150 day fetuses as compared to 4 hours in the newborn and yearling animals. The sequential pattern of responsiveness was demonstrated with other irritants and clearly

TABLE 3.
Cells in Peripheral Blood and Cellular Infiltrate
To Irritants in Rhesus Fetuses

	Peripheral Blood Cells cu mm.		Character of 24 hours Intradermal Lesions with Irritants			
	Mononuclears	Neutrophils	Turpentine	LPS	Killed Staph	Immune Complex
Day of Gestation 90	1550	172	NC*	NC	NC	NC
120	2416	100	M	M	NC	NC
150	997	524	M,N	M	M,N	M,N
165 Newborn	2138	18,511	N	N	N	N
Yearling	5958	4809	N	N	N	N

*NC - No cells, M - Mononuclear, N - Neutrophil

(Schwartz and Osburn, 1974)

demonstrates that factors associated with the inflammatory response are not present in their full complement until after birth.

Lesions associated with fetal infections demonstrate the sequential maturation of host defense systems in the fetus. Brucella ovis is a bacterial infection of low pathogenicity in adult sheep. It seldom if ever causes death; instead it has a predilection for the reproductive tract. The most serious aspect of disease is in rams where it is the cause of epididymitis and subsequently testicular atrophy. B. ovis rarely causes abortions in ewes. Lesions in the male sheep are confined to the epididymis and testes, while in female sheep the lesions are confined to inflammatory infiltrate including neutrophils at the site of placentation. The lesions in the fetal lamb are primarily mononuclear and neutrophils are present only at the maternal-fetal interface in the cotyledon and placenta. Fetal lambs infected with B. ovis prior to 50 days gestation respond with loose collections of mononuclear cells in the lungs by 54 days gestation followed by organized aggregates resembling granulomas at 80 days gestation (Table 4) (Osburn, 1975). Lymphoid hyperplasia in lymphoid organs and lymphocytic infiltrates in the mononuclear aggregates of the lungs were present at 80 days. Immunoglobulins were detected in serum followed by specific complement-fixing antibody at 91 days gestation. Infection occurring after 100 days gestation (or at the beginning of the last one-third of gestation) causes lymphoid hyperplasia with no lesions observed in other visceral organs. A similar pattern of inflammatory responses occurs with bluetongue virus infection. The major exceptions are the fetal age at which lesions appear (Table 4).

ROLE OF NON-IMMUNOLOGIC FACTORS IN CONGENITAL DISEASE

There are other factors which contribute to the success of infectious agents in fetuses. Biochemical products of fetal and placental metabolism may enhance microbial growth. Erythritol, a by-product of placental and fetal metabolism, has been shown to greatly enhance the growth of Brucella spp. (Smith et al., 1962). In the case of viral infections, there are a number of tissues which are undifferentiated during fetal development. Undifferentiated cells are a favored site for viral

TABLE 4.
ONTOGENY OF HOST DEFENSE SYSTEM DURING FETAL INFECTION

Day of Gestation	Normal Development	*Brucella Ovis* Infection	Bluetongue Virus Infection
32	Blood		
	Lymphocytes in blood		
41	Lymphocytes in thymus		
45	Lymphocytes in lymph nodes		
54		Lung Macrophages Aggregates	
56	Lymphocytes in spleen		Lung Mononuclear/ Macrophage in loose granuloma
58	Ig bearing cells in blood monocytes		
60	Neutrophils		
63	IgM in serum		
65			Lymphoid hyperplasia Interferon

(Continued)

TABLE 4.
ONTOGENY OF HOST DEFENSE SYSTEM IN FETAL LAMBS

Day of Gestation	Normal Development	Brucella Ovis Infection	Bluetongue Virus Infection
75	Lymphocytes in gut		
80		Granulomas and Lymphoid Hyperplasia	
95		Complement-Fixing Antibody	Germinal centers Plasma cells IgM & IgG neutralizing antibody
110			Immune clearance of virus
112	Eosinophils		
123	Hemolytic complement activity		
135	Esterase positive neutrophils		
Birth	Lipase positive macrophages		

(Osburn, 1975; Osburn, 1977)

infection and replication. Organ systems which are not fully differentiated include the nervous, skeletal, endocrine and urogenital systems. Viral infections of these systems often lead to destruction of tissues and teratogenic lesions. Viral infections of the nervous system may result in anencephaly, cerebellar hypoplasia, hydrocephalus, etc. Other changes associated with congenital viral infections include arthrogryposis, kyphosis, scoliosis, renal hypoplasia and small, unthrifty newborn animals.

IMMUNE TOLERANCE

Another system which is not fully differentiated is the lymphoid/immune system. Infection with viruses which have a predilection for lymphoid tissue may lead to "immune tolerance." The condition has been described with the pestiviruses, bovine virus diarrhea virus, border disease virus and hog cholera virus. If these viruses infect fetal calves, lambs or pigs before they develop immune competence to the respective viruses, they become immunologically compromised (Sawyer et al., 1986). The newborn remains persistently viremic, and demonstrable immune responses to the respective viruses are nonexistent or equivocal at best. There is some evidence that the cell mediated immune responses are somewhat compromised as well. In contrast to fetuses infected after immune competence to the virus comes about, they develop an immune response that clears the infection and produces neutralizing antibodies.

SUMMARY

There are a number of factors which contribute to the large number of congenital infections which occur in domestic animals. The more important factors include: 1) The agammaglobulinemic fetus because of a lack of transplacental transfer of maternal immunoglobulins, 2) An immature immune and accessory immune system, and 3) Undifferentiated cells in a number of developing organ systems in the fetus. The immune and accessory immune systems and other organ systems develop in a sequential manner. The types of lesions associated with a microbial agent depends upon the status of the target organ, immune response and accessory immune response at the particular moment of the insult. Once immune competence is attained, the fetus clears infection. Immune tolerance occurs with certain pestiviruses which have a predilection for lymphoid cells. Infection must occur before immune competence to these viruses is attained.

REFERENCES

Barta O, Barta V, Ingram DG, Hubbert WT (1972). Bactericidal activity of bovine fetal serum against smooth and rough strains of Escherichia coli. Am J Vet Res 33:731-740.

Culbertson MR (1976). Bovine hemostatic and complement systems. I. Ontogenic studies. II. Fetal response to bacterial endotoxin. Ph.D. Thesis, University of California, Davis.

Enright FM, Osburn BI (1979). Cytokine production by bluetongue virus-infected fetal sheep cells. Infect Immun 25:403-407.

Gorham SL, Enright FM, Snider TG, Roberts ED (1986). Morphologic lesions in Brucella abortus infected ovine fetuses. Vet Path 23:331-335.

MacLachlan JJ, Schore CE, Osburn, BI (1984). Antiviral responses of bluetongue virus-inoculated bovine fetuses and their dams. Am J Vet Res 45:1469-1473.

Osburn BI (1975). Animal models for the study of immunologic modulation of fetal infectious disease processes. In Neter E, Milgrom F (eds): "Immune Systems and Infectious Diseases," Buffalo: S. Karger, pp 25-32.

Osburn BI (1977). Sequential resistance to congenital infection. In Solomon JB, Horton JD (eds): Amsterdam: Elseiver/North Holland Biomedical Press pp 427-432.

Osburn BI (1981). The ontogeny of the ruminant immune system and its significance in the understanding of maternal-fetal-neonatal relationships. In Butler JE (ed): "The Ruminant Immune System," New York: Plenum pp 91-103.

Osburn, BI, MacLachlan NH, Terrell TG (1982). Ontogeny of the immune system. J Am Vet Med Assoc 181:1049-1052.

Rice CE, Silverstein AM (1964). Hemolytic complement activity of sera of foetal and newborn lambs. Can J Comp Med 28:34-37.

Sawyer MM, Moe JB, Osburn BI (1978). Ontogeny of

immunity and leukocytes in the ovine fetus and elevation of immunoglobulins related to congenital infections. Am J Vet Res 39:643-648.
Sawyer MM, Schore CE, Menzies PI, Osburn BI (1986). Border disease in a flock of sheep: epidemiologic laboratory, and clinical finding. J Am Vet Med Assoc 189:61-65.
Schwartz LW, Osburn BI (1974). An ontogenic study of the acute inflammatory reaction in the fetal rhesus monkey. I. Cellular response to bacterial and nonbacterial irritants. Lab Invest 31:441-453.
Silverstein AM, Uhr J, Kraner KL, Lukes RJ (1963). Fetal response to antigenic stimulus II. Antibody production by the fetal lamb. J Ex Med 117:799-805.
Smith H, Williams AE, Pearce JH, Keppie J, Harris-Smith PW, Fitz-George RB, Witt K (1962). Foetal erythritol, a cause of the localization of Brucella abortus in bovine contagious abortion. Nature 193:47-49.

DISCUSSION

DR. ROSA: You seem to concur with Dr. Sever's hypothesis that placental infections are hematogenous in origin. In the case of chronic viremias in humans, some are not spread transplacentally, but spread through breast-feeding (HTLV-1) or during birth (most hepatitis B). Is there a similar mechanism for the spread in animals?

DR. OSBURN: Yes, most of the infections that I described here are spread primarily by the hematogenous route. There are some exceptions, such as those that are involved in the early embryonic period. For example, vibriosis and trichomoniasis are probably spread by coitus. We do have a number of animal viruses that are spread through the milk in the neonatal period. For example, some of the retroviruses, such as caprine arthritis-encephalitis virus and bovine leukemia virus, are present in milk and can be spread through feeding milk. We also believe that mycoplasmas are spread to the newborn through milk.

DR. HEMMING: Have you looked specifically for the presence of virus or viral antigens or Brucella in the granulomas in the lungs of young sheep? One suspects that if the animal is infected hematogenously, the lung acts as a trap, and these agents are trapped in the unexpanded lung. Thus, you have a nidus of active infection to which the animal responds. If that is true, you might be able to recover virus or bacteria from the granulomas.

DR. OSBURN: We have cultured these organs and have isolated bacteria from the lungs. We have been able to isolate bluetongue virus from the lungs of some of the fetal lambs in early gestation . It seems to be a very transient event since fetal lambs can clear virus from the lungs. There seems to be a predilection of the virus to localize in the brain where it causes considerable damage.

Interestingly enough, in many congenital viral infections, the fetus will actually clear the virus before birth. The only way that we can actually identify the congenital infection is by taking serum and looking for specific antibody activity.

DR. HEMMING: What if the infection were to occur very late in gestation? Is it possible that if infection were to occur 3 to 5 days prior to delivery of the animal that the animal may suffer clinical infection that would express itself minutes or hours or days after delivery and yet the mechanism be the same?

DR. OSBURN: In a study which we have completed recently, different strains of bluetongue virus that are genetically different were inoculated into late term calves. One strain of the virus caused premature delivery and elevated cortisol levels. In addition, there was a mild meningoencephalitis. The newborn calves were very weak and had a reduced birth weight. The other strain of virus did not cause early delivery nor were there any lesions in the brain.

DR. HADDOW: I wonder whether the virus infecting the fetus is more likely to go directly across the placenta or if there is any chance of its going transamniotically?

DR. OSBURN: Our indications are that the infection will actually cross the placenta, probably enter the blood vasculature system and be transmitted by hematogenous route of placental vessels to the fetal organs. With some of the bacterial infections, we know that the bacteria is in the chorioallantois as well as in the amniotic and allantoic fluids, and also in the stomach or abomasal fluids. This indicates that the fetuses are becoming infected by swallowing fluid.

DR. QUINN: One of the infections that you have not discussed is the ureaplasmal infections which occur in both cattle and sheep. About 14% of field abortions in cattle are associated with this infection. In the experimental studies done by Miller and colleagues at the University of Guelph, they have infected pregnant heifers and followed the development of the infection, which is associated with early pregnancy loss and later losses with chorioamnionitis and alveolitis in the fetus. It is also associated with premature delivery. I wondered if this would not be a model for a comparative study in the sense that these infections don't seem to be hematogenous. When you examine all the organs in the stillborn calf, only the lung and placenta carry these organisms. They are not found in the other organs. The same phenomenon is found in human stillbirths. This suggests that the infection is probably not hematogenous. More likely the infection occurs in the placenta, then passes through the amniotic fluid and into the respiratory tract of the fetus. Would you please comment?

DR. OSBURN: We have considered the pathogenesis of the lung lesions. In the early fetal lamb there is very little respiratory movement and the fluid in the bronchi, bronchioles, and trachea is a transudate from the blood vascular system. If the trachea is severed it is possible to see a flow of fluid emanating from the lung. I am not saying that these microorganisms cannot get into the lung through some respiratory movement, but they are swimming upstream, particularly in early gestation. In the later gestation, there may be some respiratory movement, particularly with distress associated with anoxia and that caused by placentitis. It may be possible that respiratory inspirations may lead to mixing some of these agents and their eventual aspiration into the lung.

DR. QUINN: That might be very important because it is in the losses after 20 weeks of gestation that this organism is playing a role. The organisms also may be moving along the mucus layer among the tracheal cilia and be protected in some way.

DR. OSBURN: That is correct.

DR. L. ROBINSON: Could you comment on strain differences with respect to the response to the individual agents?

DR. OSBURN: We are at the point where we are beginning to understand strain differences. We do have strains of bluetongue virus that have different pathogenic patterns in both the neonatal mouse and in the fetal calf. In fact, we have strains of bluetongue virus that, if inoculated into a newborn mouse, will cause no mortalities or no lesions whatsoever. If we take another strain, it is possible to get 80 to 90% mortalities along with neurologic changes. There is evidence of strain differences with other agents, such as those in pestivirus groups, that give different pathogenic properties.

DR. MUELLER: I think you answered part of my question already. I also wanted to point out that in many of the bacterial infections resulting in placentitis in the ruminant, you have the advantage of having several placental implantations. This will result in a hypoxic state rather than death of the fetus because some reserve blood supply remains. That is the situation where you most likely will get the inhalation of fluid. It may be, therefore, quite specific for the ruminant to show this primary pulmonary involvement with bacterial infections if you compare ruminants with other mammals that have different placentations.

Transplacental Effects on Fetal Health, pages 33–47

CONGENITAL BLUETONGUE VIRUS INFECTION

N. James MacLachlan and Bennie I. Osburn

Department of Microbiology, Pathology, and Parasitology, School of Veterinary Medicine, North Carolina State University, Raleigh, NC 27606 USA (NJM) and Department of Veterinary Pathology, School of Veterinary Medicine, University of California, Davis, CA 95616 USA (BIO)

INTRODUCTION

Bluetongue is an insect-transmitted viral disease of domestic and wild ruminants. The causative agent, bluetongue virus (BTV), is a member of the Reoviridae and the prototype virus of the genus Orbivirus (Matthews 1982). At least 24 serotypes of BTV have been recognized and 5 of these occur in the United States. The virion consists of an icosahedral particle with an outer shell of virus proteins 2 and 5, and a core containing proteins 1, 3, 4, 6, and 7 (Mertens et al 1984). The genome consists of 10 segments of double stranded RNA (Verwoerd et al 1979). Genetic reassortment and genetic drift are responsible for considerable genetic heterogeneity of BTV in nature (Samal et al 1987; Sugiyama et al 1982; Stott et al 1987).

In the United States, BTV infection of ruminants is highly seasonal, usually occurring in late summer and fall (Osburn et al 1981). Bluetongue disease, which is characterized by widespread endothelial injury and consumptive coagulopathy, occurs most commonly in sheep and white-tailed deer (Hoff, Trainer 1978; Howell, Verwoerd 1971). Although infection of cattle is very common (Metcalf et al 1981), clinical disease is rare. The absence of clinical disease in the vast majority of BTV-infected cattle, and the prolonged viremia that characteristically occurs in this species, has led some investigators to propose that cattle are a reservoir host of BTV in nature (Du Toit

1962; Nevill 1971). It is proposed that BTV "overwinters" in infected cattle when the vector of BTV, which is *Culicoides variipennis* in the United States, is absent. When the vector returns in warmer periods, it then transmits BTV from cattle to more susceptible ruminant species.

Cases of natural and experimental BTV infection of fetal cattle and sheep have been described (Barnard, Pienaar 1976; Brown, MacLachlan 1983; MacLachlan, Osburn 1983; MacLachlan et al 1984a; MacLachlan et al 1985b; MacLachlan et al 1985a; Osburn et al 1971a; Osburn et al 1971b; Richards, Cordy 1967; Richards et al 1971; Thomas et al 1986; Young, Cordy 1964), including an outbreak of abortion and teratogenic defects associated with the use of a modified live BTV vaccine amongst pregnant ewes (Cordy, Shultz, 1961; Shultz, DeLay 1955). Infection of fetal ruminants with BTV is important for at least two reasons: First, such infections can impair reproductive performance as a consequence of fetal death and teratogenic defects in animals that survive *in utero* infection. Second, persistent postnatal infections of lambs and calves have been described after *in utero* infection (Gibbs et al 1979; Luedke et al 1970; Luedke et al 1977a; Luedke et al 1977b). Persistently infected ruminants would obviously provide an ideal virus reservoir.

We have studied the pathologic effects of BTV infection of the bovine fetus, and antiviral responses of fetuses to this infection.

RESULTS

Bluetongue Virus Induced Teratogenesis

Twelve bovine fetuses at 85-125 days of gestation were inoculated with BTV, and two received a placebo. Eight fetuses were inoculated with BTV serotype 10, two with serotype 11, and individual fetuses with serotypes 13 and 17. The viruses used to inoculate fetuses were partially purified by ether and fluorocarbon extraction (MacLachlan et al 1984a). Fetuses were inoculated intramuscularly, through the uterine wall after a laparotomy had been done on their dams. Five of the fetuses that received BTV serotype 10 (at 125 days of gestation), and 2 placebo-inoculated fetuses of similar gestational age, were delivered by cesarean section at regular intervals after inoculation; BTV-inoculated fetuses were delivered at post-inoculation days 4, 8, 12, 20, and 50, and placebo-inoculated fetuses were delivered at postinoculation days 20 and 50. Gestation of the 7 remaining fetuses was allowed to progress until parturition.

Three of the fetuses inoculated with BTV early in gestation died prior to delivery and were either aborted or resorbed; all 3 of these fetuses were inoculated at 85-90 days of gestation, two with serotype 11 and one with serotype 10. All four BTV-inoculated fetuses that survived until term had extensive cerebral malformations. The brain of the calf inoculated with BTV serotype 17 at 85 days of gestation was most severely affected. The cerebral hemispheres were totally replaced by membranous fluid-filled sacs that freely communicated through a ruptured septum pellucidum. Only remnants of the cerebellum and midbrain were present. The brain stem and spinal cord were of normal size. Two calves that were inoculated with BTV serotype 10 at gestation day 125 had extremely dilated lateral ventricles and thin-walled cerebral hemispheres which consisted of cerebral cortex with a narrow underlying zone of subcortical white matter (Fig 1). Cysts were present in the persisting cerebral tissue and usually were located within the subcortical white matter. The remainder of the brains of these 2 calves grossly were normal. The brain of the calf inoculated with serotype 13 at 85-90 days of gestation had dilated lateral ventricles, reduced subcortical white matter, and a single, bilaterally symmetrical cyst was present in the lateral aspects of the persisting parenchyma of each hemisphere. These cysts extended from the anterior aspects of the frontal lobes to the caudal aspects of the temporal lobes.

The histologic development of BTV-induced cavitating encephalopathy was characterized in fetuses inoculated with BTV serotype 10 at gestation day 125; these fetuses were delivered at 4, 8, 12, 20, and 50 days after inoculation. Extensive necrosis was present within the cerebrum of BTV-inoculated fetuses as soon as 12 days after inoculation (Fig 2). Discrete areas of hemorrhagic necrosis were present throughout the hemispheres, especially the rostral portions. Vessels in affected areas were prominent because of hypertrophy and hyperplasia of vascular

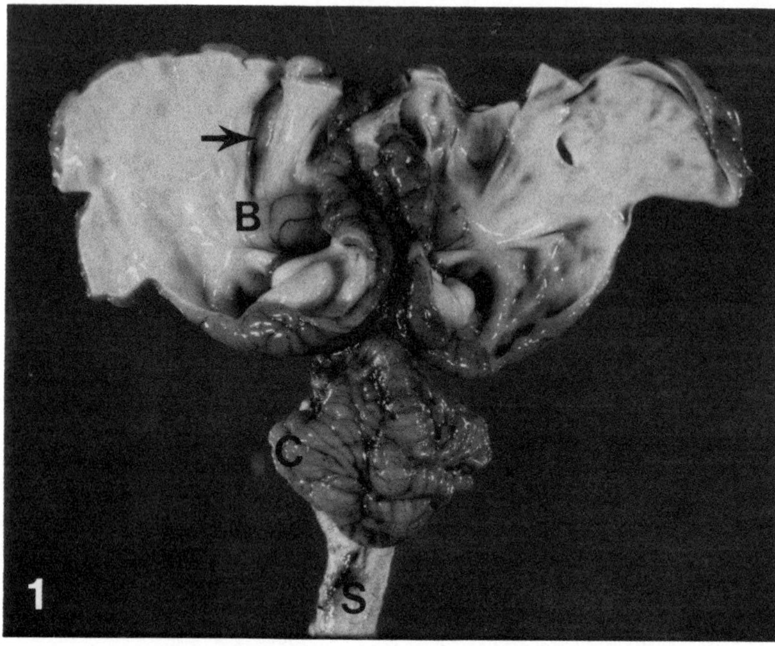

Fig 1. Brain of calf inoculated with BTV serotype 10 at gestation day 125. Note extreme dilation of lateral ventricles and cysts in persisting cerebral tissue (arrow). Basal nuclei (B), cerebellum (C), and brain stem (S) appear normal.

endothelium. Perivascular hemorrhage was common. Mononuclear cells were present in considerable number in the meninges by 20 days after infection and gitter cells were abundant within foci of cerebral necrosis and cavitation. Necrosis of cells within the subventricular zone also was prominent.

To further characterize the pathogenesis of the cavitating encephalopathy induced by BTV, newborn suckling mice were intracerebrally inoculated with BTV. Some mice were also inoculated with a polyclonal sheep antisera to mouse L cell interferon prior to BTV infection. Mouse brains were collected at various intervals after infection

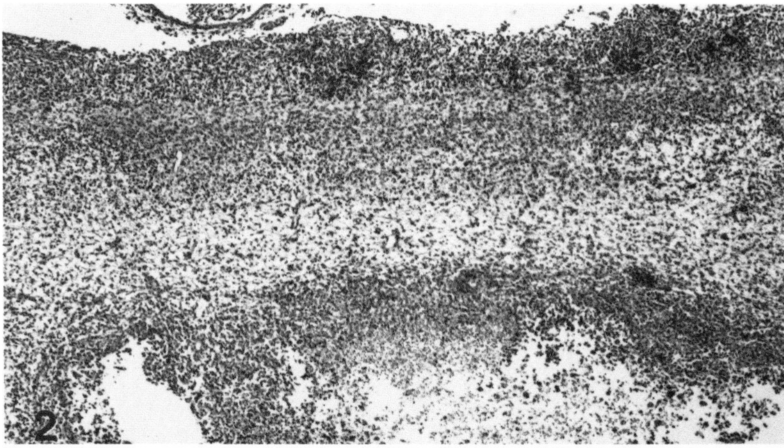

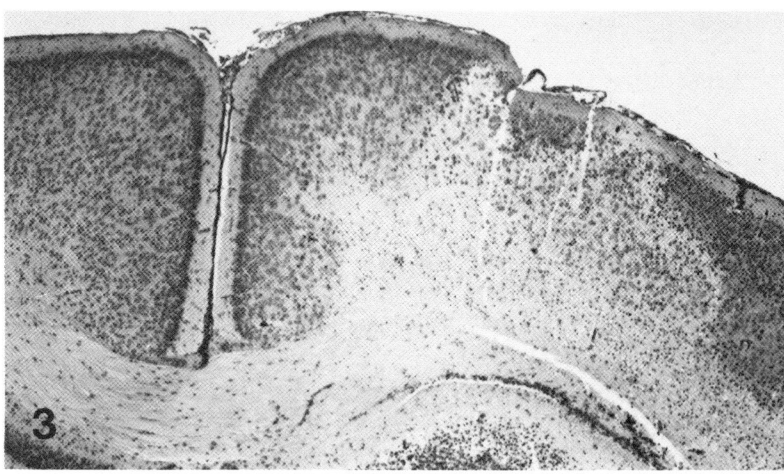

Fig 2. Hemorrhagic necrosis within cerebrum of 137 day fetus, 12 days after inoculation with BTV serotype 10.

Fig 3. Necrosis within the cerebrum of BTV-infected suckling mouse. Note extensive necrosis within one hemisphere but not the other.

and fixed in Bouin's solution. In addition, some brains were frozen in liquid nitrogen, and stained with a fluoroscein isothiocyanate-conjugated monoclonal antibody specific for protein 7 of BTV.

Suckling mice inoculated with BTV succumbed in 5-7 days. Administration of an antiserum to mouse interferon had no beneficial effect. Lesions within the brains of BTV infected mice commenced as focal areas of necrosis and rapidly progressed to involve extensive areas (Fig 3). Particularly susceptible areas include the hemispheres, basal ganglia, hippocampus, and internal granular layer of the cerebellum. Necrosis of the ependymal lining of the lateral ventricles was extensive. Although blood vessels within and adjacent to areas of necrosis were prominent, infection of vascular endothelium was not demonstrated by immunofluorescence staining. However, fluorescent staining did reveal extensive infection of cells throughout susceptible areas of the brain, prior to appearance of necrosis within these areas.

Antiviral Responses of Bovine Fetuses to Bluetongue Virus

Interferon in sera and tissues was quantitated by vesicular stomatitis virus plaque reduction assay in primary cultures of ovine testicular cells (MacLachlan et al 1984a). The BTV-infected fetuses produced interferon, although serum interferon was detected only at 4 and 8 days after inoculation. Titers of interferon in fetal sera were higher than those that we have detected in the serum of BTV-infected calves (MacLachlan, Thompson 1985). High titers were present within the cerebrum at 12 days after inoculation so the susceptibility of the bovine central nervous system to the teratogenic effects of BTV is not due to inability of the fetal brain to produce interferon. Interferon production within virus infected fetuses apparently ceased long before virus clearance occurred.

Bluetongue virus specific serum antibody was detected by the agar gel immunodiffusion test and a microtiter neutralization assay. Immunoglobulin G and M in fetal sera were quantitated by radial immunodiffusion. Fetuses produced antibody in response to BTV infection. Increased levels of IgM (200 mg/dl) were present at 12 and 20 days after inoculation, and levels were low (15-40 mg/dl) in the serum of a fetus delivered 50 days after inoculation, and in 2 fetuses that were delivered at term. Levels of IgG, on the other hand, increased from 12 days after inoculation (40 mg/dl) through term (240-600 mg/dl).

Precipitating and neutralizing antibody were first detected at 20 days after inoculation (145 days of gestation), although titers of neutralizing antibody were low (4) at 20 and 50 days after inoculation (Table 1).

Table 1. IMMUNE RESPONSES OF BOVINE FETUSES INOCULATED AT GESTATION DAY 125 WITH BTV OR PLACEBO

	Humoral Immunity*		Cellular Immunity**			
			Mitogens			Antigen
PID†	Neut. Ab	AGID Ab	PHA	Con A	PKW	BTV
BTV-Inoculated Fetuses						
4	<4	-	2.0	16.5	8.1	<2.0
8	<4	-	7.0	21.6	8.8	<2.0
12	<4	-	3.9	7.2	5.9	<2.0
20	4	+	4.9	<2.0	2.5	<2.0
50	4	+	124.6	132.2	54.1	<2.0
150	128	+	31.8	102.5	11.9	<2.0
150	1024	+	14.0	6.4	7.7	<2.0
Placebo-Inoculated Fetuses						
20	<4	-	24.2	20.7	18.0	<2.0
50	<4	-	40.7	43.8	14.7	<2.0

*Humoral immune responses assayed by plaque reduction assay (Neut Ab) and agar gel immunodiffusion test (AGID Ab).

** Cellular immune responses assayed by lymphocyte blastogenesis assay measuring uptake of tritiated thymidine by stimulated lymphocytes. Mitogens included phytohemagglutinin (PHA), Conconavalin A (Con A), and pokeweed mitogen (PKW). Results reported as peak Stimulation Index induced by mitogens and a variety of BTV antigen preparations. A stimulation index > 2.0 was considered significant.

† Post inoculation day, (time of delivery).

Sera collected from calves that survived _in utero_ infection invariably contained high titers of neutralizing antibody (128-1024). Fetal humoral responses occurred independently of maternal responses as the epitheliochorial cotyledonary placenta of ruminants does not facilitate transfer of maternal immunoglobulin (Osburn et al 1982).

Cellular immune responses to BTV were assayed by culturing fetal peripheral blood lymphocytes and lymph node cells in the presence of a variety of BTV antigen preparations (MacLachlan et al 1984a; MacLachlan et al 1984b). Blastogenic responses were quantitated by uptake of tritiated thymidine by lymphocyte cultures. Cellular immune responses to BTV were not detected by lymphocyte blastogenesis assay. Peripheral blood lymphocytes from all fetuses and calves consistently underwent blast transformation after mitogen stimulation (Table 1).

Tissues and blood of calves and fetuses were inoculated into embryonating chicken eggs and cultures of bovine fetal bone marrow cells. Virus was isolated from all BTV-inoculated fetuses delivered prior to term; that is through postinoculation day 50, which was gestation day 175. In contrast, BTV was not isolated from any of the calves that survived *in utero* infection. Virus clearance occurred, therefore, between gestation day 175 and delivery (approximately gestation day 275). Particularly high titers of BTV were isolated from the cerebrum of the fetus delivered 12 days after inoculation, and this coincided with the onset of extensive necrosis within the cerebrum and the presence of high titers of interferon.

CONCLUSIONS

The cavitating encephalopathy that occurs in BTV-infected bovine fetuses is dependent upon the presence of susceptible cell populations within the developing brain. During the first half of gestation, stem cell populations within the ventricular and subventricular zones divide and immature neuronal and glial cells then migrate to populate the cerebral cortex and subcortical white matter (Angevine et al 1970). The severity of the cavitating encephalopathy that occurs in fetal ruminants clearly is age-related as this lesion does not occur in fetuses inoculated after midgestation. The most severe lesions in our study were present within the brain of the calf inoculated with serotype 17 at 85 days of gestation and we have previously described similar lesions in calves inoculated early in gestation with epizootic hemorrhagic disease virus, an *Orbivirus* closely related to BTV (MacLachlan et al 1985b). Fetuses inoculated later in gestation develop less extensive lesions. In addition, it is likely that strains of BTV differ in their pathogenicity and in our study serotype 13 appeared less virulent than the other serotypes used.

Neonatal rodents provide an extremely convenient model system with which to study BTV-induced cavitating encephalopathy (Becker et al 1974; Narayan, Johnson 1972; Narayan et al 1972; Richards, Cordy 1967; Waldvogel et al 1986; Waldvogel et al 1987). Despite the hemorrhagic nature of the cerebral necrosis that occurs in BTV-infected neonatal rodents, and ruminant fetuses, virus infection of vascular endothelium was not demonstrated in this nor other investigations (Waldvogel et al 1987). Vascular changes that occur in BTV-infected brains, then, probably occur as a consequence of cerebral necrosis, rather than initiating the necrosis as previously proposed (MacLachlan, Osburn 1983).

Bluetongue virus is an exceptionally potent inducer of interferon in laboratory animals (Jameson 1982), and interferon has recently been implicated in the pathogenesis of fatal infections of neonatal mice with lymphocytic choriomeningitis virus (Riviere, Oldstone 1986) and Pichinde virus (Clark et al 1986). Furthermore, high titers of interferon were present within the cerebrum of a BTV-infected fetal calf delivered 12 days after inoculation, and extensive necrosis also was present within the cerebrum of this fetus. We were unable, however, to alter the course of BTV infection of newborn mice with a polyclonal sheep antisera to murine interferon suggesting that interferon is not important in the pathogenesis of BTV-induced encephalopathy in suckling mice. It has previously been established that abrogation of immune responses in neonatal mice does not influence the severity of BTV infection (Narayan et al 1972). Seemingly, BTV-induced necrosis within the brains of neonatal mice, and likely fetal cattle as well, is the result of direct virus-mediated destruction of susceptible populations of glial and neuronal cells.

Results of this study strongly suggest that bovine fetuses infected in early gestation are unlikely to be virus reservoirs, as has previously been proposed. The fetal malformations that consistently occur in fetuses infected in early gestation are incompatible with life. Furthermore, fetuses that survived in utero infection invariably had cleared infection by the time they were born. These observations are consistent with results of an extensive epidemiologic study of BTV infection conducted in California (Osburn et al 1981); in this study, BTV was never isolated from calves born in late winter and spring, yet this is the time of year when any fetuses infected during the previous bluetongue season would be born. Interestingly, BTV has been isolated from newborn calves in the bluetongue season of early summer and fall suggesting that infection in late gestation can occur. Sheep fetuses infected in late gestation remain viremic for up to 2 months after birth (Gibbs et al 1979), and viremia of similar duration occurs in newborn calves inoculated with BTV (MacLachlan, Fuller 1986; MacLachlan et al 1987). Failure to isolate BTV from ruminants throughout the winter months does, however, suggest that ruminants, including animals infected during late gestation, are not the reservoir host in which BTV "overwinters" in much of the United States.

REFERENCES

Angevine JB, Bodian D, Coulombre AJ, Edds MV, Hamburger V, Jacobson M, Lyser KM, Prestige MC, Sidman RL, Varon S, Weiss PA (1970). Embryonic vertebrate central nervous system: Revised terminology. Anat Rec 166:257.

Barnard BJH, Pienaar JG (1976). Bluetongue virus as a cause of hydranencephaly in cattle. Onderstepoort J Vet Res 43:155.

Becker LE, Narayan O, Johnson RT (1974). Comparative studies of the developing forebrain. 1. Pathogenesis of rat virus and bluetongue vaccine virus infections in neonatal hamsters. J Neuropathol Exp Neurol 33:519.

Brown CC, MacLachlan NJ (1983). Congenital encephalopathy in a calf. Vet Pathol 20:770.

Clark T, Gresser I, Peau C, Moss J, Woodrow D (1986). Antibody to mouse alpha/beta interferon abrogates Pichinde virus-induced liver lesions in suckling mice. J Virol 59:728.

Cordy DR, Shultz G (1961). Congenital subcortical encephalopathies in lambs. J Neuropathol Exp Neurol 20:554.

DuToit RM (1962). The role played by bovines in the

transmission of bluetongue in sheep. J S Afr Vet Med Assoc 153:662.

Gibbs EPJ, Lawman MJP, Herniman KAJ (1979). Preliminary observations on transplacental infection of bluetongue virus in sheep - a possible overwintering mechanism. Res Vet Sci 27:118.

Hoff GL, Trainer DO (1978). Bluetongue and epizootic hemorrhagic disease viruses: Their relationships to wildlife species. Adv Vet Sci Comp Med 22:111.

Howell PG, Verwoerd DW (1971). Bluetongue virus. In Gard S, Hallauer C, Meyer KF (eds): "Virology Monographs," ed 9, Vienna: Springer Verlauf, p 35.

Jameson P (1982). Induction of the interferon protein in vivo: antiviral inducers. Tex Rep Biol Med 41:135.

Luedke AJ, Jochim MM, Bowne JG, Jones RH (1970). Observations on latent bluetongue virus infection in cattle. J Am Vet Med Assoc 156:1871.

Luedke AJ, Jochim MM, Jones RH (1977a). Bluetongue in cattle: Effects of _Culicoides variipennis_ transmitted bluetongue virus on pregant heifers and their calves. Am J Vet Res 38:1687.

Luedke AJ, Jones RH, Walton TE (1977b). Overwintering mechanism for bluetongue virus: Biological recovery of latent virus from a bovine from bites of _Culicoides variipennis_. Am J Trop Med Hyg 26:313.

MacLachlan NJ, Fuller FJ (1986). Genetic stability in calves of a single strain of bluetongue virus. Am J Vet Res 47:762.

MacLachlan NJ, Heidner HW, Fuller FJ (1987). Humoral immune response of calves to bluetongue virus infection. Am J Vet Res 48:1031.

MacLachlan NJ, Osburn BI (1983). Bluetongue virus-induced hydranencephaly in calves. Vet Pathol 20:563.

MacLachlan NJ, Osburn BI, Ghalib HW, Stott JL (1985a). Bluetongue virus-induced encephalopathy in fetal cattle. Vet Pathol 22:415.

MacLachlan NJ, Osburn BI, Stott JL, Ghalib HW (1985b). _Orbivirus_ infection of the bovine fetus. In: Barber TL, Jochim MM (eds): "Bluetongue and Related Orbiviruses." New York: Alan R. Liss, p 79.

MacLachlan NJ, Schore CE, Osburn BI (1984a). Antiviral responses of bluetongue virus-inoculated bovine fetuses and their dams. Am J Vet Res 45:1469.

MacLachlan NJ, Schore CE, Osburn BI (1984b). Lymphocyte blastogenesis in bluetongue virus or _Mycobacterium bovis_-inoculated bovine fetuses. Vet Immunol

Immunopathol 7:11.
MacLachlan NJ, Thompson J (1985). Bluetongue virus-induced interferon in cattle. Am J Vet Res 46:1238.
Matthews REF (1982). Classification and nomenclature of viruses. Intervirology 17:1.
Mertens PPC, Brown F, Sangar DV (1984). Assignment of the genome segments of bluetongue virus type 1 to the proteins which they encode. Virology 135:207.
Metcalf HE, Pearson JE, Klingsporn AL (1981). Bluetongue in cattle: A serologic survey of slaughter cattle in the United States. Am J Vet Res 42:1057.
Narayan O, Johnson RT (1972). Effects of viral infection on nervous system development. 1. Pathogenesis of bluetongue virus infection in mice. Am J Pathol 68:1.
Narayan O, McFarland HF, Johnson RT (1972). Effects of viral infection on nervous sytem development. 2. Attempts to modify bluetongue virus induced malformations with cyclophosphamide and antithymocyte serum. Am J Pathol 68:15.
Nevill EM (1971). Cattle and Culicoides biting midges as possible overwintering hosts of bluetongue virus. Onderstepoort J Vet Res 38:65.
Osburn BI, Johnson RT, Silverstein AM, Prendergast RA, Jochim MM, Levy SE (1971b). Experimental viral-induced congenital encephalopathies. II. The pathogenesis of bluetongue virus infection of fetal lambs. Lab Invest 25:206.
Osburn BI, MacLachlan NJ, Terrell TG (1982). Ontogeny of the immune system. J Am Vet Med Assoc 182:1047.
Osburn BI, McGowan B, Heron B, Loomis E, Bushnell R, Stott JL, Utterback W (1981). Epizootiologiv study of bluetongue: Virologic and serologic results. Am J Vet Res 42;884.
Osburn BI, Silverstein AM, Prendergast RA, Johnson RT, Parshall CJ (1971a). Experimental viral-induced congenital encephalopathies. I. Pathology of hydranencephaly and porencephaly caused by bluetongue vaccine virus. Lab Invest 25:197.
Richards WPC, Cordy DR (1967). Bluetongue virus infection: pathologic responses of nervous systems in sheep and mice. Science 156:530.
Richards WPC, Crenshaw GL, Bushnell RB (1971). Hydranencephaly associated with natural bluetongue virus infection. Cornell Vet 61:336.
Riviere Y, Oldstone MBA (1986). Genetic reassortants of lymphocytic choriomeningitis virus: Unexpected disease

and mechanism of pathogenesis. J Virol 59:363.
Samal SK, Livingstone CW, McConnell S, Ramig RF (1987). Analysis of mixed infection of sheep with bluetongue virus serotypes 10 and 17: Evidence for genetic reassortment in the vertebrate host. J Virol 61:1086.
Shultz G, DeLay PD (1955). Losses in newborn lambs associated with bluetongue vaccination of pregnant ewes. J Am Vet Med Assoc 127:224.
Stott JL, Oberst RD, Channell MB, Osburn BI (1987). Genome reassortment between two serotypes of bluetongue virus in a natural host. J Virol 61:1270.
Sugiyama K, Bishop DHL, Roy P (1982). Analyses of the genomes of bluetongue viruses recovered from different states of the United States and at different times. Am J Epidemiol 115:332.
Thomas FC, Randall GCB, Myers DJ (1986). Attempts to establish congenital bluetongue virus infections in calves. Can J Vet Res 50:280.
Verwoerd DW, Huismans HW, Erasmus BJ (1979). Orbiviruses. In: Fraenkel-Conrat H, Wagner RR (eds): "Comprehensive Virology, Vol 14." New York: Academic Press, p 285.
Waldvogel AS, Anderson CA, Higgins RJ, Osburn BI (1987). Neurovirulence of the UC-2 and UC-8 strains of bluetongue virus serotype 11 in newborn mice. Vet Pathol 24:404.
Waldvogel AS, Stott JL, Squire KRE, Osburn BI (1986). Strain-dependent virulence characteristics of bluetongue virus serotype 11. J Gen Virol 67:765.
Young S, Cordy DR (1964). An ovine fetal encephalopathy caused by bluetongue vaccine virus. J Neuropathol Exp Neurol 23:635.

DISCUSSION

DR. ROSA: Interferons have a pretty broad spectrum of effects on reproducing cells. Would it be worthwhile looking to see if interferon had any effect?

DR. MACLACHLAN: That is an excellent point. We have injected pregnant mice with recombinant murine interferons in some very preliminary studies. Progeny appeared normal at birth, but I have not examined them histologically.

DR. NAEYE: Is there any possibility that this agent could infect humans? I have seen several cases of cerebral palsy over the years with lesions in the central nervous system that resembled those you have just demonstrated.

DR. MACLACHLAN: There is no evidence whatsoever that BTV is a human pathogen. I think it is very valid to point out that there are multiple ways to produce hydranencephaly. There are many agents that can destroy the CNS stem cell populations and the end results may be similar.

DR. SCARPELLI: Is it known why the virus is neurotropic?

DR. MACLACHLAN: No, but obviously one would have to look for specific receptors, and that is probably going to be the way that it can be followed in the future. Dr. Osburn's group has identified strains of bluetongue viruses that do not affect the CNS of suckling mice when inoculated subcutaneously. Most strains, like ours, affect the CNS following subcutaneous inoculation; both strains replicate when inoculated directly into the brain. This suggests viral entry into the brain is probably receptor-mediated.

DR. CAPEN: In your experience, are other areas of the brain affected, particularly the brain stem or the hypothalamus, and are affected lambs ever retained _in utero_ for intervals beyond the length of the normal gestation period?

DR. MACLACHLAN: I will confine my comments to cattle; our animals were delivered normally except one that had, unfortunately, severe hydranencephaly. I induced parturition in that animal with prostaglandins. In the others there were lesions throughout the brain, and the more immature the fetus at infection, the more extensive were the lesions. Whether these lesions are sufficient to induce prolonged gestation by interfering with the pituitary-hypothalamic axis, I am not sure. Dr. Osburn may want to comment on this question.

DR. OSBURN: We don't have good evidence for this, but usually the brain stem is intact, and the pituitary appears to have developed normally.

DR. LAMMER: The illustrations in your presentation suggest that the pathogenesis underlying much of the brain injury might actually be secondary to vasculitis, as opposed to a primary effect on the neurons.

DR. MACLACHLAN: That was the point that we were trying to establish with the fluorescent antibody studies. The lesions look like infarcts, and we have gone on record as saying that. However, all the studies that have been done have shown that there is diffuse infection of cell populations throughout the cerebrum before necrosis appears, and specific infection of vascular endothelium has not been identified. So there is no experimental evidence that infarction occurs; in addition, there was one ultrastructural study done a long time ago, and virus was not observed in vascular endothelium. I agree, the lesions look like infarcts, but no one has been able to prove that; in fact, quite the opposite.

DR. SEVER: Venezuelan equine encephalitis in humans produces CNS pathology, and this can be reproduced in monkeys by inoculating them *in utero*. There is also ocular damage associated with this infection. Do you see any such findings in your animals?

DR. MACLACHLAN: Ophthalmic lesions are well described in BTV-infected sheep. We looked at the eyes from all our animals, and there were no retinal lesions of the type described in sheep. If we looked at more animals infected earlier in gestation, I am sure we would find retinal lesions in those animals.

Transplacental Effects on Fetal Health, pages 49–58

CONGENITAL PESTIVIRUS DISEASE (BOVINE VIRUS DIARRHEA) OF CATTLE

J.F.L. Pohlenz, G. Trautwein, S. Bolin and V. Moennig

Institute for Pathology, (J.F.L.P., G.T.), Institute for Virology, Tierärztliche Hochschule Hannover, D-3000 Hannover, (V.M.), and National Animal Disease Center, Ames, IA 50010 (S.B.)

INTRODUCTION

Bovine virus diarrhea (BVD) was first described in 1946 as an apparently new transmissible enteric disease of cattle in the United States (Olafson et al 1946). Within a few years this disease spread throughout the U.S., and due to the lesions produced in the upper digestive tract (erosive to ulcerative stomatitis, esophagitis, rumenitis) and the lower digestive tract (ulcerative abomasitis, severe fibrinonecrotic to diphtheric enteritis and necrosis of Peyer's patches), it was named mucosal disease (MD) (Ramsey and Chivers, 1953; Ramsey, 1956). During the past four decades the disease has been observed in many countries around the world and has been frequently referred to as the BVD-MD disease complex. Further disease syndromes have been described in association with the BVD virus infection. They include subclinical infection with or without growth retardation, virus diarrhea, immunosuppression associated with high susceptibility to secondary respiratory tract infection, abortion, mummification, and early embryonic death, congenital defects, acute and chronic mucosal disease, and persistent infection with immunotolerance (Baker, 1987). Calves infected intrauterinely with most BVD virus strains during the first trimester of gestation will be born persistently infected and are immunotolerant to this virus (Malmquist, 1968; Coria and McClurkin, 1978) without any signs of disease. Those animals persistently infected are, under special circumstances, potential candidates to succumb to MD (Liess et al., 1974; Liess et al., 1983; Malmquist, 1968; Roeder and Drew, 1984; Steck et al., 1980). Most recent research has focused on those cattle which are born immunotolerant to BVD and persistently infected. One to two percent of the cattle population is known to be persistently infected and in some selected herds this may be much higher (Baker, 1987). Independently, Brownlie et al (1984) and Bolin et al (1985a) have elaborated the hypothesis that only those animals will develop MD which are infected in utero by a noncytopathogenic biotype of BVD before the fetus develops its own immune system. Those animals are born persistently infected and later in life exposed to, or superinfected by, a similar or homologous cytopathogenic strain of the virus. This observation was furthermore supported by the fact that Bolin et al (1985a) and McClurkin et al (1985) were able to reisolate two different viruses (a noncytopathogenic and a cytopathogenic) from spleens of animals having succumbed to acute or chronic MD. Thus, MD today must be considered a congenital infection though it often occurs at no earlier than 4 months of age or as late as 4 years of age, or later (see chart).

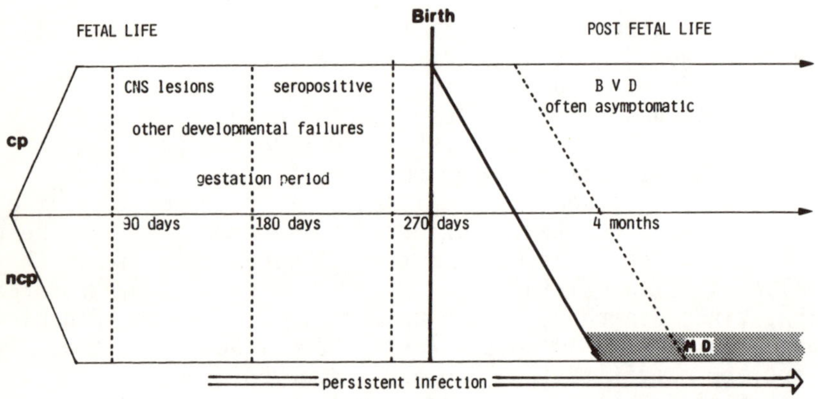

Schematic explanation of the current understanding of different disease complexes in BVD infection

BVD = Bovine Virus Diarrhea
cp = cytopathogenic
ncp = noncytopathogenic
CNS = Central Nervous System
MD = Mucosal Disease

The objectives of this presentation from the point of view of the pathologist are:

1. To describe briefly a few characteristics of the BVD virus which appear necessary for the understanding of the current hypothesis of the pathology and pathogenesis of this disease.

2. To review the most recent results of experimental and accidental infections <u>in utero</u> describing teratogenic lesions associated with a BVD infection.

3. To contribute to the established hypothesis of dual infection with some further results of experimentally produced MD in a gnotobiotic calf and in four 10-month-old bovines.

SOME VIRUS PROPERTIES

BVD virus is a pestivirus currently belonging to the family of Togaviridiae. Antigenetically it is closely related to the hog cholera virus and the Border disease virus (BD) of sheep. BVD and BD, however, appear to be more closely related to one another than to hog cholera. (Moennig et al., 1987). The virus is transmitted by contact through virus-containing body fluids (Duffell and Harkness, 1985) including semen of infected bulls, uterine secretions, placenta containing virus (Stöber, 1984) and contaminated vaccines, or it is iatrogenically transmitted by contaminated needles (Roeder and Harkness, 1986). In infected pregnant animals, the virus will pass the placenta and infect the fetus (Done et al., 1980). The outcome of this infection appears to depend upon the time of infection (as will be discussed later), the strain of the virus, its antigenicity (Hafez et al., 1976), and its behaviour in cell culture. It is important to realize that two biotypes, namely a noncytopathogenic and cytopathogenic do exist. Special strains grown in cell culture will not produce a cytopathogenic effect, and they are detectable only by indirect techniques. Basically both biotypes are indistinguishable except for one difference in their respective polypeptide pattern. The 115 KD nonstructural protein of pestiviruses is found to be degraded to a 80 KD protein in cells infected with cytopathogenic strains of BVD (Moennig et al., 1987). It still is questionable which factors are involved in the change of cytopathogenicity and whether this may occur in infected animals or during passage of virus through cell cultures. Several viruses used for vaccine production, however, have been derived from cytopathogenic strains only.

TERATOGENIC EFFECTS ON THE FETUS

The virus can be transmitted transplacentally (Duffell and Harkness, 1985; Kahrs, 1981; Roeder and Harkness, 1986). The outcome of a diaplacental infection depends on the time of gestation when a pregnant cow is infected, the type of virus strains infecting the animals, its characteristics, whether the infecting virus is a cytopathogenic or a noncytopathogenic one, and the immune status of the cow. Much has been learned over the past years and a broad spectrum of congenital alterations has been described: mononuclear infiltration in hepatic portal areas, myocarditis, necrosis in spleen and lymph nodes, thymic hypoplasia, growth arrest lines in bones, partial alopecia, hypoplasia of hair follicles, cystic distension of adnexal glands and a broad spectrum of lesions in the central nervous system, consisting of varying degrees of cerebellar atrophy, porencephaly, hydranencephaly, microencephaly, hydrocephalus, cystic septum pellucidum, dysmyelinization, and ocular lesions including retinal dysplasia and atrophy, cataracts, heterochromasia of the iris, optic neuritis and atrophy, microphthalmia and persistent pupillary membrane (Jubb et al., 1985). Much remains to be learned from detailed experimental work on the development of these alterations mentioned above, but it is generally accepted that early infections between days 50 and 100 of gestation will result in fetal abortion or mummification. Infections occurring at the time of organogenesis of the central nervous system (100 to 150 days of gestation) seem to be hazardous, but only until the fetus begins to develop its immune competence between day 130 and 200 of gestation (Baker, 1987). Immune responses of fetuses, however, may be possible earlier, since Ohmann (1982) and Ohmann et al (1982) reported on specific virus neutralizing antibodies in two fetuses infected 135 to 150 days of gestation.

Results of two more recent experimental studies are considered in order to exemplify a few data on present knowledge of the diaplacental BVD infection.

a) Done et al (1980) infected 15 pregnant antibody-free heifers intramuscularly at day 100 of gestation with an inoculum produced from 10 different strains of cytopathogenic viruses isolated from field cases with BVD-MD. Seven animals were given a low dose of this virus mixture. Eight were infected with a high dose (one of these 8 heifers was pregnant with twins). None of the animals became sick, but all seroconverted between day 136 and 154 of pregnancy. Six fetuses died in utero and 10 fetuses were born alive but developed different congenital defects. Most striking are the varying degrees of decreased weight of thymus, gastrocnemium muscle, lung, body, cerebellum and brain, and reduced length of tibia and of crown to anus. Three of the calves born alive were clinically abnormal; they were unable to stand, showed abnormal stance or astasia, dysmetria or tremors. Four of the liveborn animals had severe morphological CNS defects, two of them showed malformations and two had spinal cord hypoplasia. From 8 of the 10 liveborn calves, noncytopathogenic BVD virus was reisolated; 2 of the calves developed neutralizing antibody titers.

b) From a group of 22 seronegative cattle vaccinated between day 51 and day 123 of pregnancy with a commercial modified live virus vaccine containing mostly cytopathogenic BVD virus (Liess et al., 1984), Trautwein et al (1986) described the central nervous system malformations which occurred in calves from cows vaccinated between day 90 and 118 of gestation. Out of the 13 calves from cows vaccinated earlier than 90 days of gestation, 10 were persistently infected and two of them showed growth retardation. The others were clinically normal and had been sold persistently infected. Two calves vaccinated on days 110 and 123 were not infected and sold healthy. Out of the 7 animals with CNS lesions, 5 showed clinical signs of astasia, opisthotonus or torticollis. Upon pathologic examination severe cerebellar hypoplasia associated with hydranencephaly was discovered in 4 calves, cerebellar hypoplasia alone was found in one calf and mild internal hydrocephalus in two animals.

MD RESULTING FROM AN INTRAUTERINE INFECTION OF NONCYTOPATHOGENIC VIRUS AND A SECOND INFECTION WITH A CYTOPATHOGENIC VIRUS

As pointed out earlier, MD must be considered a congenital disease. It is a sporadic severe disease in young cattle in the age group ranging from 6 months to 2 years. Generally 3% to 5% of the animals in a herd may be clinically severely affected. Animals which develop MD rarely survive. The morphological changes which characterize this disease, whether acute of chronic, involve the gastrointestinal tract, the respiratory tract, the integumentary system, and the lymphoid tissues. To study the pathogenesis of the intestinal lesions involved and to find out why MD is an intractable fatal disease, similar experiments were used as previously described (Bolin et al., 1985a) in order to reproduce MD in a gnotobiotic calf and in 4 ten-month-old heifers. Some of these results have been discussed (9th International Symposium on Infections of the Reproductive System of some Domestic Animal Species, Perugia, Italy, 1986).

All animals were derived from artificially inseminated heifers which were serologically negative against BVD virus and negative for virus isolation from blood samples before impregnation. Between day 90 and 100 the animals were intravenously infected with 10^6 TCID 50 of the noncytopathogenic (ncp) BVD virus strain 7443. One calf was obtained by cesarean section at term and transferred into an isolator. The other calves were born alive and healthy and raised in a closed unit until they reached ten months of age. All calves were shown to be persistently infected with the ncp strain 7443 and to be seronegative before being challenged with a cytopathogenic (cp) BVD strain, TGAC, the gnotobiotic calf at day 1 of life, the others at 10 months of age. The animals were killed sequentially (day 6,12,17, and 24) and the gnotobiotic calf on day 9, when it was moribund. All animals showed lesions comparable to those described in MD, however, varying in degree as well as intensity. They were less intense on day 6 and day 12 and more advanced on day 17 and day 24. The lesions consisted of progressing depletion of follicles in Peyer's patches, hemorrhages and focal necrosis of the mucosa over Peyer's patches, indentation of Peyer's patches in the later stage of infection, and herniation of intestinal mucosa into the depleted lymph follicles. Colonic lesions were present in areas of aggregated lymphoid follicles at the ileocecal entrance, the proximal colon, and rectum. Histologically, there was prominent lymphangiectasia in the ileum with an increase of intraepithelial cells of which there were even more present in colonic tissue. A decreased number of goblet cells in colonic crypts and crypt hyperplasia with immature mucosal surface was a common finding. These lesions suggest that mechanisms are involved which disturb the regular turnover rate in the mucosal renewal system. Observations that the intestinal immune system may be involved in the disease process had been reported earlier (Ohmann, 1983; Ramsey, 1956).

In general, these results are consistent with the hypothesis of dual infection (Brownlie et al., 1984). However, there is a gap in this hypothesis since Bolin et al (1985b) and Harkness et al (1984) observed some cases in which a second infection with a modified live virus (cp) did not result in disease. Those cases were observed by others. Littlejohns and Walker (1985) are discussing whether other trigger factors are necessary to reproduce MD. Trautwein et al (1987) indicated that there is some evidence that in persistently infected animals without clinical disease, the virus is hidden in neurons in special areas of the brain. Pohlenz et al (1987) have observed in animals persistently infected and developing mucosal disease that intramural ganglia do harbour the virus. Further investigations are urgently needed to obtain a better understanding of this intriguing disease.

REFERENCES

Baker JC (1987). Bovine viral diarrhea virus: a review. J Am Vet Med Assoc 190:1449-1458.

Bolin SR, McClurkin AW, Cutlip RC, Coria MF (1985a). Severe clinical disease produced in cattle persistently infected with noncytopathic bovine viral diarrhea virus by superinfection with cytopathic bovine viral diarrhea virus. Am J Vet Res 46:573-576.

Bolin SR, McClurkin AW, Cutlip RC, Coria MF (1985b). Response of cattle persistently infected with noncytopathic bovine viral diarrhea virus to vaccination for bovine viral diarrhea and subsequent challenge exposure with cytopathic bovine viral diarrhea virus. Am J Vet Res 46:2467-2470.

Brownlie J, Clarke MC, Howard CJ (1984). Experimental production of fatal mucosal disease in cattle. Vet Rec 114:535-536.

Coria MF, McClurkin AW (1978). Specific immune tolerance in an apparently healthy bull persistently infected with bovine viral diarrhea virus. J Am Vet Med Assoc 172:449-451.

Done JT, Terlecki S, Richardson C, Harkness JW, Sands JJ, Patterson DSP, Sweasey D, Shaw IG, Winkler CE, Duffell SJ (1980). Bovine virus diarrhoea-mucosal disease virus: pathogenicity for the fetal calf following maternal infection. Vet Rec 106:473-479.

Duffell SJ, Harkness JW (1985). Bovine virus diarrhea-mucosal disease infection in cattle. Vet Rec 117:240-245.

Hafez SM, Liess B, Frey HR (1976). Studies on the natural occurrence of neutralizing antibodies against six strains of bovine viral diarrhea virus in field sera of cattle. Zentralbl Veterinärmed (B) 23:669-677.

Harkness JW, Roeder PL, Wood L (1984). Mucosal disease in cattle. Vet Rec 115:186.

Jubb KVF, Kennedy PC, Palmer N (1985). "Pathology of Domestic Animals." 3rd ed Vol 2. New York: Academic Press, pp 95-100.

Kahrs RF (1981). "Viral Disease of Cattle." Ames: Iowa State University Press, pp 89-103.

Liess B, Frey HR, Kittsteiner H, Baumann F, Neumann W (1974). Observations and investigations on mucosal disease of cattle, a late stage of BVD-MD virus infection with immunobiologic explanation and criteria of a slow virus infection? Dtsch Tierärztl Wschr 81:481-487.

Liess B, Frey HR, Orban S, Hafez SM (1983). Bovine Virus-diarrhoe (BVD) -"Mucosal Disease": Persistente BVD-Feld-virusinfektionen bei serologisch selektierten Rindern. Dtsch Tierärztl Wschr 90:249-296.

Liess B, Orban S, Frey HR, Trautwein G, Wiefel W, Blindow H (1984). Studies on transplacental transmissibility of a Bovine Virus Diarrhoea (BVD) vaccine virus in cattle. Zentrabl Veterinarmed [B] 31:669-681.

Littlejohns IR, Walker KH (1985). Aetiology and pathogenesis of mucosal disease of cattle: current concepts, observations and speculation. Aust Vet J 62:101-103.

Malmquist WA (1968). Bovine viral diarrhea-mucosal disease: etiology, pathogenesis and applied immunity. J Am Vet Med Assoc 152:763-768.

McClurkin AW, Bolin SR, Coria MF (1985). Isolation of cytopathic and noncytopathic bovine viral diarrhea virus

from the spleen of cattle acutely and chronically affected with bovine viral diarrhea. J Am Vet Med Assoc 186:568-569.
Moennig V, Bolin SR, Coulibaly COZ, Kelso-Gourley NE, Liess B, Mateo A, Peters W, Greiser-Wilke I (1987). Investigation of the antigenic structure of pestiviruses using monoclonal antibodies. Dtsch Tierärztl Wschr 94:572-576.
Ohmann HB (1982). Experimental fetal infection with bovine viral diarrhea virus II. Morphological reactions and distribution of viral antigen. Can J Comp Med 46:363-369.
Ohmann HB (1983). Pathogenesis of bovine viral diarrhoea-mucosal disease: distribution and significance of BVDV antigen in diseased calves. Res Vet Sci 34:5-10.
Ohmann HB, Jensen MH, Sorensen KJ, Dalsgaard K (1982). Experimental fetal infection with bovine viral diarrhea virus I. Virological and serological studies. Can J Comp Med 46:357-362.
Olafson P, MacCullum Ad, Fox FH (1946). An apparently new transmissible disease of cattle. Cornell Vet 36:205-213.
Pohlenz J, Liebler EM, Hewicker M, Trautwein G, Liess B, Stahl C (1987). Morphologic lesions in the intestinal mucosa in cattle persistently infected with bovine viral diarrhea virus (BVDV). Summer Meeting Brit Soc for Immunol, Cambridge, Aug 6 and 7, 1987.
Ramsey FK (1956). Pathology of a mucosal disease of cattle. Monograph, Iowa State Univ, Vet Med, Ames, Iowa.
Ramsey FK, Chivers WH (1953). Mucosal disease of cattle. North Am Vet 34:629-633.
Roeder PL, Drew TW (1984). Mucosal disease of cattle: A late sequel to foetal infection. Vet Rec 114:309-313.
Roeder PL, Harkness JW (1986). BVD virus infection: Prospects for control. Vet Rec 118:143-147.
Steck F, Lazary S, Fey H, Wandeler A, Huggler Chr, Oppliger G, Baumberger H, Kaderli R, Martig K (1980). Immune responsiveness in cattle fatally affected by bovine virus diarrhea-mucosal disease. Zentralbl Veterinärmed (B) 27:429-445.
Stöber M (1984). Current knowledge of the BVD syndrome of cattle: agent, immune response, course and spread, control. Bovine Pract 19:49-60.
Trautwein G, Hewicker M, Liess B, Orban S, Grunert E (1986). Studies on transplacental transmissibility of a bovine virus diarrhea (BVD) vaccine virus in cattle III. Occurrence of central nervous system malformations in calves born from vaccinated cows. J Vet Med B 33:260-268.

Trautwein G, Hewicker M, Fernandes A, Liess B, Stahl C, Pohlenz J (1987). Central nervous system lesions in cattle persistently infected with bovine viral diarrhea virus. Summer meeting Brit Soc Immunol, Cambridge, Aug 6 and 7, 1987.

DISCUSSION

DR. OSBURN: You mentioned that there is some possibility that humans have antibodies to the bovine viral diarrhea virus. Do you have any idea how they may have acquired this antibody?

DR. POHLENZ: I don't know. This information was published by Dr. Potts, National Institutes of Health, in a report about 6 or 8 months ago. I would suggest that it is possible that it occurs from contact with infected bovine material. I don't know how else it would be possible. But if you consider the broad spectrum of viruses in ruminants and pigs, you can imagine that contact with sheep or pigs may lead to exposure from which antibodies against pestivirus will result. Dr. Potts has, to my knowledge, demonstrated only pestivirus antibodies of the Togaviridae family.

DR. OSBURN: The other possibility may be through human vaccination with modified live virus vaccines where bovine serum was used as enrichment for the cell cultures. Also there may be a human pestivirus acting similarly to those in animals.

Transplacental Effects on Fetal Health, pages 59–70

HYPOMYELINATION IN BORDER DISEASE: THE ROLES OF THYROID HORMONES, GROWTH HORMONE, AND VIRUS INFECTION OF THE CNS

Charles A. Anderson, Robert J. Higgins, Marion E. Smith, Mary M. Sawyer, and Bennie I. Osburn

Merck Sharp and Dohme Research Laboratories, West Point, Pennsylvania 19486 (C.A.A.), Department of Pathology, School of Veterinary Medicine, University of California Davis, Davis, California 95616 (R.J.H., M.M.S., B.I.O.), and the Department of Neurology, Veterans Administration Medical Center, Palo Alto, California 94304 (M.E.S.)

INTRODUCTION

Border disease (BD) is a congenital disorder of sheep, first described in 1959 (Hughes et al 1959). It is caused by a pestivirus in the Togaviridae, which is closely related to bovine viral diarrhea virus and hog cholera virus (Terpstra 1985). Affected lambs display a spectrum of lesions, including intrauterine growth retardation, hairy birthcoat, and various central nervous system (CNS) abnormalities (Terpstra 1985).

Hypomyelination in Border Disease

The most characteristic defect in the CNS is diffuse hypomyelination, generally without accompanying inflammation (Barlow 1982). Despite extensive research, the mechanism by which border disease virus (BDV) causes the hypomyelination is not known. It has been shown that affected lambs have fewer mature oligodendrocytes, and greater numbers of immature glial cells of indeterminate origin than do healthy lambs (Barlow 1982; Barlow et al 1977). Therefore, it has been assumed that BDV interferes with the differentiation of oligodendrocytes. There is no clear evidence, however, that this interference with differentiation is the result of viral infection of oligodendrocytes.

Studies to detect BDV antigen in the CNS of affected lambs have led to conflicting results. In one study, in which newborn and 5-month-old lambs experimentally infected in utero with a BDV-containing brain homogenate were examined, widespread infection was detected in many cells in the CNS (Gardiner 1980). However, the antiserum used to detect BDV antigen was obtained from ewes inoculated with the same brain suspension, and although the antiserum was absorbed with dried brain powders, there may have been residual antibodies to CNS tissue.

In another study in which the central nervous systems of naturally infected lambs from 2 to 52 weeks of age were examined (using conjugated antiserum from a ewe which had given birth to BD lambs), minimal BDV antigen was detected. There were no BDV antigen-containing cells in the cervical and lumbar portions of the spinal cord, in any of the lambs, and only scattered infected cells were present in the cerebral cortex and cerebellum of the 2- and 4-week old lambs (Terpstra 1978).

In addition to investigating how extensively BDV infects cells in the CNS, researchers have also tried to determine whether BDV has a selective affinity for oligodendrocytes. Neither of the above studies definitively identified the infected cells. However, in a recent abstract BDV antigen was reported to be in neurons, astrocytes, oligodendrocytes, and endothelial cells of affected lambs, although the extent of infection in the CNS was not described (Potts et al 1986). These results agree with studies in vitro which indicated that although BDV will infect some oligodendrocytes in primary fetal ovine brain cell cultures, it definitely does not have a selective tropism for them (Anderson et al 1987b).

Proposed Pathogenesis for the Hypomyelination in BD

In light of the possibly minimal viral infection of oligodendrocytes in lambs with BD, we decided to investigate another possible mechanism by which BDV might cause the diffuse hypomyelination so characteristic of the disease. Previous work demonstrated that the thyroid and pituitary glands of BD lambs are consistently infected with BDV (Terpstra 1978). Since both thyroid hormones and growth hormone (GH) are essential for normal myelination (Balazs et al 1969; Noguchi et al 1982b; Pelton et al 1974) we felt that the hypomyelination in BD may be due to perturbations in the circulating levels of these hormones secondary to infection of the pituitary and/or thyroid glands.

The importance of thyroid hormones in myelin formation has been known for some time. In 1969 it was reported that neonatal thyroidectomy in rats resulted in a reduced amount of cerebral myelin (Balazs et al 1969). In addition, hypomyelination has been demonstrated in the congenitally hypothyroid mouse, where it can be prevented by the administration of thyroxine (T_4) in the dam's breast milk (Noguchi et al 1985a).

Growth hormone is also critical for normal myelination. The congenitally GH-deficient mouse has hypomyelination (Noguchi et al 1985b), as does the Snell dwarf mouse, which has severely reduced levels of GH, thyroid stimulating hormone (TSH), and other anterior pituitary hormones (Noguchi et al 1982a). The hypomyelination in the Snell dwarf mouse can be prevented by giving both GH and T_4 (Noguchi et al 1982b; Sugisaki et al 1985).

A critical aspect of our investigation was the measurement of 2',3'-cyclic nucleotide-3'-phosphodiesterase (CNP) activity in CNS tissue from BD lambs. CNP is an enzyme found in oligodendrocytes (Snyder et al 1983) and myelin (Kurihara et al 1967) and its activity increases in parallel with myelination both _in vivo_ (Sprinkle et al 1978) and _in vitro_ (Fry et al 1973). However, it was measured in this study not only to confirm the hypomyelination, but because CNP is dependent on both thyroid hormones and GH for maximum activity (Sarlieve et al 1983).

We present evidence that neonatal lambs with BD have 1) minimal infection of the CNS by BDV, 2) a myelin deficiency with reduced activity of CNP, and 3) a depression in circulating thyroid hormone levels, associated with an extensive, noninflammatory, and noncytolytic infection of the thyroid gland by BDV.

EXPERIMENTAL DESIGN

Detailed descriptions of the materials and methods for this work have already been published (Anderson et al 1987a; Anderson et al 1987c). Briefly, border disease was experimentally induced in nine lambs by inoculation of their dams with BDV isolate #31 at 50 days gestation. These lambs were studied in parallel with three age-matched control lambs, whose dams had received an inoculum of virus-free cell culture supernatant.

The lambs were euthanized 48 hours after birth. The weight, crown-rump length, and length of the right tibia and right radius were recorded. Aliquots of serum and plasma were collected at that time and subsequently assayed for L-3,3',5-triiodothyronine (T_3), T_4, GH, and TSH. Samples of thyroid and pituitary glands were also obtained. Indirect immunofluorescence techniques were used to detect BDV antigen in the thyroid glands. In the pituitary glands, double immunofluorescence techniques were used to simultaneously demonstrate BDV antigen and various pituitary hormones, including luteinizing hormone (LH), GH, TSH, adrenocorticotrophic hormone (ACTH), and prolactin.

Portions of cervical (C_6), thoracic (T_6), and lumbar (L_3) spinal cord were also obtained at necropsy. Sections of spinal cord from each of these 3 levels were later stained immunocytochemically for myelin associated glycoprotein (MAG) and myelin basic protein (MBP), histochemically with hematoxylin and eosin and luxol fast blue/cresyl Echt violet (LFB/CEV), and by immunofluorescence for BDV antigen. Finally, homogenates of whole spinal cord, again from the same three levels, were assayed for CNP.

Statistical analyses were done by using the two-sided Student's t-test. For the GH values, a Mann-Whitney test was performed as there was such a wide range in values. In both cases a probability value less than 0.05 was used as the level of significance.

RESULTS AND DISCUSSION

The results of this study have been previously published (Anderson et al 1987a; Anderson et al 1987c). All of the control lambs were normal. The lambs with border disease had variable clinical signs (Table 1). Eight had abnormally hairy birthcoats, and all but one lamb had a constant tremor. Some lambs were weak; one was unable to stand. There was a statistically significant

TABLE 1. Clinical Signs, Weights, Crown-rump Lengths, and Long Bone Lengths of BD and Control Lambs.

Lamb No.	Sex	Clinical signs	Weight (kg)	Crown-rump length (cm)	Long bone length rt tibia/rt radius (cm)
LAMBS FROM EWES WHICH WERE GIVEN BDV					
1-1	M	Weak, moderately hairy birthcoat	2.3	40	10/7.5
1-2	M	Weak, mild shaking, moderately hairy birthcoat	2.7	45	11/8.1
2	F	Stillborn	ND	ND	ND
3-1	F	Moderate shaking	3.6	45	10.6/7.5
3-2	F	Moderate shaking, moderately hairy birthcoat	3.6	50	11/8
4-1	M	Moderate shaking, moderately hairy birthcoat	2.9	42.5	10.7/8.3
4-2	M	Stillborn	ND	ND	ND
5	M	Severe shaking, mildly hairy birthcoat	4.3	45	12.7/9.5
6	M	Mild shaking, mildly hairy birthcoat	4.1	43	12/9
7	M	Severe shaking, moderately hairy birthcoat	2.9	42	11.7/8.9
8	M	Severe shaking, unable to stand, markedly hairy birthcoat	2.9	46	11.5/8.7
LAMBS FROM CONTROL EWES					
9	M	Normal	5.7	47	13/9.8
10	M	Normal	4.1	44	12/9.1
11	F	Normal	4.8	46.5	12.5/9.5
		Control means	4.8 ± 0.8	45.8 ± 1.6	12.5 ± 0.5/9.5 ± 0.3
		Affected lamb means	3.2 ± 0.7	44.3 ± 2.9	11.2 ± 0.8/8.4 ± 0.7
		P value	0.01	0.38	0.04/0.03

ND = not done.

reprinted from American Journal of Veterinary Research 48:502, 1987 difference between the mean body weight of the nine affected lambs and that of the three control lambs. Similarly statistically significant differences were seen in the mean lengths of their right tibiae and radii. There was no significant difference in the mean crown-rump lengths between the two groups; however, crown-rump length is considered a less accurate indicator of skeletal growth (Richardson et al 1976). These clinical signs, including the growth retardation, are typical of BD (Terpstra 1985).

Spinal Cords

At all three levels of spinal cord (C_6, T_6, and L_3) in the affected lambs there was diffuse hypomyelination (Table 2), which was not accompanied by inflammation. This was relatively mild in 3 lambs, moderate in 2 lambs, and severe in 4 lambs. The hypomyelination was documented with the LFB/CEV stains, as well as with the stains for MAG and MBP. In all the BD lambs, the hypomyelination involved all white matter tracts, and was slightly more severe in lumbar and thoracic sections than in cervical sections. There was no hypomyelination or inflammation in the spinal cords of control lambs.

The hypomyelination in the affected lambs was accompanied by decreased activity of the myelin-associated, thyroid hormone-dependent enzyme, CNP (Table 2). The mean activity of this enzyme was statistically significantly reduced in the affected lambs as compared to the control lambs in the lumbar samples and the thoracic samples. At the cervical level, the difference in mean CNP activity was not significant in a two-sided t-test at the 0.05 level, although it was at the 0.1 level. However, this was not unexpected since histologically the hypomyelination was less severe at the cervical level than at lower levels in the spinal cord.

Staining for BDV antigen in the C_6, T_6, and L_3 sections of spinal cord revealed very small numbers of infected cells at all three levels in the affected lambs, and no infected cells in the control lambs. The percentage of cells infected in these sections varied from 0.01% to 0.3%. This limited infection of CNS tissue agreed with the work of Terpstra (Terpstra 1978) who had found little BDV antigen in the CNS of naturally infected lambs. It also

TABLE 2. Levels of Circulating Thyroid and Pituitary Hormones and Spinal Cord CNP Activity in BD and Control Lambs

Lamb number	BD-affected (BD) or control (C) lamb	Overall severity of hypomyelination based on MAG and MBP staining	CNP activity (μmoles phosphate released/μg of protein in 30 min			Serum T_3 (ng/dl)	Serum T_4 (μg/dl)	Plasma GH (ng/ml)	Plasma TSH (ng/ml)
			C_6	T_6	L_3				
1-1	BD	+	0.179	0.155	0.140	169	6.9	22.4	ND[a]
1-2	BD	+	0.172	0.156	0.156	137	6.6	34.0	ND
3-1	BD	+++	0.145	ND	0.160	343	7.2	12.6	ND
3-2	BD	+	0.174	0.144	0.132	330	7.4	26.0	ND
4-1	BD	+++	0.129	0.105	0.111	256	8.1	10.2	17.6
5	BD	++	0.140	0.146	0.127	250	7.6	15.6	22.9
6	BD	++	0.150	ND	0.155	385	9.1	10.0	36.9
7	BD	+++	0.154	0.096	0.093	195	10.3	150.0	ND
8	BD	+++	0.115	0.124	0.120	203	7.6	124.0	36.7
9	C	NA[a]	0.162	0.166	0.211	420	9.4	13.0	21.4
10	C	NA	0.196	0.194	0.213	447	11.2	14.4	12.9
11	C.	NA	0.177	0.204	0.187	395	11.5	31.6	31.2
BD lamb means			0.151 ±0.021	0.132 ±0.024	0.133 ±0.022	252.0 ±85.0	7.87 ±1.16	45.0 ±53.2	28.53 ±9.80
C lamb means			0.178 ±0.017	0.188 ±0.019	0.204 ±0.014	420.7 ±26.0	10.70 ±1.14	19.7 ±10.4	21.83 ±9.16
p value			0.089	0.018	0.002	0.022	0.006	NS[a]	NS

[a] ND, not done; NA, not applicable; NS, not significant.

reprinted from Laboratory Investigation 57:172, 1987

indicated that infection of oligodendrocytes, with subsequent cytolysis or functional modulation, may not be the mechanism by which BDV induces hypomyelination.

Thyroid and Pituitary Glands

Histologically, the thyroid glands of the BD and control lambs were normal. In both cases most of the parenchyma consisted of fairly uniformly sized follicles with only small numbers of interfollicular cells. The follicles were lined with cuboidal, nonhypertrophied cells. There was no inflammation in any of the glands. Immunofluorescence staining for BDV antigen demonstrated extensive infection of thyroid follicular epithelial cells in all the BD lambs, but no infection in controls.

The pituitaries of the affected and control lambs were also histologically normal. There were BDV antigen-positive cells in the pituitaries of all the affected lambs, but the number of infected cells was much less than in the thyroids. BDV antigen-positive cells were not found in the pituitaries of the controls.

In both BD and control lambs, the majority of cells in the pituitaries were positive for prolactin and GH with slightly fewer LH- and ACTH-containing cells. TSH-positive cells were rare, with none detected in pituitary sections from the three control lambs and from four of the affected lambs. In the remaining five affected lambs only a few TSH-positive cells were seen.

Double labeling revealed that the few BDV antigen-containing cells in the pituitaries were positive for prolactin, ACTH, GH, or LH. However, the virus had no apparent predilection for any one of these cell types. None of the TSH cells were positive for BDV antigen.

Hormone Levels

There were statistically significant reductions in the mean serum levels of T_3 and T_4 in the BD lambs as compared to the controls (Table 2). Similar significant differences in the mean plasma concentrations of GH and TSH were not found between the affected and control lambs (Table 2).

Combined with the extensive infection of the thyroid follicular cells and the only mild infection of pituitary cells, these results indicate that infection of the thyroid, but not of the pituitary, may be important in the pathogenesis of the hypomyelination in BD.

CONCLUSION

Although not definitive, these results indicate that the hypomyelination in BD may not be due to infection of oligodendrocytes by BDV, but instead may be due to depressed levels of circulating thyroid gland hormones secondary to a noninflammatory and noncytolytic infection of the thyroid gland _in utero_ by BDV.

REFERENCES

Anderson CA, Higgins RJ, Smith ME, Osburn BI (1987a). Border disease: Virus-induced decrease in thyroid hormone levels with associated hypomyelination. Lab Invest 57:168-175.

Anderson CA, Higgins, RJ, Waldvogel AS, Osburn BI (1987b). Tropism of border disease virus for oligodendrocytes in ovine fetal brain cell cultures. Am J Vet Res 48:822-827.

Anderson CA, Sawyer M, Higgins RJ, East N, Osburn BI (1987c). Experimentally induced ovine border disease: Extensive hypomyelination with minimal viral antigen in neonatal spinal cord. Am J Vet Res 48:499-503.

Balazs R, Brooksbank BWL, Davison AN, Eayrs JT, Wilson DA (1969). The effect of neonatal thyroidectomy on myelination in the rat brain. Brain Res 15:219-232.

Barlow RM (1982). Neuropathology of affected sheep. In Barlow RM, Patterson DSP (eds): "Border Disease of Sheep: A Virus-Induced Teratogenic Disorder", Berlin and Hamburg: Verlag Paul Parey, p 22.

Barlow RM, Storey IJ (1977). Myelination of the ovine CNS with special reference to border disease. I. Qualitative aspects. Neuropathol Appl Neurobiol 3:255-265.

Fry JM, Lehrer GM, Bornstein MB (1973). Experimental inhibition of myelination in spinal cord tissue cultures: enzyme assays. J Neurobiol 4:453-459.

Gardiner AC (1980). The distribution and significance of border disease viral antigen in infected lambs and

foetuses. J Comp Pathol 90:513-518.
Hughes LE, Kershaw GF, Shaw IG (1959). "B" or border disease: an undescribed disease of sheep. Vet Rec 71:313-317.
Kurihara T, Tsukada Y (1967). The regional and subcellular distribution of 2', 3'-cyclic nucleotide-3'-phosphohydrolase in the central nervous system. J Neurochem 14:1167-1174.
Noguchi T, Sugisaki T, Satoh I, Kudo M (1985a). Partial restoration of cerebral myelination of the congenitally hypothyroid mouse by parenteral or breast milk administration of thyroxine. J Neurochem 45:1419-1426.
Noguchi T, Sugisaki T, Takamatsu K, Tsukada Y (1982a). Factors contributing to the poor myelination in the brain of the Snell dwarf mouse. J Neurochem 39:1693-1699.
Noguchi T, Sugisaki T, Tsukada Y (1982b). Postnatal action of growth and thyroid hormones on the retarded cerebral myelinogenesis of Snell dwarf mice (dw). J Neurochem 38:257-263.
Noguchi T, Sugisaki T, Tsukada Y (1985b). Microcephalic cerebrum with hypomyelination in the growth hormone-deficient mouse (lit). Neurochem Res 10:1097-1106.
Pelton EW, Young E, Bass NH, Grindeland RE (1974). Defective myelinogenesis in developing rat cerebrum induced by selective growth hormone deficiency. Neurology 24:377.
Potts B, Elder G, Sever J, Sawyer M, Osburn B (1986). Border disease of sheep: an animal model for virus-induced hypomyelination (abstr). Neurology 36:204.
Richardson C, Hebert C, Terlecki S (1976). Estimation of the developmental age of the ovine fetus and lamb. Vet Rec 99:22-26.
Sarlieve LL, Bouchon R, Koehl C, Neskovic NM (1983). Cerebroside and sulfatide biosynthesis in the brain of Snell dwarf mouse: effects of thyroxine and growth hormone in the early postnatal period. J Neurochem 40:1058-1062.
Snyder DS, Zimmerman TR Jr, Farooq M, Norton WT, Cammer W (1983). Carbonic anhydrase, 5'-nucleotidase, and 2',3'-cyclic nucleotide-3'-phosphodiesterase activities in oligodendrocytes, astrocytes, and neurons isolated from the brains of developing rats. J Neurochem 40:120-127.
Sprinkle TJ, Zaruba ME, McKhann GM (1978). Activity of 2',3'-cyclic nucleotide-3'-phosphodiesterase in regions

of rat brain during development: quantitative relationship to myelin basic protein. J Neurochem 30:309-314.
Sugisaki T, Noguchi T, Tsukada Y (1985). Cerebral myelinogenesis in the Snell dwarf mouse: Stimulatory effects of GH and T_4 restricted to the first 20 days of postnatal life. Neurochem Res 10:767-778.
Terpstra C (1978). Detection of Border disease antigen in tissues of affected sheep and in cell cultures by immunofluorescence. Res Vet Sci 25:350-355.
Terpstra C (1985). Border disease: A congenital infection of small ruminants. Prog Vet Microbiol Immunol 1:175-198.

DISCUSSION

DR. SEVER: Does T3, T4, or TSH cross between the ewe and the lamb, and if so, do you have comparative maternal-fetal levels?

DR. C. ANDERSON: The ovine placenta is impermeable to T3, T4, and TSH, thus none of them cross the placenta.

DR. MOSER: Have you had an opportunity to determine whether the axons are normal in number, and is it truly a primary demyelination, or a failure of myelination?

DR. C. ANDERSON: We did not specifically stain for axons or specifically examine them. However, I did look at hemotoxylin and eosin stained sections of spinal cord, and the axons appeared normal. In addition, in the past, other investigators have done considerable work on that topic, and the axons have always been reported as normal.

DR. CAPEN: I was wondering if you had another control group in which you used a thyroid blocking drug to comparably lower T4 and T3 levels in order to determine whether you could produce similar hypomyelinosis with low thyroid hormone levels without ever exposing lambs to the virus?

DR. C. ANDERSON: We didn't do that, although it would be an interesting experiment. Work has been done on fetal thyroidectomy in lambs, though, in the past. Since, as I just mentioned, there is no transfer of T3, T4, or TSH across the ovine placenta, these lambs are born with very low levels of thyroid gland hormones. Investigators who did this work never really specifically looked at myelination, but they did document that brain weights were less in these lambs and that they contained less DNA, RNA, and protein than normal brains. Hypothyroidism does therefore appear to affect brain development.

DR. SCARPELLI: The evidence of localizing virus in the thyroid is indirect. Has anyone tried to infect follicular cells *in vitro* and shown an impairment of hormone secretion?

DR. C. ANDERSON: To my knowledge, no, and I didn't do that. I did do some work infecting fetal sheep brain cell cultures with the virus but never thyroid follicular cell cultures.

DR. APOSTOLOU: Have you seen any similar changes with sulfonamides at high doses which are also supposed to lower thyroid activity?

DR. C. ANDERSON: No, I have not.

II. CONGENITAL BACTERIAL AND OTHER INFECTIONS

Transplacental Effects on Fetal Health, pages 73–86

ACUTE BACTERIAL CHORIOAMNIONITIS

Richard L. Naeye, M.D.

Department of Pathology, M.S. Hershey Medical Center, The Pennsylvania State University College of Medicine, Hershey, Pa. 17033

INTRODUCTION

Acute chorioamnionitis is a disorder in which bacteria or mycoplasmas gain access and grow in the amniotic fluid. It is a frequent cause of preterm delivery, stillbirth and neonatal death in every population group where it has been studied (Benirschke, 1960; Emig, Napier and Grazie, 1961; Naeye & Tafari, 1983). It is particularly important as a cause of poor pregnancy outcome in those with low socioeconomic status (Naeye et al, 1977; Ross et al, 1982). Populations that have impaired amniotic fluid defense mechanisms have a particularly high frequency of chorioamnionitis (Appelbaum et al, 1977; Tafari et al, 1977), suggesting that the remaining defense mechanisms in these populations are unable to control the infections. Chorioamnionitis is responsible, directly or indirectly, for nearly a third of the high perinatal mortality rates in African societies where it has been studied (Table 1).

TABLE 1 - Perinatal deaths in two African locations.

	----Perinatal Deaths/100 Births----	
	Durban, South Africa	Addis Ababa, Ethiopia
Acute chorioamnionitis	14.2	17.5
Disorders sometimes caused by acute chorioamnionitis		
Abruptio placentae	8.1	4.5
Premature membrane rupture	1.1	
Other disorders	31.2	30.3
Total Perinatal Mortality Rate	54.6	53.4

Chorioamnionitis is identified by the presence of an acute inflammatory process in the extraplacental membranes, plate of the placenta, decidua and umbilical cord. These inflammatory processes are usually collectively termed chorioamnionitis because the first signs of the inflammation are found beneath the amnion and along the surface of the chorion in the extraplacental membranes. The disorder is a continuum that extends from a very mild inflammatory process in the fetal membranes to a severe inflammatory process that involves the fetus as well as the fetal membranes, the placenta and the umbilical cord. The inflammatory process can be absent in individual sections taken from the umbilical cord and fetal membranes, but it is reliably found in the chorionic plate of the placenta in those places where the plate is very thin and where there is little or no blood clot attached to the underside of the plate (Naeye, 1987). Some of the consequences of acute chorioamnionitis can be long term, including bronchopulmonary dysplasia and psychomotor impairments (Naeye, 1978; Hardt et al, 1985).

Acute chorioamnionitis most often starts as an ascending infection that reaches the fetal membranes through the cervical os, but at times it reaches the placenta and amniotic fluid by crossing the placenta, by fetoscopy, during an intrauterine transfusion or during amniocentesis (Blanc,1981; Naeye, 1979). It is this transplacental passage that qualifies it for inclusion in this transplacental infection symposium.

ETIOLOGY

In spite of many studies there is still debate about the pathogenesis of chorioamnionitis. Some doubt that it is infectious in origin because a number of studies have failed to culture microorganisms from many of the placentas with chorioamnionitis, and the disorder is often unassociated with any clinical evidences of infection in mothers, their fetuses or their newborns (Naeye and Tafari, 1983; Svensson, 1986). Recent studies, using up-to-date culture techniques, have shown that bacteria or myoplasmas can be recovered from over 70% of extraplacental membranes and placentas that have the histological findings of chorioamnionitis (Naeye et al, 1977, Pankuch GA et al, 1984). About two-thirds of the cultures yield a single organism. Many of the organisms are difficult to culture because they are anaerobes with fastidious growth characteristics. Many culture studies have not found organisms because they failed to use isolation techniques for mycoplasmas. In various studies mycoplasmas have constituted from 0 to 20% of the organisms isolated from the inflammatory process.

Results of experimental studies have added evidence that infectious agents are the cause of chorioamnionitis. Lauweryns et al (1973) showed that all features of chorioamnionitis could be produced in experimental animals by introducing various species of bacteria into the amniotic fluid, whereas adding non-bacterial substances, including meconium, gastric juice and amniotic fluid debris, did not produce acute chorioamnionitis in the absence of bacteria. Evaldson (1982) has shown that the bacteria that cause chorioamnionitis travel along the surface of the chorion in the extraplacental membranes. Naeye and Ross (1982) showed that these bacteria traverse this route around the entire uterine circumference in 12-48 hours.

Fetal neutrophils in the umbilical vessels are often attracted by bacterial chemotactic substances in the amniotic fluid to migrate toward the amniotic cavity. This produces funisitis. Maternal neutrophils in the intervillous blood are attracted to migrate through the chorionic plate of the placenta by these same chemotactic substances. In the first day or two these neutrophils stick to the underside of the placental plate (stage 1) (Blanc, 1981; Naeye & Ross, 1982). In the next several days the neutrophils migrate into the plate (stage 2). When they reach the amnion, the process is classified stage 3. We have found no relationship between chorioamnionitis and increasing maternal gestational antibody titers to ten viruses that can infect the fetus, so it appears that rarely, if ever, are viruses a cause of chorioamnionitis (Naeye & Tafari, 1983).

PATHOGENESIS

As previously mentioned, chorioamnionitis most often starts in the fetal membranes, adjacent to the cervical os. Early in its course bacteria are shed into the amniotic fluid and inactivate antibacterial systems that are normally present there. The fetus can be infected by inhaling this infected amniotic fluid. In many cases the infection extends into the decidua basalis, from which bacteria probably reach the fetus by being shed into the intervillous blood. Cooperman et al (1980) found almost as high an incidence of bacterial colonization in the decidua in cases of chorioamnionitis as in the membranes and in the amniotic fluid. This raises the possibility that hematogenous spread from the decidua is nearly as frequent a route for bacteria reaching the fetus as is aspiration of bacteria that have been shed into the amniotic fluid.

Acute chorioamnionitis almost always starts labor, presumably because the neutrophils and bacteria that are present release phospholipase, which enzymatically releases arachidonic acid from the fetal membranes (Bejar et al, 1981; Romero et al, 1986). The arachidonic acid rapidly converts to prostaglandin E_2 and to F_{2a}. Prostaglandin E_2 causes the cervix to dilate and F_{2a} initiates uterine contractions. There is also some evidence that bacterial products induce or increase prostaglandin E_2 production by amnion cells (Lamont et al, 1985). Unlike oxytocin which initiates contractions only in term or near term uteruses, prostaglandin F_{2a} causes the uterus to contract at any stage of gestation. In a recently completed study at our institution acute chorioamnionitis appeared responsible for nearly 70% of spontaneous preterm deliveries between 24-26 weeks of gestation. From that point the proportion of preterm deliveries that could be attributed to acute chorioamnionitis progressively decreased to about 30% at 34-36 weeks of gestation. In another recent study at our institution hydration, rest and tocolytic therapy failed to stop a single preterm labor in which bacterial products were identified in the amniotic fluid by gas chromatography, whereas many preterm labors were successfully stopped by tocolytic therapy when the products of infection were absent from the amniotic fluid.

EFFECTS ON THE FETUS

Infants born preterm as the result of bacterial-initiated chorioamnionitis are often ill in the neonatal period as the result of antenatal hypoxia and their immaturity (Naeye et al, 1983). Such infants usually develop the respiratory distress syndrome due to hyaline membrane disease shortly after birth. This is due to the combined effects of lung immaturity, antenatal hypoxic damage to their lungs and a destruction of surfactant by aspirated bacteria (Naeye et al, 1983). Most of the neonatal morbidity and mortality associated with chorioamnionitis are in fact due to antenatal hypoxia.

The hypoxia is manifest by low umbilical arterial pH values, low Apgar scores, the need to resuscitate, the aforementioned respiratory distress syndrome and recurrent apneic episodes (Naeye et al, 1983; Naeye & Tafari, 1983). These findings correlate much more strongly with the extent and severity of placental villous edema than with the stage and severity of chorioamnionitis (Table 2) (Naeye & Tafari, 1983; Naeye et al, 1983). The edema presumably impedes the movements of gases and nutrients into the fetal circulation by compressing capillaries and other blood vessels inside the placental villi (Naeye et al, 1983).

TABLE 2. The relationship of villous edema to mean 1-minute Apgar scores in newborns born before 32 weeks of gestation who had chorioamnionitis.

Villous Edema	Mean Apgar Scores	
Mild	6.0≠0.8	
Moderate	3.8≠1.9	$P<.001$
Severe	1.6≠1.2	

Clinical findings of infection in the gravida or neonate are present in only about 10% of cases in which histologic evidences of chorioamnionitis are present. It surprises many that evidences of clinical infection are not present in a higher proportion of fetuses and neonates who have chorioamnionitis, particularly since most have aspirated infected amniotic fluid. Signs of infection are usually absent because the aspirated bacteria are usually low in virulence. The aspiration does occasionally lead to pneumonia, particularly in preterm fetuses who do not have mature defense mechanisms. When the bacteria are virulent, fetal breathing movements can become infrequent and tachycardia can appear (Hager & Pauly, 1985; Vintzileos et al, 1986).

A few neonates with congenital aspiration pneumonia develop bacteremia or septicemia, often accompanied by neutropenia. An even smaller proportion develop otitis media, meningitis, septic arthritis or other evidence of disseminated infection (Russell, 1979). Death can occur when the infecting agent is very virulent as is the case with beta streptococcus (Novak & Platt, 1985).

DIAGNOSIS

The most reliable method for making the diagnosis of acute chorioamnionitis is by the histologic identification of polymorphonuclear leukocytes in the plate of the placenta. In about one third of such cases infectious agents can be found by smear. Very few of the organisms can be found by the widely used Brown and Brenn (1931) stain. Silver stains are often more successful. Several methods have been proposed to make a rapid diagnosis of the disorder. These include frozen section of the umbilical cord, examination of fluid from the ear canal, cytology of gastric aspirate and smears of the amnion and chorion. The cytologic examination of gastric aspirate and fluid from the ear canal can be either falsely negative or positive. Frozen sections of the umbilical cord are often falsely negative because funisitis frequently skips segments of the cord. A smear taken between the amnion and chorion for the presence of polymorphonuclear leukocytes is the most reliable rapid method for diagnosing chorioamnionitis.

FACTORS PREDISPOSING TO THE DEVELOPMENT OF CHORIOAMIONITIS

There are great variations in the frequency of chorioamnionitis among various population groups. Some of this difference may be due to differing levels of antimicrobial activity in the amniotic fluid and to differing coital practices during pregnancy. Normally, antimicrobial activity first appears in the amniotic fluid in the second trimester of pregnancy, progressively increases in titer to term and is active against a wide spectrum of aerobic and anaerobic bacteria. When this antimicrobial activity is absent, bacteria and mycoplasmas normally present in the vagina and cervix can invade and spread through the fetal membranes and freely grow in the amniotic fluid. Over 90 percent of malnourished gravidas in some third-world populations lack antimicrobial activity in their amniotic fluid, often due to a deficiency of zinc which must be present for antimicrobial activity to be operative (Appelbaum et al, 1977; Tafari et al, 1977). Between 10-15% of U.S. whites and blacks also have abnormally low levels of this antimicrobial activity during late gestation (Appelbaum et al, 1980). None of these U.S. women were likely zinc-deficient, so they presumably had non-zinc abnormalities in their antimicrobial system. A prospective study will be needed to determine if such women are particularly vulnerable to chorioamnionitis.

There are other mechanisms that also protect against the development of chorioamnionitis and fetal infection. These include a low vaginal pH, the cervical mucous plug, various cellular and humoral defense mechanisms in the fetal membranes and the various defense mechanisms in the fetus. The fetus may be more vulnerable to infection before than after 32 weeks of gestation because maternal IgG does not pass the placenta in significant quantities until about the 32nd week of gestation (Sidiropoulos et al, 1986).

Coitus appears to have a role in the genesis of chorioamnionitis. Our most recent, unpublished studies show that women who discontinue coitus during pregnancy for a month or more and then resume it before term have a high rate of preterm labors, many of which are due to chorioamnionitis. The responsible mechanisms are a matter of speculation. Coitus could be introducing new organisms into the vagina. This could explain why chorioamnionitis is more frequent when women have more than one coital partner during pregnancy. Another possibility is that seminal fluid and sperm aid the passage of bacteria through the mucous plug in the cervix. Seminal fluid has proteolytic enzymes that facilitate the passage of sperm through this mucous plug (Lundquist et al, 1955; Moghissi, 1971). This mucous becomes more resistant to penetration by sperm during pregnancy, but the resistance may not be absolute. Mycoplasmas and some bacteria attach themselves to sperm and thus may be transported at least some distance through the cervical mucous (Gnarpe & Friberg, 1973). The older literature reports that seminal fluid is strongly antibacterial. More recent studies show that over 80% of seminal fluids will kill _S. aureus_ whereas only half will kill _E. coli_. _E. coli_ is a much more frequent cause of chorioamnionitis than is _S. aureus_ (Appelbaum et al, 1980).

There are other predisposing factors to the development of chorioamnionitis. The frequency of the infection increases with the duration of labor, starting at about 10 hours. This can occur without membrane rupture, so it presumably is the result of exposure of the fetal membranes to bacteris from the cervical canal. This takes place when the cervix is dilated and its mucous plug has dropped out. The same thing happens before the onset of labor, late in gestation, in some multigravida. Partial opening of the cervix leads to a loss of the mucous plug after which bacteria have ready access to the fetal membranes. This latter mechanism is presumably responsible for the sharp increase in the frequency of chorioamnionitis after 37 weeks of gestation in the general population (Naeye and Tafari, 1983).

PREMATURE RUPTURE OF THE FETAL MEMBRANES

This is defined as fetal membrane rupture before the onset of labor. There has long been uncertainty about the nature and causes of the membrane damage that predisposes to premature ruptures. In the laboratory, membranes that have ruptured prematurely usually resist rupture by pressures as high as those generated during labor. Most of this strength is in a zone of connective tissue beneath the amnion and little difference has been found between the elastin and collagen content of membranes that ruptured prematurely and those that ruptured normally after the onset of labor. The simplest explanation is that the rupture passed through and destroyed the localized membrane abnormalities in which the ruptures started (Bourne, 1962). Acute chorioamnionitis appears to be the most frequent cause of this localized membrane damage. Evidence for this is derived from a large study in which chorioamnionitis was twice as frequent when fetal membranes ruptured within four hours before the onset of labor as when they ruptured after labor began (Naeye & Tafari, 1983). This indicates that chorioamnionitis may have antedated up to half of the premature ruptures because four hours is too short a time for chorioamnionitis to develop after membrane rupture. Collagenase and elastase released by acute inflammatory cells are the suspected causes of the local membrane damage that leads to premature membrane ruptures (Sibille et al, 1986).

Cooperstock et al (1987) have provided additional evidence that chorioamnionitis has a major role in the genesis of premature membrane rupture. They found that such ruptures have a highly circadian incidence, reaching a peak in the hours just after midnight. When chorioamnionitis was present there was no peak, post-midnight or at any other time.

Coital-induced orgasm appears to be an important cofactor with acute chorioamnionitis in the genesis of some premature membrane ruptures. Goodlin et al (1972) showed that orgasm can induce uterine contractions. We showed, in a prospective study, that coital-generated orgasm was followed by a high frequency of premature membrane ruptures when chorioamnionitis was present (Naeye, & Ross, 1982). When chorioamnionitis was absent, the frequency of premature membrane rupture after coitus-generated orgasm was low.

ABRUPTIO PLACENTAE

Abruptio placenta is defined as the separation of all or part of the placenta from the wall of the uterus before the fetus has been delivered. The retroplacental hemorrhages that start most placental abruptions presumably originate in the rupture of a decidual arteriole or small artery. This can occur when the vessel is damaged by necrosis or infection. In the course of chorioamnionitis, bacteria or mycoplasmas can invade the decidua where blood vessel damage can lead to hemorrhage and an abruption (Cooperman et al, 1980; Naeye, 1981).

LONG TERM CONSEQUENCES OF ACUTE CHORIOAMNIONITIS

Chorioamnionitis can have long term effects on mental and motor development. Neonatal bilirubin levels are higher when chorioamnionitis is present than when it is absent (Naeye, 1978). The neurotoxicity of bilirubin is also potentiated by chorioamnionitis (Naeye, 1978). This neurotoxicity is evident both in measurements of cognitive performance and in the frequency of neurologic abnormalities in older children.

Chorioamnionitis also often affects long term psychomotor development by initiating the development of placental villous edema. We have recently found that placental villous edema has a major role in the genesis of severe cerebral intraventricular hemorrhages in preterm-born neonates. Up until now most intraventricular hemorrhage has been considered the result of impaired autoregulation of the cerebral circulation caused by a combination of immaturity and the neonatal respiratory distress syndrome (Lou et al, 1979; Volpe, 1981). This loss of autoregulation has usually been attributed to the hypoxia, acidosis and hypercarbia that are produced by the respiratory distress syndrome. Our findings indicate that placental villous edema is the factor that initiates these events by making fetuses hypoxic before birth. The severity and extent of the villous edema correlate much better with the development of severe intraventricular hemorrhage than do any of the other factors that have been linked to the hemorrhages. Morales (1987) has also found an association between acute chorioamnionitis and cerebral intraventricular hemorrhage. Hardt et al (1985) recently reported that children who had chorioamnionitis with premature membrane ruptures subsequently had lower Bayley mental scores than did children who had premature membrane rupture without chorioamnionitis.

REFERENCES

Appelbaum PC, Holloway Y, Ross SM, Dhupelia I (1977). The effect of amniotic fluid on bacterial growth in three population groups. Am J Obstet Gynecol 128:868-871.

Appelbaum PC, Shulman G, Chambers NL, Simon NV, Granados JL, Fairbrother PF, Naeye RL (1980). Studies on the growth-inhibiting property of amniotic fluid from two U.S. population groups. Am J Obstet Gynecol 137:579-582.

Bejar P, Curbelo V, Davis C, Gluck L (1981). Premature labor, II Bacterial sources of phospholipase. Obstet Gynecol 57:479-482.

Benirschke K (1960). Routes and types of infection in the fetus and newborn. Am J Dis Child 99:714-721.

Blanc WA (1981). Pathology of the placenta, membrane and umbilical cord in bacterial, fungal and viral infections in man. In Naeye R, Kissane JM, Kaufman N (eds): "Perinatal Diseases," Baltimore: Williams & Wilkins.

Bourne G (1962). The Human Amnion and Chorion. London: Lloyd-Luke, p 175.

Brown JH, Brenn L (1931). A method for the differential staining of gram-positive and gram-negative bacteria in tissue sections. Bull Johns Hopkins Hosp 48:69-73.

Cooperman NR, Kasin M, Rajaschekazaiah KR (1980). Clinical significance of amniotic fluid, amniotic membranes and endometrial biopsy cultures at the time of caesarean section. Am J Obstet Gynecol 137:536-541.

Cooperstock M, England JE, Wolfe RA (1987). Circadian incidence of premature rupture of the membranes in term and preterm birth. Obstet Gynecol 69:936-941.

Emig OR, Napier JV, Brazie JV (1961). Inflammation of the placenta correlation with prematurity and perinatal death. Gynaecology 17:743-750.

Evaldson GR, Malmborg AS, Nord CE (1982). Premature rupture of the membranes and ascending infection. Br J Obstet Gynaecol 89:793-801.

Gnarpe H, Friberg J (1973). T-mycoplasmas on spermatozoa and infertility. Nature 245:97-98.
Goodlin RC, Schmidt WR, Creevy DC (1972). Uterine tension and fetal heart rate during maternal orgasm. Obstet Gynecol 39:125-127.
Hager WD, Pauly TH (1985). Fetal tachycardia as an indicator of maternal and neonatal morbidity. Obstet Gynecol 66:191-194.
Hardt NS, Kostenbauder M, Ogburn M, Behnke M, Resnick M, Cruz A (1985). Influence of chorioamnionitis on Long-term prognosis in low birth weight infants. Obstet Gynecol 65:5-10.
Lamont RF, Rose M, Edler MG (1985). Effect of bacterial products on prostaglandin E production by amnion cells. Lancet 2:1331-1333.
Lauweryns J, Bernat R, Lerut A, Detournay G (1973). Intrauterine pneumonia: an experimental study. Biol Neonate 22:301-318.
Lou HC, Lassen NA, Friis-Hansen B (1979). Impaired autoregulation of cerebral blood flow in the distressed newborn infant. J Pediatr 94:118-121.
Lundquist F, Thorsteinsson T, Buss O (1955). Purification and properties of some enzymes in human seminal plasma. Biochem J 59:69-70.
Moghissi KS (1971). Sperm migration through cervical mucus. In Sherman AI (ed): "Pathways of Conception. The Role of the Cervix and Oviduct in Reproduction," Springfield IL: Charles C. Thomas, p 214-236.
Morales WJ (1987). The effect of chorioamnionitis on the developmental outcome of preterm infants at one year. Obstet Gynecol 70:183-186.
Naeye RL (1978). Amniotic fluid infections, neonatal hyperbilirubinemia and psychomotor impairment. Pediatrics 62:497-503.
Naeye RL (1979). Causes of the excessive rates of perinatal mortality and prematurity in pregnancies complicated by maternal urinary tract infections. N Engl J Med 300:819-823.
Naeye RL (1981). Coitus and antepartum hemorrhage. Brit J Obstet Gynecol 88:765-770.
Naeye RL (1987). Functionally important disorders of the placenta, umbilical cord and fetal membranes. Hum Pathol 18:680-691.
Naeye RL, Maisels MJ, Lorenz RP (1983). The clinical significance of placental villous edema. Pediatrics 71:588-594.
Naeye RL, Ross SM (1982). Coitus and chorioamnionitis, a prospective study. Early Hum Dev 6:91-97.

Naeye RL, Tafari N (1983). Risk Factors in Pregnancy and Diseases of the Fetus and Newborn. Baltimore: Williams & Wilkins.

Naeye RL, Tafari N, Judge D, Gilmour D, Marboe C (1977). Amniotic fluid infections in an African city. J Pediatr 90:965-970.

Novak RW, Platt MS (1985). Significance of placental findings in early-onset group B streptococcal neonatal sepsis. Clin Pediatr 24:256-258.

Pankuch GA, Appelbaum PC, Lorenz RP et al (1984). Placental microbiology and histology and the pathogenesis of chorioamnionitis. Obstet Gynecol 64:802-806.

Romero R, Emamian M, Quintero R, Wan M, Hobbins JC, Mitchell MD (1986). Amniotic fluid prostaglandin levels and intra-amniotic infections. Lancet 1:1380.

Ross SM, MacPherson TA, Naeye RL, Khantree MHD, Wallace J (1982). Causes of fetal and neonatal mortality in a South African Black community. S Afr Med J, 61:905-908.

Russell P (1979). Inflammatory lesions of the human placenta. I. Clinical significance of acute chorioamnionitis. Am J Diag Gynecol Obstet 1:127-137.

Sibille Y, Lwebugam JS, Polonski L, Merrill W, Ingbar DH (1986). An in-vitro model for polymorphonuclear leukocyte induced injury to extracellular matrix. Am Rev Respir Dis 134-140.

Sidiropoulos D, Herrmann U, Morell A, Von Muralt G, Barandun S (1986). Transplacental passage of intravenous immunoglobulin in the last trimester of pregnancy. J Pediatr 109:505-508.

Svensson L., Ingermarsson I, March PA (1986). Chorioamnionitis and the isolation of microorganisms from the placenta. Obstet Gynecol 67:403-409.

Tafari N, Ross SM, Naeye RL, Galash RP, Zaar B (1977). Failure of bacterial growth inhibition by amniotic fluid. Am J Obstet Gynecol 128:187-189.

Vintzileos AM, Campbell WA, Nochimson DJ, Weinbaum PJ (1986). Fetal breathing as a predictor of infection in a premature rupture of the membranes. Obstet Gynecol 67:813-817.

Volpe JJ (1981). Neonatal intraventricular hemorrhage. N Engl J Med 304:886-891.

DISCUSSION

DR. OSBURN: Are most of the neutrophils involved in this condition of fetal origin or of maternal origin?

DR. NAEYE: Most of the neutrophils in the amniotic fluid are of maternal origin. A few originate from the fetus, mainly from the umbilical vein.

DR. WAHL: Can you define your villous edema score?

DR. NAEYE: The score is based on microscopic point counting. It takes into account both the severity and the extent of villous edema.

DR. SERTICH: What are the more common organisms that are associated with this condition?

DR. NAEYE: In most populations, about 60% of the bacteria are aerobes and 40% anaerobes. Many of the anaerobes have fastidious growth characteristics so it can take days to weeks to isolate them. Common aerobes are streptococci from the intestinal tract and E. coli. Over the years we have isolated more than 100 types of bacteria from placentas with acute chorioamnionitis, almost every bacteria that can be found in the vagina and cervix. A few bacteria are never or almost never found with acute chorioamnionitis. They include the gonococcus and group B streptococcus. Mycoplasmas are found in from 0-15% of placentas with acute chorioamnionitis. Populations of women living at the poverty level often have high rates of mycoplasma isolations.

DR. V. ANDERSON: Has the Gram's stain helped you?

DR. NAEYE: Gram's stain, and Brown and Brenn stain will demonstrate very few of the bacteria. In about one quarter of the cases, bacteria can be demonstrated by silver stains.

DR. QUINN: The microorganisms may not be detectable because the bacteria have been phagocytized in the placenta or the organisms, such as mycoplasmas, are too small to clearly identify by light microscopy.

DR. NAEYE: I doubt that explanation. All or almost

all of the bacteria can be demonstrated by fluorescent labeled antibodies against the various specific bacterial strains.

Transplacental Effects on Fetal Health, pages 87–106

CONGENITAL SYPHILIS

David M. Judge, M.D.

Pathology Department, Baylor College of Medicine, Houston, Texas 77030

INTRODUCTION

This report places congenital syphilis in its proper national and global context, describes the pathology in an effort to elucidate the pathogenesis, and suggests future research. Congenital syphilis is an infectious disease caused by a spirochete, *Treponema pallidum*, that is acquired transplacentally. Almost 500 years ago syphilis appeared as a "new" disease causing a large epidemic with severe morbidity and heavy mortality (Zinsser, 1934) reminiscent of the tragedy of the HIV epidemic of our own time. Awareness of newborn infections was immediate, but the congenital nature of this phenomenon took another 350 years (Ingall and Musher, 1983).

Sexually transmitted disease is one of the Surgeon General's fifteen priority areas (Parra and Cates, 1985) and congenital syphilis is a key target. It is a major factor in the high infant mortality of the preindustrialized world (Larson and Larson, 1970). In the U.S. it remains a small but important factor (Ingall and Musher, 1983). Congenital syphilis has already been increasing since 1983 (Centers for Disease Control, 1983) and it is under-reported (Mascola et al., 1985). The 268 reported cases in 1985 do not include the macerated stillborn with syphilis. Reported cases probably represent only one third of the actual cases (Ingall and Musher, 1983). Primary and secondary syphilis rose dramatically in the first three months of 1987; therefore, a further increase in congenital syphilis is expected to follow (Wilder et al., 1987).

Congenital syphilis becomes a recognizable disease in the fetus in conjunction with the appearance and maturation of the immune system (Silverstein, 1962). The interaction of organism and fetus varies with the gestational age and the immunocompetence of the fetus. This has led to some confusion in the previous morphologic descriptions. A second variability involves late gestational maternal syphilis leading to very mild or no discernible disease in the newborn. Another apparent source of confusion in the literature is the frequent conjunction of other diseases such as amniotic fluid infections (Naeye et al., 1977) and other disease processes such as the placental changes of intrauterine death. Congenital syphilis appears to be a manifestation of immune and/or inflammatory response rather than a toxic effect of the organism (Silverstein and Lukes, 1962).

Researchers must develop and characterize animal models and show their relevance to the human disease. Study of congenital syphilis in humans is incomplete since there remains some confusion about the nature of the response of the human fetus to this infection. Acquired immunodeficiency syndrome (AIDS) and syphilis occur together with great frequency (Tramont, 1987). Study of the conjunction of AIDS and syphilis, especially in the fetus, can give us a great deal of information about the development and interaction of the immune system and the inflammatory response.

PATHOLOGY

First Trimester

The first trimester embryo with syphilis shows no histologic changes. There are no foci of necrosis, no inflammation, and spirochetes are rare enough that silver stains alone are insufficient to assure demonstration (Harter and Benirschke, 1976). Syphilis is not a cause of first trimester fetal loss. This lack of effect in the early stages of pregnancy is the basis of a discredited theory, that the Langhans' cell layer of the placenta is a barrier to transplacental passage of the spirochete (Dippel, 1944).

Second Trimester

It is somewhat difficult to describe the pathology of second trimester syphilis since 85% of the second trimester fetuses in our study were stillborn and 30% of these were severely macerated (Judge et al., 1986). The second trimester fetus, even when liveborn, has very subtle changes that may go undetected (Braunstein, 1978). Spirochetes are usually scarce in fetuses of 24 weeks or less (Judge et al., 1986) but the Warthin-Starry silver stain is sufficient to demonstrate them. By 26 weeks, organisms are numerous. These infected second trimester fetuses have occasional plasma cells, minimal intimal proliferation in small arteries, and mild interstitial fibrosis. The most obvious change at this stage is a gross enlargement of the placenta (a placental/fetal ratio of 0.52 compared to 0.3 overall). The placenta is histologically unremarkable. McCord observed in 1934: "It seems ... that the more premature the placenta, the more difficult it is to make a diagnosis of syphilis" (McCord, 1934).

Third Trimester

Prematures make up the bulk of congenital syphilitics. The pathologic changes become more obvious or classical. There is intimal proliferation in small arteries, diffuse fibrosis, depletion of lymphocytes from thymus and lymph nodes with decreased thymic size, enlarged spleens and livers due mostly to increased hematopoiesis, and both diffuse and focal infiltration of tissue with plasma cells and monocytes. There is no apparent interference with fetal growth (Naeye, 1971). The percentage of stillborn is less than that in the second trimester, 66% vs. 85%, but more of the stillborn are severely macerated, 55% vs. 30%.

Lungs: The lungs appear more immature than expected for gestational age with thicker alveolar walls and minimal persistence of hematopoiesis. Pulmonary arteries have prominent perivascular cuffing of connective tissue and chronic inflammation [Fig. 1]. The inflammation consists of plasma cells, lymphocytes, and macrophages [Fig. 2].

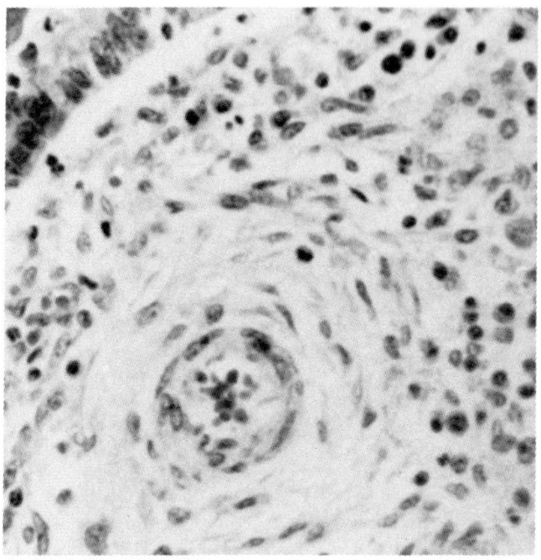

Figure 1. Lung, perivascular fibrosis and inflammation. H&E, x250.

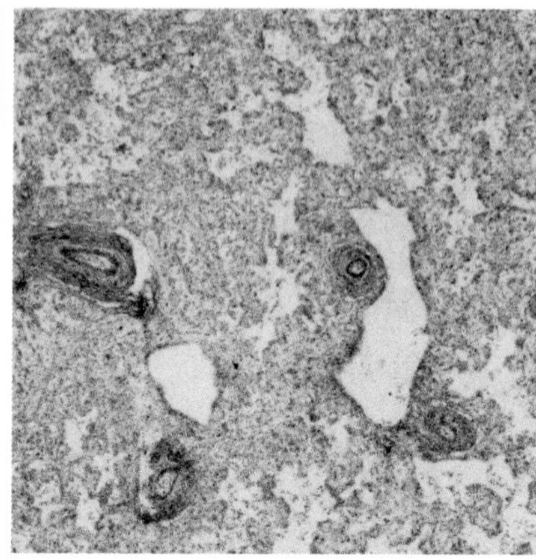

Figure 2. Lung, severely macerated stillborn, prominent pulmonary arteries. H&E, x50.

Polymorphonuclear leukocytes do not appear to be a part of the response to this infection. Occasionally there is more diffuse interstitial fibrosis but this is a microscopic, not a gross finding. Pneumonia alba, a grossly visible fibrosis, is a term frequently encountered in the literature (Whipple and Dunham, 1938). This entity must be uncommon or is the manifestation of a different and superimposed disease process. Small foci of necrosis can occur accompanied by fibrosis.

Usually there will be evidence of terminal amniotic fluid aspiration in the stillborn. Occasionally patients with congenital syphilis also have superimposed amniotic fluid infection and fetal pneumonia since both conditions occur more frequently in the same population. It is important to distinguish the pathology of the one from the other. Acute inflammation almost always indicates superimposed bacterial infection in these patients. The presence of acute inflammation does not affect the ability to detect spirochetes [Fig. 3].

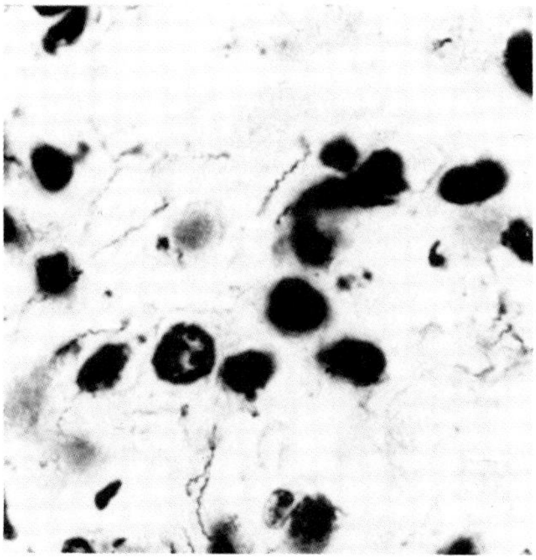

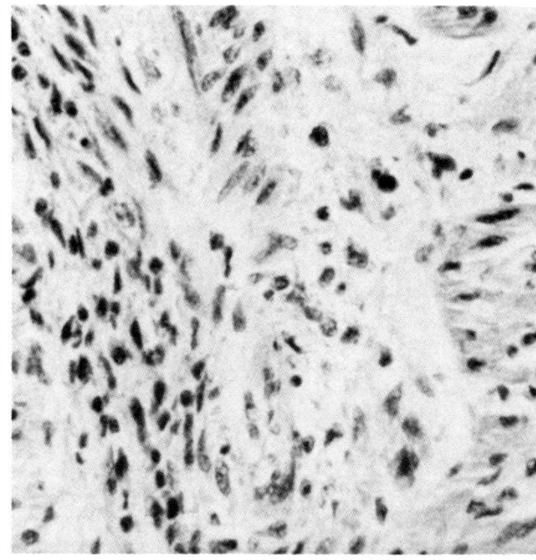

Figure 3. Lung, superimposed amniotic fluid infection. Warthin-Starry, x900.

Figure 4. Heart, periarterial chronic inflammation and fibrosis in epicardium. H&E, x250.

Heart: The vascular change described above is also present in the heart accompanied by interstitial fibrosis [Fig. 4]. Since the arteries are the target of the inflammation, the most prominent changes are in the epicardium. The perivascular inflammation and fibrosis extend into the myocardium. Fully developed lesions in well-preserved tissue contain activated fixed cardiac macrophages, so-called Anitschow myocytes. In the severely macerated stillborn, the vascular changes in the lungs and in the epicardium remain identifiable long after other tissues become unrecognizable.

Lymph Nodes: The lymph nodes have a variable appearance. Some show lymphoid depletion and diffuse fibrosis and others show early nodule formation. The nodes usually contain a few plasma cells.

Thymus: There is a sharp decrease in the number of cells in the thymus and a concomitant increase in fibrous tissue [Fig. 5]. Plasma cells are plentiful. Edematous fibrous septa are prominent. Necrosis is uncommon. Dubois abscesses, which are microscopic foci of necrosis and acute inflammation, are uncommon. Reports of these microabscesses are more frequent in older literature.

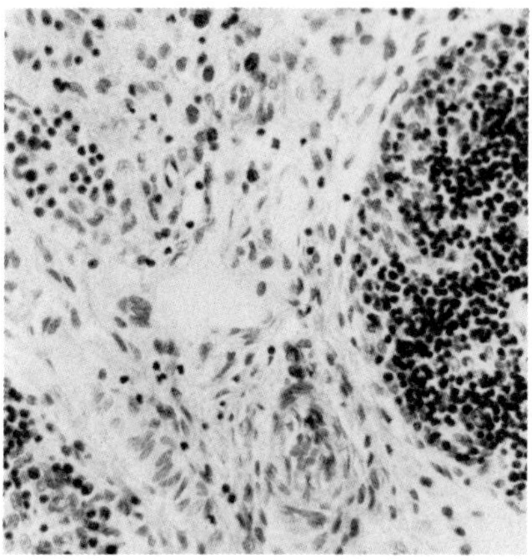

Figure 5. Thymus, fibrous septa with chronic inflammation. H&E, x125.

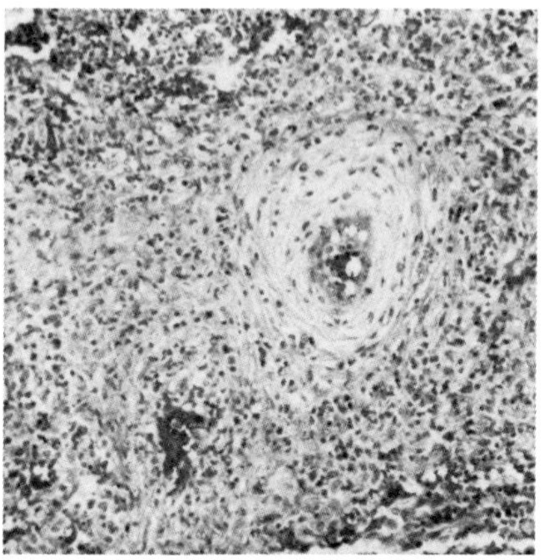

Figure 6. Spleen, "onion skin" appearance of penicillar artery. H&E, x60.

Spleen: The spleen is enlarged by extensive hematopoiesis. Chronic inflammation with plasma cells and macrophages are diffusely scattered through the parenchyma. The most obvious change is the presence of layers of fibrous tissue and chronic inflammation surrounding the arterioles [Fig. 6]. The arteries also have intimal proliferation. These arteriolar changes resemble the "onion skin" lesions of systemic lupus erythematosus. Reaction centers are uncommon and there is some diminution of the prominence of the lymphocytic cuff about the arterioles.

Liver: There is more hematopoiesis than expected for gestational age (Naeye, 1971). It is distributed both in the portal areas and parenchymally. There is a mild diffuse chronic inflammation. Fibrosis is minimal.

Kupffer cells are prominent. There is very little evidence of necrosis or hepatocellular dropout. Infarcts occur in the liver as they occasionally do in other organs of the congenital syphilitic. In general, the inflammation and fibrosis in the liver is less prominent than in many of the other organs [Fig. 7], despite the fact that the liver contains many more T. pallidum organisms than any other organ. The organisms are predominantly interstitial as they are in other tissues (Brooks and Audretsch, 1978).

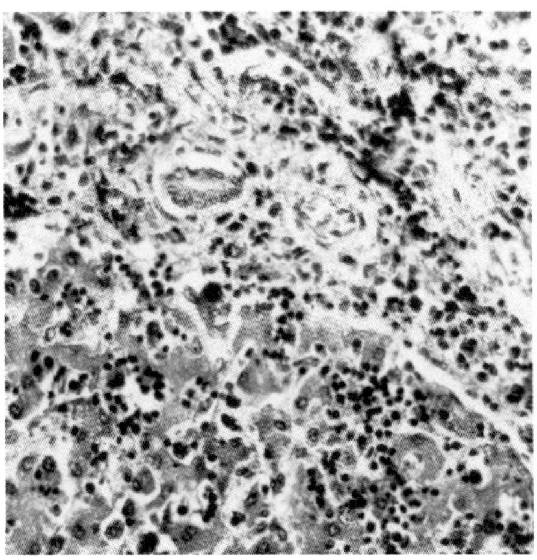

Figure 7. Liver, portal tract with chronic inflammation and parenchymal hematopoiesis. H&E, x125.

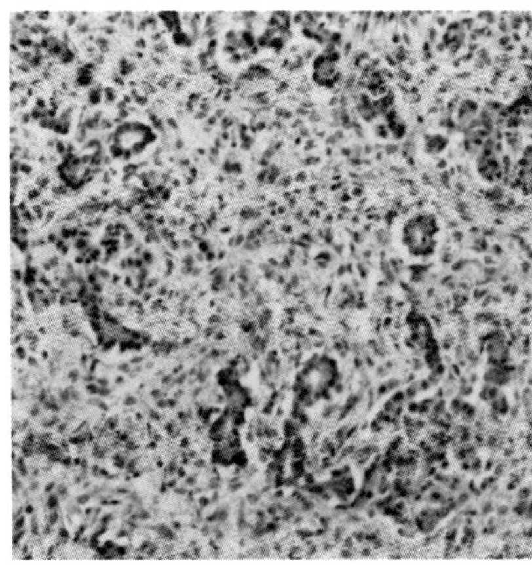

Figure 8. Pancreas, interstitial fibrosis and chronic inflammation. H&E, x125.

Pancreas: Histologically, the changes in this organ resemble severe chronic pancreatitis with chronic inflammation, fibrosis, and acinar atrophy [Fig. 8]. Extra-medullary hematopoiesis is more prominent than usual at this stage of development. The major ducts are unremarkable. Development of the islets appears normal and islets are not decreased. Acute inflammation and necrosis are not part of the picture.

Gastrointestinal Tract: There is diffuse chronic inflammation and fibrosis of the lamina propria [Fig. 9] and occasionally extensive focal fibrosis (Oppenheimer and Hardy, 1971). Reports of peritoneal inflammation and fibrosis suggest that small infarcts may be present and be associated with perforation (Oppenheimer and Dahms, 1981).

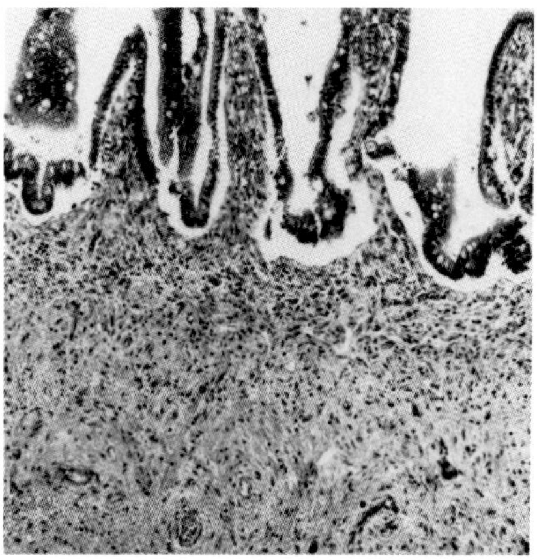

Figure 9. Jejunum, fibrosis of lamina propria. H&E, x60.

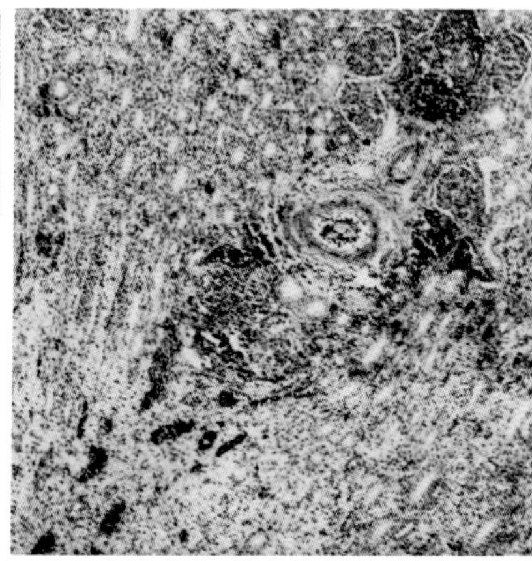

Figure 10. Kidney, prominent artery at junction of cortex and medulla. H&E, x50.

Kidneys: The perivascular fibrosis and chronic inflammation is prominent about arcuate arteries [Fig. 10] but may also involve smaller cortical arteries. There is minimal interstitial fibrosis in some patients. Glomeruli and tubules are unremarkable. Glomerular damage is undetectable at this stage.

Bone: The bone changes are striking in these third trimester prematures but less so than they are in the full-term. Small infarcts occur in this tissue as they do in others. Roentgenographs may show irregular widened physeal spaces, metaphyseal arrest lines near the physis indicating the time of the maximum growth disturbance, and complete or partial cuffs of periosteal new bone.

Predictably, the changes are most prominent at the knee joint since maximum bone growth occurs in this location.

Small arteries have intimal proliferation, perivascular chronic inflammation, and fibrosis. The inflammation and thus the morphologic changes are most prominent where ossification is most active and thus where vessels are most numerous. Such affected vessels are more common in metaphyseal aspect of the physis, known as the epiphyseal growth zone, and in the periosteum (Pick, 1920). There is disruption of the calcification of the physeal cartilage and thus of the orderly maturation of the growth zone of the physis. Disruption of the calcification of the columns of proliferating cartilage stops its degeneration and its orderly ossification. The growth zone will continue to widen when calcification and degeneration cease. All vessels are not uniformly involved so the growth disturbances are not uniform [Fig. 11]. Macroscopically the normally smooth, thin gray line between the physis and the metaphysis becomes wider and irregular with yellow discoloration. Occasionally there is periosteal new bone formation associated with involvement of the periosteal vessels. New bone may encircle the original cortex.

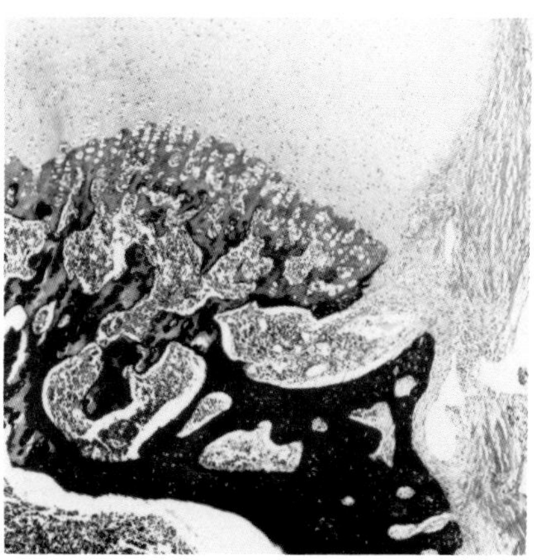

Figure 11. Bone, irregularity of physis and periostitis. H&E, x25.

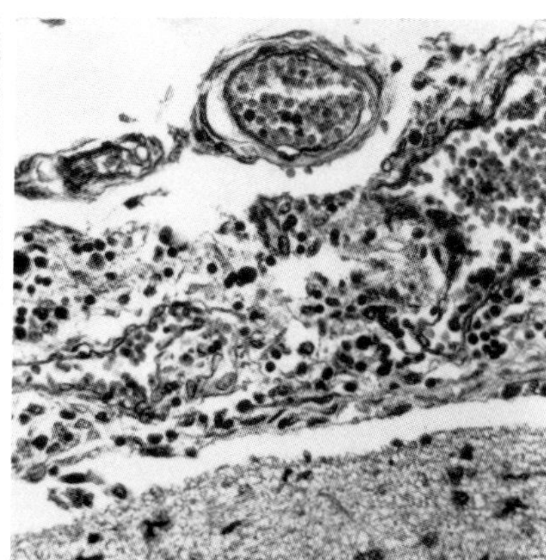

Figure 12. Brain, inflammation and fibrosis or meninges at base of brain. H&E, x125.

Brain: The brain itself is relatively unaffected at this stage. Grossly there may be some thickening of the meninges, particularly at the base of the brain. Microscopically, there is fibrosis and chronic inflammation which is predominantly perivascular [Fig. 12].

Placenta: Much has been written about the changes of congenital syphilis in the placenta. McCord probably said it all in 1929 (McCord, 1929). "Increasing experience has caused me to form gradually the opinion that the histologic diagnosis of syphilis of the placenta is laden with many difficulties and to question its practical value as a routine method of determining congenital syphilitic infection." The changes of intrauterine death, especially the vascular changes, must not be attributed to syphilis. Amniotic fluid infection, chorioamnionitis, herpetic lesions, and other diseases more common in the same population as those with gestational syphilis should be searched for and excluded. The placenta is somewhat more immature than expected. Villi have a slight increase in cellularity [Fig. 13].

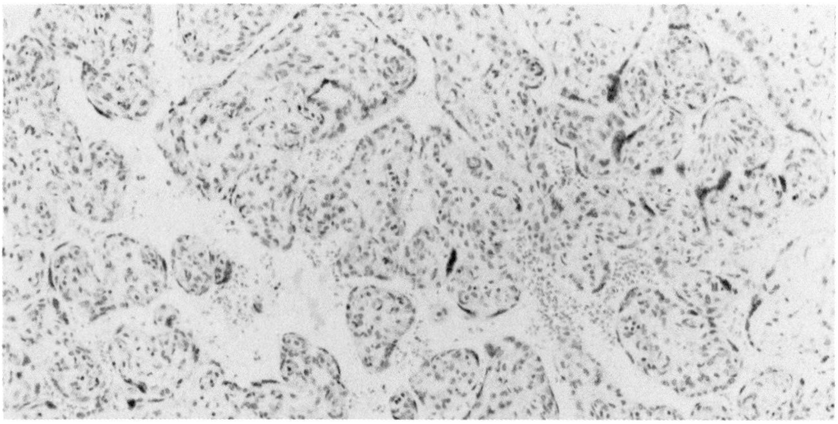

Figure 13. Placenta, increased cellularity, 40 week gestation stillborn with moderate maceration. H&E, x60.

A few Hofbauer cells may be present and the plumpness of interstitial cells gives the impression of increased fluid. Occasionally, focal villitis with chronic inflammatory cells, including plasma cells, is present. Spirochetes are present but even in the face of overwhelming numbers of spirochetes in the fetus, the number of organisms in the placenta is very limited. The size of the placenta relative to the fetus remains large but the ratio drops as full term approaches. The placental/fetal ratio in this premature group drops to 0.3, about twice the expected value (Little, 1960).

Full Term

The pathologic changes in the full term infant form a continuum with those of the premature stillborn. Chronic inflammation, necrosis, and fibrosis become more severe. Bone changes continue, become radiographically evident, and may become diagnostic (Sachdev et al., 1982). The most common bone changes are metaphyseal dystrophy and periosteal reaction, e.g., saber shins. Saddle nose is one of the classic changes and is caused by focal inflammation and necrosis of the nasal bones and cartilage. Hydrarthrosis and pseudoparesis are reported. Skin rashes and chronic inflammation in the dermis become evident. "Snuffles," one of the classic signs, is secondary to chronic inflammation of the nasal epithelium. Occasionally immune complex glomerulonephritis develops (Kaplan et al., 1972). Those that die frequently have superinfections with gram negative bacilli. There are reports of gummas in congenital syphilis (Oppenheimer and Dahms, 1981). Gummas are areas of necrosis with granulomatous inflammation and are usually thought of as part of tertiary syphilis. There are focal areas of necrosis or infarcts in congenital syphilis, especially in the liver. Since the immature liver frequently reacts to injury by forming giant cells, these infarcts may appear to be granulomatous inflammation with necrosis. The exact nature and pathogenesis of gummas is not established with certainty and the presence or absence of gummas in congenital syphilis also remains somewhat uncertain.

DIAGNOSTIC CRITERIA

The criteria for establishing the diagnosis of congenital syphilis are clear. These include, but are not confined to, demonstrating organisms, or the presence of a combination of findings such as condyloma, osteochondritis, snuffles, hepatosplenomegaly, and hemolytic anemia (Kaufman et al., 1977). All such diagnostic criteria rightfully stress making the diagnosis in the living patient but may mislead us in doing so. Congenital syphilis is a cause of perinatal mortality and most patients with the disease are macerated stillborn. Diagnosis based on clinical criteria will not identify these patients. All intrauterine pregnancies are potential victims of this disease. Thus the really important diagnostic criteria is a positive serology in the mother. The only meaningful intervention in the disease involves early and continued prenatal care including syphilis serology. Weigh the placenta as well as the baby at birth (Thomson et al., 1969). A placental/fetal ratio of 0.3 or more would suggest a special search for syphilis.

In addition, much emphasis must be placed on detection of syphilis in the stillborn. We cannot determine the extent that syphilis contributes to perinatal mortality if we ignore the premature, macerated stillborn. No matter how macerated, an autopsy should include histologic examination of the lungs and heart (Judge et al., 1986).

ANIMAL MODELS

It has been difficult to do research on congenital syphilis because early efforts failed to establish congenital infections in an animal model (Festenstein and Bokkenheuser, 1961). Recent efforts report success inducing fetal disease in the rabbit with *T. pallidum*, Nichols strain (Fitzgerald, 1985), and in the Syrian hamster with *T. pallidum, endemicum* (Kajdacsy-Balla et al., 1987). The relevance of these models to the human disease remains uncertain at this point. One of the major efforts to determine this relevance must be to compare the ontogeny of the immune system in the various animals with that in humans since the development of this system appears to be critical to the development of the disease (Osburn et al., 1982). Second, researchers familiar with the human disease must evaluate and compare the morphologic changes, the pathology, of the congenital disease in animals with that in humans.

PATHOGENESIS

Certain facts are established. *T. pallidum* crosses the placenta in all trimesters including the first (Harter and Benirschke, 1976). Some maternal immunoglobulin crosses the placenta starting near the end of the first trimester (Spiegelberg, 1974). The passage of IgG across the placenta accelerates after 32 weeks because of active transport. Early complement production in the fetus begins in the first trimester but the alternate pathway with its opsonic, chemotactic and cytolytic activities may be delayed (Goldman et al., 1985). There is no association between congenital syphilis and first trimester fetal loss or congenital anomalies. Second trimester fetal losses occur late in the trimester and are associated with few organisms and minimal morphologic changes. The most severe disease is associated with the largest number of organisms. The morphologic changes of congenital syphilis are directly proportional to the number of organisms and the maturity of the fetal immune system (Judge et al., 1986). The element of the immune system that appears to be operative in pathogenesis may be something other than, or in addition to, the plasma cell and immunoglobulin since some maternal immunoglobulins, presumably including maternal anti-syphilitic antibody, are present late in the first trimester. It may involve the development of the complement system, the maturation of monocytic inflammatory cells and the production of fibroblast activating factors, and/or it may be a maturation of receptors in the target tissues allowing an inflammatory reaction to take place. Syphilis inhibits T-cell function and cell-mediated immunity which could aid in establishing and maintaining the disease (Levene et al., 1971) but would not explain the timing of the onset of disease.

Just as the appearance of the disease concomitantly with the maturation of the immune system suggests that the pathogenesis of the disease is related to that immune response, many of the morphologic changes fit together to suggest a final common pathway. The major change is in the arteries with intimal proliferation and perivascular fibrosis. Small infarcts are relatively common and large infarcts occasionally occur. Metaphyseal enchondral ossification is disturbed. Extramedullary hematopoiesis is very prominent. The placenta is large. The final common pathway appears to be vascular insufficiency and hypoxia. The mild hemolytic anemia that occurs may contribute to the systemic changes. Since the organism appears to have a hematogenous route of spread and the vascular and perivascular changes are not uniformly distributed throughout the body, it is likely that there are local factors in the tissue that govern the capacity to react.

FUTURE RESEARCH

We need to understand more about the nature and ontogeny of the human immune response and the nature and ontogeny of the inflammatory response to immune reactions (Ward, 1978). We also need to know more about the organism to understand how it elicits the particular type of immune response. With immunoblot and gene cloning technology it should be possible to produce large quantities of *T. pallidum* gene products and selectively test those products for toxicity and for effect on the immune system. Secondly, it should be possible to work out the ontogeny of the immune system to determine not only the timing but also the adequacy of mediator release. As part of that study, it must be shown that the target tissues, including fibroblasts, have receptors and the capacity to respond to those mediators. Additionally a good animal model of congenital syphilis must be established and used to study the hypotheses derived from the study of the chemistry of *T. pallidum* and the ontogeny of the immune system.

AIDS presents a new clinical opportunity to gain more insight into the nature of congenital syphilis. Women with HIV infection are more likely to also have syphilis and vice versa. Pregnant women with AIDS may deliver an infant with HIV. Occasionally the neonatal HIV infection is far enough advanced to be accompanied by immune deficiency. Since HIV and syphilis occur with greater frequency in the same population, an effort must be made to find fortuitous conjunction of AIDS and syphilis in pregnant women to determine in what way the decreased immunocompetence of the mother, and separately of the fetus, affects the development of congenital syphilis. The study of such a patient could shed much light on the pathogenesis of congenital syphilis. Much new information about the workings of the immune system will come out of this tragedy known as AIDS. Any and all of this information is likely to be helpful in the study and understanding of syphilis (Tramont, 1987).

ACKNOWLEDGEMENTS

I would like to acknowledge the assistance of Drs. Richard Naeye, Nebiat Tafari, Charles Marboe, and David Gilmour in the planning and performance of the 1000+ autopsies of the Ethiopian perinatal mortality study (65 autopsies from this group form the basis of the congenital syphilis study).

REFERENCES

Braunstein H (1978). Congenital syphilis in aborted second trimester fetus: diagnosis by histologic study. J Clin Pathol 31:265.

Brooks SEH, Audretsch JJ (1978). Hepatic ultrastructure in congenital syphilis. Arch Pathol Lab Med 102:502.

Centers for Disease Control (1983). Annual summary 1982: reported morbidity and mortality in the United States. MMWR 31:82.

Dippel AL (1944). The relationship of congenital syphilis to abortion and miscarriage and the mechanism of intrauterine protection. Am J Obstet Gynecol 47:369.

Festenstein H, Bokkenheuser V (1961). Attempted induction of immunologic tolerance in rabbits using living Treponema pallidum. Br J Exp Pathol 42:158.

Fitzgerald TJ (1985). Experimental congenital syphilis in rabbits. Can J Microbiol 31:757.

Goldman AS, Ham Pong AJ, Goldblum RM (1985). Host defenses: development and maternal contributions. Adv Pediatr 32:71.

Harter CA, Benirschke K (1976). Fetal syphilis in the first trimester. Am J Obstet Gynecol 124:705.

Ingall D, Musher D (1983). Syphilis. In Remington JS, Klein JD (eds): "Infectious Diseases of the Fetus and Newborn Infant," Philadelphia: W.B. Saunders, pp 335-374.

Judge DM, Tafari N, Naeye RL, Marboe C (1986). Congenital syphilis and perinatal mortality. Pediatr Pathol 5:411.

Kajdacsy-Balla A, Howeedy A, Bagasra O (1987). Syphilis in the Syrian hamster: a model of human venereal and congenital syphilis. Am J Pathol 126:599.

Kaplan BS, Wiglesworth FW, Marks MI, Drummond KN (1972). The glomerulopathy of congenital syphilis: an immune deposit disease. J Pediatr 81:1154.

Kaufman RE, Jones OG, Blount JH, Wiesner PJ (1977). Questionnaire survey of reported early congenital syphilis: problems in diagnosis, prevention, and treatment. Sex Transm Dis 4:135.

Larson Y, Larson V (1970). Congenital syphilis in Addis Ababa. Ethiop Med J 8:163.

Levene GM, Wright DJM, Turk JL (1971). Cell-mediated immunity and lymphocytic transformation in syphilis. Proc R Soc Med 64:14.

Little WA (1960). The significance of placental/fetal weight ratios. Am J Obstet Gynecol 79:134.

Mascola L, Pelosi R, Blount JH, Alexander CE, Cates W (1985). Congenital syphilis revisited. Am J Dis Child 139:575.

McCord JR (1929). A study of two hundred autopsies made on syphilitic fetuses. Am J Obstet Gynecol 18:597.

McCord JR (1934). Syphilis of the placenta. Am J Obstet Gynecol 28:743.

Naeye RL (1971). Fetal growth with congenital syphilis: a quantitative study. Am J Clin Pathol 55:228.

Naeye RL, Tafari N, Judge D, Gilmour D, Marboe C (1977). Amniotic fluid infections in an African city. J Pediatr 90:965.

Oppenheimer EH, Dahms BB (1981). Congenital syphilis in the fetus and neonate. Perspect Pediatr Pathol 6:115.

Oppenheimer EH, Hardy JB (1971). Congenital syphilis in the newborn infant: clinical and pathological observations in recent cases. Johns Hopkins Med J 129:63.

Osburn BI, MacLachlan NJ, Terrell TG (1982). Ontogeny of the immune system. J Am Vet Med Assoc 181:1049.

Parra WC, Cates W (1985). Progress toward the 1990 objectives for sexually transmitted diseases: good news and bad. Public Health Rep 100:261.

Pick L (1920). Angeborene Knochensyphilis. In Henke VF, and Lubarsch, O (eds): "Handbuch der speziellen pathologisch Anatomie und Histologie," Berlin: Springer, IX (pt1), p. 240.

Sachdev M, Bery K, Chawla S (1982). Osseous manifestations in congenital syphilis: a study of 55 cases. Clin Rad 33:319-323.

Silverstein AM (1962). Congenital syphilis and the timing of immunogenesis in the human fetus. Nature 194:196.

Silverstein AM, Lukes RJ (1962). Fetal response to antigenic stimulus: I. Plasmacellular and lymphoid reactions in the human fetus to intrauterine infection. Lab Invest 11:981.

Spiegelberg HL (1974). Biological activities of immunoglobulins of different classes and subclasses. Adv Immunol 19:259.

Thomson AM, Billewicz WZ, Hytten FE (1969). The weight of the placenta in relation to birth weight. J Obstet Gynaecol Br Commonw 76:865.

Tramont EC (1987). Syphilis in the AIDS era. N Engl J Med 316:1600.

Ward PA (1978). Mediators of inflammatory responses. In Cohen S, Ward PA, McCluskey RT (eds): "Mechanisms of Immunopathology," New York: John Wiley & Sons, p. 1.

Whipple DV, Dunham EC (1938). Congenital syphilis: Part I. Incidence, transmission, and diagnosis. J Pediatr 12:386.

Wilder MH, Schultz S, Fannin S, Acree K (1987). Increases in primary and secondary syphilis - United States. MMWR 36:393.

Zinsser H (1934). "Rats, Lice and History." New York: Little Brown, p. 55.

DISCUSSION

DR. OSBURN: You mentioned that immune complex glomerulonephritis can occur. When does this occur in the third trimester?

DR. JUDGE: Immune complex glomerulonephritis, or glomerular changes in general, occur only postnatally. I have not seen nor have I read about any glomerular damage developing *in utero*.

DR. POHLENZ: Do you have any suggestions why the arteries in the heart are the most affected?

DR. JUDGE: No, but cardiac arteries are not the only ones. The arteries that are most prominent, the ones I wanted to stress, were those in the heart and lungs because so many of these patients are macerated. I don't know about your pathologists, or how you might do an autopsy, but most pathologists look at the macerated infant with little interest, assuming that all pertinent information has been lost. That is why I emphasized the vessels of the heart and lungs. One can see those vessels and can identify their component cells longer than the cells of other tissue. I am trying to get people to pay more attention to macerated infants. The vessels of the spleen, kidney, and other organs of the body are also affected in a similar fashion.

The heart vessels may be retained because they may get some passive flow of blood from the placenta. Blood from the placenta would still have some oxygen, so that the death of the heart and lung cells might be delayed.

The pathologic changes in congenital syphilis parallel the maturation of the immune system. The earlier involvement of some vessels such as those in the lung, heart, and spleen suggests an earlier maturation of the capacity to respond to an inflammatory stimulus.

DR. NAEYE: I have two questions. First, I have compared the findings presented by Dr. Judge from Ethiopian patients with findings in newborns at the Johns Hopkins Hospital in the years just before the introduction of penicillin. The differences were striking, with congenital syphilis being much more severe in the Ethiopian newborns than in those born in Baltimore. Most of the Ethiopians had striking lesions in the pancreas, and often in the liver and lungs as well, whereas lesions of such severity were rare in children born with congenital syphilis in Baltimore. Would you like to speculate on why the lesions were so much more severe in Ethiopia than in Baltimore? Second, I have had a chance recently to review the neonatal clinical course and placentas of a number of children born with congenital syphilis in South Africa. Some of these children have all of the neonatal findings of severe intrapartum asphyxia including persistent low Apgar scores, the neonatal respiratory distress syndrome, neonatal apnea, severe cerebral intraventricular hemorrhage, and necrotizing enterocolitis. Some of these children now have severe neurologic impairments. This raises the possibility that some of the central nervous system abnormalities in children with congenital syphilis may be due to severe antenatal hypoxia caused by placental villous edema. Such villous edema is a common cause of the severe antenatal hypoxia experienced by some non-syphilitic preterm-born infants in the U.S. and elsewhere.

DR. JUDGE: Your second question was a comment. To answer your first question, I also compared the Ethiopian findings with the Johns Hopkins findings. I discussed this with Dr. Ellen Oppenheimer and decided that the difference in the pathologic changes of Addis Ababa and the Baltimore cases was not extreme and was probably nutritional in nature. The average nutrition of the Ethiopian mother was not very good. I thought the differences we were seeing were related to the nutritional status of the mother. That judgement is subjective and not based on hard scientific data.

DR. OSBURN: I was wondering whether the mothers had HIV infection and if that may have been responsible for the severe disease?

DR. JUDGE: In Ethiopia, at that time? I hope not. During my first stay in Ethiopia, I spent almost two years working with the African green monkey (Cereopithecus aethiops). I have heard since then that the African green monkey is a reservoir of a similar virus and so I hope they didn't have AIDS in Ethiopia at that time. I did many autopsies and saw many patients in Ethiopia between 1967 and 1975, and saw nothing suggestive of AIDS.

DR. V. ANDERSON: Syphilis, like AIDS, is a great mimic and I was wondering if you had any thoughts as to why there is this great variation in the pathologic expression of the disease? It can't simply be related to nutritional status.

DR. JUDGE: To answer the first part, I have no idea why there are so many different clinical manifestations and we will have difficulty sorting it out because of a lack of an animal model. We can't do this work with a human. We can't design an experiment in which one would infect a woman at various gestational states. Until we have a good animal model which mimics the human disease, we will continue to be faced with trying to explain what we find rather than having hard data. I can think of reasons why infections of the fetus at one gestational age might differ from infections at another age but these are based on armchair research.

DR. V. ANDERSON: Do you think that the fetus that is exposed to spirochetes for the first time during the third trimester, when the mother was not previously infected, is at high risk for developing the stigma of congenital syphilis?

DR. JUDGE: I don't know. There is conflicting data on the risk to the fetus of infection acquired late in gestation.

DR. QUINN: I wonder if some of the variations you observed are due to concurrent infection with other organisms. Your studies detect syphilis, but could there be other organisms such as mycoplasmas? We have seen a number of cases of concurrent infections with ureaplasma and viruses in pneumonias. Such viruses rarely cause death in infants, yet these babies were dying. At autopsy both viral and ureaplasmal infections were evident. I think this may be one of the underlying mechanisms.

DR. JUDGE: Many of our patients with congenital syphilis had amniotic fluid infections. When I was doing the autopsies and I found polymorphonuclear leukocytes in the lungs, I knew immediately that I was dealing with something other than syphilis. The fetus had another infection superimposed on syphilis. You don't get a polymorphonuclear response to syphilis.

Transplacental Effects on Fetal Health, pages 107–151

MYCOPLASMA INFECTION OF THE FETUS AND NEWBORN

Patricia A. Quinn, M.A., Ph.D.

The Hospital For Sick Children,

555 University Ave., Toronto, Canada, M5G 1X8

INTRODUCTION

Over the past ten years, there have been significant advances in our knowledge of genital mycoplasmas as a cause of infection in pregnancy. The spectrum of poor pregnancy outcome ranges from infertility and early abortion through stillbirth, premature birth, amnionitis at term, neonatal respiratory disease and neonatal death. The objectives of this presentation are to discuss evidence supporting the concept that the genital mycoplasmas, *Ureaplasma urealyticum* and *Mycoplasma hominis* are a cause of infection in the fetus and neonate; to discuss the contribution of bovine studies to our understanding of intrauterine and neonatal ureaplasma infection in humans; to challenge our thinking regarding the pathogenic mechanisms by which ureaplasmas could cause disease and to highlight the need for development of new methods to diagnose women at risk of intrauterine ureaplasma infection.

Perinatal mortality is a major health care problem. Technical advances have seen increased survival of premature neonates but the prevention of stillbirths has been less successful. Morrison (1985) reported that the decrease in stillbirths between 1977 and 1981 was only 10% compared to 46% for neonatal deaths. He also observed that 59% of stillbirths occurred at less than 1500 gm compared to 33.4% of neonatal deaths. Among the list of causes of stillbirths and categories of hypoxia, no mention is made of intrauterine or placental infection as a causal factor.

The concept of intrauterine mycoplasma infection certainly warrants consideration as a cause of stillbirth and neonatal death. As will be discussed, the focus of poor outcomes associated with *U.urealyticum* infection is the fetus-neonate of less than 1500 grams or 32 weeks of gestation, a portion of which have respiratory disease. This is the very group which contributes significantly to perinatal health care costs.

Since mycoplasmas as a group are very host specific, animal models of infection have been limited. One learns only so much by observing the human situation when there are high carriage rates and multiple strains for the organisms in question. Thus application of the basic science approach to delineate virulence factors and pathogenic mechanisms will increase our understanding of the effects of ureaplasma in the human host.

The etiological causes of early pregnancy loss, i.e. miscarriage or abortion in the first trimester are well documented. The majority of losses are associated with chromosomal abnormalities, and an infectious etiology may play a role in about 15% of miscarriages. However, in stillbirths, the cause of *in utero* death can be determined in only one third of cases even after extensive autopsies (Mueller et al, 1983; Naeye, 1983; Ontario Registrar General, 1983; Ornoy et al, 1981; Quinn et al, 1985a). Maternal or fetal infection was identified as the cause of death in less than 1% of stillbirths in Ontario (Ontario Registrar General, 1983).

Two reasons for the lack of identification of infectious causes of death are that the placenta is often not examined at the time of autopsy and appropriate cultures are not done routinely for fastidious organisms such as genital mycoplasmas, anaerobic bacteria, and viruses. Swabs of tissue submitted are considered negative for all organisms when in fact they were cultured for only common bacteria.

The isolation of genital mycoplasmas from the placenta of stillbirths with chorioamnionitis was first reported by Kundsin et al (1967) and Jones (1967). The first isolation of *M. hominis* from a case of respiratory failure associated with amnionitis was reported by Brunell et al (1969) However, the concept of genital mycoplasma infection in pregnancy loss and neonatal disease has remained controversial.

Neonates acquire the organism at birth from the maternal genital tract. Approximately 25% of neonates were born with surface colonization (Taylor-Robinson and McCormack, 1979) and 15-20% have mycoplasmas in the nasopharynx (Rudd et al, 1984). Children tend to lose these organism by 1 year of age so that less than 5% of female children and 1% of male children carry the organism in their genital. The prevalence of colonization rises in the population after puberty. The rate of genital colonization with *U. urealyticum* in the female population is high ranging from 10% to 80% (Taylor-Robinson and McCormack,

1979). This has made it difficult to accept that in some patients mycoplasmas are pathogenic, while in others there is no evidence of infection. However, it is well documented that people are colonized with *E. coli* in the gut but only specific strains are associated with gastrointestinal disease.

In our local population, 25% of normal fertile couples were colonized with genital mycoplasmas in the early seventies (Quinn et al, 1983b). By the late eighties, 45% of normal fertile women were colonized, 48% of women with a history of abortion, and 73% of women who had perinatal deaths (Quinn et al, 1987c). Among sexually active adolescents presenting with vaginitis at our hospital, 85% are colonized with *U. urealyticum* (Kaufman et al 1985). Since these organisms can persist (Taylor-Robinson and McCormack, 1979) potential for problems due to *U. urealyticum* may increase as these young women become pregnant.

The organism may also exist in a latent state or be localized in the upper genital tract. For example, in couples treated until cleared of the organism in the lower genital tract prior to conception and remaining culture negative (up to two years), ureaplasmas have been re-isolated between the second and fourth month of gestation (Quinn et al, 1981). In other cases, *U. urealyticum* has been isolated from the placenta and lung of stillbirths, yet it cannot be isolated from the lower genital tract of the untreated mother or father 6 weeks after delivery (unpublished observations).

The studies on the role of genital mycoplasmas are hampered by the fact that the infection is in the placenta, an organ which cannot be readily sampled. Presently, there is no proven method for detecting intrauterine mycoplasma infection. Thus many studies have been based on colonization of the maternal genital tract. No correlation between vaginal-cervical colonization and the risk of poor pregnancy outcome was demonstrated for *U. urealyticum* and *M. hominis* (Harrison et al, 1983). Such observations are to be expected since the studies which show a correlation are based on the isolation of the organism directly from the placenta (Embree et al 1980; Kundsin et al, 1984; Quinn et al, 1985a).

Another aspect of studies of the population at large which presents a difficulty is that less than 1% of women lose pregnancies after 20 weeks (Porter and Hook, 1980). There is increasing evidence that *U. urealyticum* is associated more with losses after 20 weeks than losses prior to 20 weeks (Embree et al, 1980; Kundsin et al, 1984; Quinn et al, 1985a, 1987a). Thus the number of women with ureaplasma-associated late pregnancy loss would be minimal, for example 60 cases among 6000 pregnancies, and these would be a subset among all the losses. It therefore is difficult to detect an association between ureaplasma colonization in pregnancy and poor outcome in the population at large.

The human mycoplasma species *U. urealyticum* and *M. hominis* are heterogeneous, consisting of multiple serotypes (Taylor-Robinson and McCormack, 1979). It is therefore possible that certain strains or serotypes would exhibit different degrees of pathogenicity. Studies on the prevalence of ureaplasma serotypes indicate a difference in the distribution of serotypes in populations but as yet no consistent pattern has emerged with a specific disease entity (Lefevre et al, 1986; Quinn and Arshoff, 1986; Lin, 1985; Shepard and Lunceford, 1978; Piot, 1976).

Thus the study of the role of genital mycoplasmas as a cause of intrauterine infection of the fetus and neonate is hindered by a number of complex factors.

ANIMAL MODELS OF GENITAL AND RESPIRATORY TRACT INFECTIONS

Mycoplasma pulmonis is a cause of reproductive failure and respiratory disease in mice and rats. It causes infertility, resorption of fetuses, and reduction in litter size in laboratory rats. Respiratory disease occurs in neonates as well as adult animals. The pathogenesis and immunology of *M. pulmonis* infection has been extensively studied in rat and mouse models (reviewed in Cassell, 1982; Lindsey and Cassell, 1973).

In bovines, there is a spectrum of genital tract infections associated with *Ureaplasma diversum* including granular vulvitis, endometritis, salpingitis, spontaneous abortion, premature delivery and respiratory disease in the newborn calf (Doig et al, 1979; 1980a,b; 1981; Doig and Ruhnke, 1984; Miller et al, 1983; Ruhnke et al, 1977; 1984) which is comparable to the spectrum of infections in humans (Taylor-Robinson and McCormack, 1979). A similar pattern of infection is under study in sheep (Doig and Ruhnke, 1977; Ball and McCaughey, 1982; Howard, 1984).

It was first observed that heifers which developed a vaginal discharge after insemination had reduced conception rates (Ruhnke et al, 1977). With the discovery of the presence of ureaplasmas in bovine semen, granular vulvitis, endometritis and salpingitis were observed in the field and reproduced experimentally in heifers infected with a primary ureaplasma isolate (Doig et al, 1979; 1980a,b). In the bull seminal vesiculitis and impaired sperm motility have been documented (Jurmanova and Sterbova, 1977; Doig et al, 1981).

To assess the role of *U. diversum* in infertility and early pregnancy loss, two studies were carried out. Heifers in estrus were inoculated with *U. diversum* directly into the uterus and immediately inseminated. The experiment confirmed a significant reduction in the fertility rate (Kreplin et al, 1987). In the second approach, it was demonstrated that *U. diversum* adhered to the outer surface of the zona pellucida of infected bovine morulae (comparable to the human ovum in development) (Britton et al, 1987). This suggested that the morulae has receptor sites on its outer membrane for the binding of *U. diversum*. Ureaplasmas were also isolated from the fluid used to flush the morulae out of the uterus in other heifers suggesting that the ureaplasmas were present in the uterine cavity prior to implantation of the morulae.

Field cases of bovine abortion and 'weak calf' syndrome (i.e. a premature calf with respiratory disease) were examined for the presence of mycoplasma infection. Evidence of an inflammatory response and isolation of ureaplasmas from the placentas and fetal-neonatal lungs were observed (Ruhnke et al, 1984). Overall, 10-12% of field abortions sent into the laboratory for investigations are associated with *U. diversum*, particularly serogroup B.

To confirm whether *U. diversum* could cause intrauterine infection, the amniotic fluid of pregnant heifers at 5 months gestation was infected with *U. diversum* and with control culture medium (Miller et al, 1983). The ureaplasmas caused both spontaneous abortion (comparable to stillbirth in humans) and a premature calf with respiratory disease. At autopsy, ureaplasmas were isolated from the placenta and fetal lung in conjunction with evidence of inflammation. The inflammatory response was localized in the alveoli. There was no evidence of infection based on the isolation of ureaplasma or inflammation in other fetal organs. This pattern of infection is very comparable to that observed in human stillbirths and neonatal respiratory disease associated with *U. urealyticum* (Embree et al, 1983; Kundsin et al, 1984; Quinn et al, 1985a,b).

Mycoplasmas are very host specific making it difficult to study pathogenicity of human ureaplasmas in animal models. The bovine model provides a comparable natural infection which can be studied experimentally. Observations from the bovine studies have proven that *U. diversum* infection in pregnancy causes infertility, early abortion, spontaneous abortion or stillbirth, prematurity and neonatal lung disease.

Recently a mouse model has been developed in which human ureaplasmas were used to infect the lung of newborn mice (Rudd et al, 1986). It was observed that following intranasal inoculation, colonization could be established in the lung concurrent with the development of an inflammatory response between 3 and 5 days of age. The inflammatory response decreased by 12 days of age. If 14-day old mice were utilized, a brief period of colonization could be demonstrated, but no inflammation developed. This model will provide an excellent opportunity to study pathogenic mechanisms of neonatal ureaplasma respiratory disease in the future.

INFERTILITY

Genital tract infection with *U. urealyticum* may be associated with human infertility from two perspectives: the inability to achieve conception and the very early loss of the embryo (reviewed in Taylor-Robinson, 1986). Ureaplasmas are known to attach to spermatozoa (Fowlkes et al 1975a; Gump et al, 1984;) or be present in the endometrium and fallopian tubes (Stray-Pedersen et al, 1978; Cassell et al, 1983b). The presence of *U. urealyticum* in semen has been associated with poor motility, low sperm count and abnormal morphology (Fowlkes et al, 1975b; Hinton et al, 1979) but these findings were not confirmed by other investigators (Gump et al, 1984). In bovines, a reduction in motility when mycoplasmas including ureaplasmas were present in semen have been reported (Jurmanova and Sterbova, 1977). *U. diversum* is also associated with a reduction in the pregnancy rate of heifers in the field and experimentally, as previously discussed.

Recently in controlled studies of sperm parameters and infectious agents in semen from infertile couples, a statistically significant correlation was demonstrated between the isolation of *U. urealyticum* and poor motility, abnormal sperm morphology and a reduction in sperm cells, but not with the other factors or other microorganisms (Naessens et al, 1986; Leader et al, 1987). This confirmed the earlier observations of abnormal semen parameters in ureaplasma-positive males (Fowlkes et al, 1975b, Swenson et al, 1979). Antibiotic therapy with doxycycline to eradicate the ureaplasmas, was reported to improve sperm morphology and motility but not low sperm concentrations (Swenson et al 1979; Comhaire et al, 1986; Naessens et al, 1986; Leader et al, 1987). Controlled studies on the efficacy of doxycycline in increasing conception among this group of infertile couples identified to be at risk, will provide valuable information.

In studies to assess the role of ureaplasmas on conception, human sperm were pre-incubated with serotypes of *U. urealyticum.* The ova penetrating capacity of sperm exposed to ureaplasmas was significantly reduced, particularly with serotype 4, 6 and 8 compared to controls in the human sperm-hamster egg fertilization test (Busolo and Zanchetta, 1985a,b). These observations are comparable to experiments in which mouse sperm exposed to *M. pulmonis* were less capable of fertilizing mouse ova (Fraser and Taylor-Robinson, 1977; Swenson, 1982).

With respect to early abortion, one can hypothesize that since ureaplasmas may be carried by the sperm to the ova (Fowlkes et al, 1975a) or may be present in the fallopian tubes (Horne et al, 1973; Cassell et al, 1983b; Stray-Pedersen et al, 1978, the toxic products produced by the ureaplasmas or the utilization of essential metabolites could damage the ovum outright or affect the chromosomes at this very early stage. *U. urealyticum* has been isolated from primary human amniotic fluid cell cultures exhibiting chromosomal errors (Rudd and Quinn, 1973; Quinn and Rudd, 1974;) and shown to cause chromosome errors in experimentally infected amniotic fluid cell cultures (Kundsin et al, 1971). Adherence of ureaplasmas to the surface of the ovum or embryo, or their localization in the endometrium, may alter implantation or development of the fetus or placenta resulting in early loss or abnormal growth.

Antibiotic studies provide conflicting evidence on the efficacy of doxycycline in preventing infertility in mycoplasma-positive couples. It is possible that those at risk cannot yet be identified among those colonized. Serological and serotyping studies may provide new insights on the association of *U. urealyticum* with infertility. Recent studies, however, confirm that ureaplasmas interact with sperm, and can reduce egg-penetrating capacity of human sperm and cause infertility in bovines.

SIGNIFICANCE OF INFLAMMATION IN THE PLACENTA

The presence of acute inflammatory cells in the placenta are frequently observed in stillbirths and neonatal deaths (Taylor-Robinson and McCormack, 1979; Embree et al, 1980; Ornoy et al, 1981; Naeye, 1983; Kundsin et al, 1984; Quinn et al, 1987a). The significance of this polymorphonuclear infiltrate is questioned. Is it related to true intrauterine infection, to ascending infection with rupture of membranes, or to non-specificity? The concept of infection has been equivocal because organisms are frequently not detected in conjunction with chorioamnionitis (Shurin et al, 1975; Blanc, 1980) and inflammation is believed to be common in first and second trimester losses (Blanc, 1980; Svensson et al, 1986).

In older studies, cultures and the detection of antibody responses for more fastidious organisms such as mycoplasmas, chlamydia, viruses and anaerobes were not done as the technology was not available. More recent studies now indicate an association between chorioamnionitis, isolation of organisms, and perinatal morbidity and mortality (Embree et al, 1980; Naeye et al, 1983; Kundsin et al, 1984; Pankuch et al, 1984; Quinn et al, 1987a).

Intact placental membranes were believed to provide a barrier to infection but isolation of organisms without rupture of membranes has now been described for bacteria (Cassell et al, 1986), *U. urealyticum* and *M. hominis* (Caspi et al, 1976; Cassell et al, 1983a) resulting in clinically silent, chronic infection characterized by an intense inflammatory response.

Acute chorioamnionitis was reported in 53% of stillbirths and early neonatal deaths by Naeye et al (1983). In studies of placentas in which care was taken to avoid vaginal contamination, the isolation of genital mycoplasmas was associated with chorioamnionitis (Embree et al, 1980; Kundsin et al, 1984; Quinn et al, 1985a; Hillier et al, 1986). Kundsin et al (1984) observed a 3 times higher odds ratio of a poor outcome when U. urealyticum was isolated from the placenta.

In our studies, chorioamnionitis was observed in 57.6% of perinatal deaths compared to 5% of placentas from normal deliveries in women with no prior history of reproductive failure, prematurity or neonatal deaths (Quinn et al, 1987a). Among the perinatal deaths, 70.8% of cases with chorioamnionitis were in deaths of no morphological cause whereas only 22% were in cases with a possible cause of death. Overall, chorioamnionitis occurred more often in women with previous pregnancies, prolonged rupture of membranes, birth weight of ≤1000 gm and gestations of 20-27 weeks. In patients with chorioamnionitis, the perinatal death rate was higher than in those without chorioamnionitis. There was also a predominance of stillbirths, particularly deaths with no morphological cause.

U. urealyticum or pathogenic bacteria, particularly anaerobes, were isolated more frequently from the villous tissue of placentas with chorioamnionitis than without, but not *M. hominis, Chlamydia trachomatis,* or viruses. Antibody responses to *U. urealyticum* were significantly elevated in the fetus-neonate and titres were four-fold higher in the neonate than in the mother, in cases with chorioamnionitis than in cases without chorioamnionitis. The presence of an inflammatory response in the placenta correlated with the isolation of microorganisms and the detection of specific antibody responses. This suggests that there is an association between infection with microorganisms such as *U. urealyticum* and/or pathogenic bacteria and chorioamnionitis.

In the study of Pankuch et al (1984), aerobic and anaerobic bacteria were isolated from 72% of placentas with chorioamnionitis, compared to 15% of placentas without chorioamnionitis. In our study, mycoplasmas or bacteria were isolated in 71.4% of chorioamnionitis positive placentas compared to 27.6% of negative placentas (Quinn et al, 1987a). In both studies the presence of anaerobic bacteria in the internal villous tissue was of significance.

However, other investigators reported no correlation between chorioamnionitis and the detection of bacteria in placentas obtained at caesarian section (Svensson et al, 1986). These results are open to question since the placenta was not decontaminated prior to sampling and appropriate cultures were not done for *M. hominis* and *U. urealyticum.* Tissue cannot be ground for the isolation of mycoplasmas as is done for bacteria. The release of toxic products from cells seriously inhibits the growth of mycoplasmas (Taylor-Robinson and Chen, 1983). In their study mycoplasmas were isolated from 0% of placentas and only 14% of patients had cervical cultures positive for *U. urealyticum.* These incidences were low since genital mycoplasmas were found in 40-80% of pregnant women (Taylor-Robinson and McCormack, 1979; Quinn et al, 1981), 9-15% of normal placentas and 25-40% of placentas associated with poor outcomes (Embree et al, 1980; Kundsin et al, 1984; Quinn et al, 1985a).

These observations support the concept that chorioamnionitis associated with *U. urealyticum* alone or in combination with bacteria is a major factor in intrauterine infections leading to perinatal morbidity and mortality in some women. The fundamental problem we face is that the means to diagnose women with intrauterine mycoplasma infection is not available. Clinical parameters such as the presence of fever or elevated white cell count did not clearly identify women with chorioamnionitis (Hillier et al, 1986; Quinn et al, 1987a). Once we can identify which women are at risk, the prevention or treatment of chorioamnionitis with antibiotic therapy is a realistic goal.

SPONTANEOUS ABORTION, STILLBIRTHS AND NEONATAL DEATH

The first reports on the isolation of genital mycoplasmas from stillbirths were based on individual cases (Jones, 1967; Kundsin et al, 1967; Brunell et al, 1969;

Caspi et al, 1971; Romano et al, 1971). In a series of studies, genital mycoplasmas were isolated more frequently from spontaneous abortions and stillbirths compared to therapeutic abortions (Driscoll et al, 1969; Caspi et al, 1972; Somplinsky et al, 1975) suggesting an association with mycoplasmas. Inflammation in the placenta and fetal lung were observed by Somplinsky et al, (1975).

Microbiological and histological studies of placentas revealed an increased prevalence of chorioamnionitis, spontaneous abortion, stillbirth and neonatal death among women with mycoplasmas isolated from the placenta compared to cases which were culture negative (Embree et al, 1980; Kundsin et al, 1984). In Kundsin's study (1984), genital mycoplasma, particularly U. urealyticum, were isolated from 20% of stillbirths, 17% of neonatal deaths and 23% of neonates requiring intensive care compared to 11% of normal term deliveries. Chorioamnionitis was found in 60% of ureaplasma-positive placentas compared to 29% of ureaplasma-negative placentas.

In preliminary serological studies of the antibody response to *U. urealyticum,* we observed elevated antibody titres in women with a history of prior pregnancy loss compared to women with normal deliveries using a modified metabolic inhibition test (Quinn et al, 1983b). The mean antibody titre in the test verus control women was significantly elevated to serotypes 4 and 8. Since the antibody was detected at delivery, it was not known when the women developed their antibody response.

A role for *U. urealyticum* in perinatal death was confirmed in our prospective study. Ureaplasmas were isolated from the placenta as well as the fetal lung in 39.4% of cases compared to 9.7% of control placentas. However, the isolation rate increased to 56.5% from the cases with no known morphological cause of death (no cause) compared to 0% of the cases with a detectable cause of death. Antibody responses ≥1:64 to at least one of the original eight serotypes of U. urealyticum were observed in 45.8% of the perinatal deaths, compared to 0% in the cord blood from normal cases. When the titres were compared by cause of death, the antibody responses were significantly higher at 58.8% of cases with no cause compared to 14.3% with cause. In the mycoplasma positive cases there was evidence of inflammation in 78.9% of the perinatal deaths compared to 11.1% of the controls. In the group which died of no cause, 83.3% of these cases had inflammation in the placenta compared to 0% of the group with a known cause of death.

There were only 4 cases in which viruses (herpes and cytomegalovirus) were detected: two isolations and two with elevated antibody titres. Three of the virus positive cases also had evidence of ureaplasma. Evidence of *C. trachomatis* was observed in only one case with an elevated antibody response and that titre was equal to the maternal titre. Thus we did not find any evidence of chlamydia infection in the pregnancy even after the investigation of over 100 perinatal deaths (Quinn et al, 1985a; unpublished observations).

There is evidence that women with chlamydial infections in pregnancy have a higher risk of poor pregnancy outcome. Ureaplasmas have been reported as the second risk factor in cervicitis of women (Paavonen et al, 1986) and are known to cause non-specific urethritis in males (Taylor-Robinson and McCormack, 1979). Thus chlamydia could be an indicator of risk due to other sexually acquired organisms such as ureaplasmas. Assessment of women with a history of two or more losses indicated a higher prevalence of detectable chlamydia antibody but not higher titres. This suggests that the women had increased past exposure to chlamydia than the control women with whom they were compared. Despite the prevalence of antibody, chlamydia were not isolated from the women before or during pregnancy and they did not develop a rise in titre (Quinn et al, 1987b). It is also possible that in the presence of chlamydial cervicitis, organisms residing in the vagina gain access to the membranes of the placenta allowing the development of intrauterine infections due to ureaplasmas, Group B streptococcus, *E. coli* or anaerobic bacteria.

A significant fact that has emerged from infection studies is that there is a mixture of organisms detected in the placenta and fetal organs of stillbirths. In our study, evidence of mycoplasma infection was observed in 83% of the bacteria-positive cases and 75% of the virus-positive cases. However, in the mycoplasma-positive cases, evidence of bacteria was found in only 50% (Quinn et al, 1985a).

In the bovine model studies, inoculation of pregnant heifers with *U. diversum* has proven that ureaplasmas can cause spontaneous pregnancy loss. These losses were associated with placentitis and an inflammatory response in the fetal lung (Miller et al, 1983; Ruhnke et al, 1984). There is also evidence of an association with ureaplasmas and pregnancy loss in other animals such as sheep (Howard, 1984).

Thus studies based on isolation of ureaplasmas, elevated antibody responses to *U. urealyticum* and experimental infections in bovines confirms that this organism causes intrauterine infection leading to perinatal death.

Among women with repeated pregnancy loss, the concept of a recurrent abortion syndrome has been proposed (Strobino et al, 1980). Characteristics associated with repeated status include cervical insufficiency, late gestation (after 16 weeks), chromosomal normality of the conceptus, prior premature livebirths and a long conception interval. All of these interface with our knowledge of mycoplasmas and pregnancy loss. Genital mycoplasmas are associated with intrauterine infection which is clinically silent and the mother has no evidence of infection in the pregnant or non-pregnant state (Cassell et al, 1983a; Quinn et al, 1985a, 1987a). Genital mycoplasmas persist (Taylor-Robinson and McCormack, 1979) or may recur in pregnancy (Quinn et al, 1981). We have observed several cases where couples were treated between pregnancies yet the organism appears to recur in each successive gestation (Quinn et al, 1981). It is therefore possible that clinically silent intrauterine infection with *U. urealyticum* is a factor in recurrent pregnancy loss.

PREMATURITY

There is growing evidence that *U. urealyticum* is associated with premature births. Early studies reported that infants born colonized with U. urealyticum had significantly lower birth weights (Braun et al, 1971; Kass et al, 1981, 1986). Studies on the association of U. urealyticum in the placenta and pregnancy outcome indicated that isolation of ureaplasmas was higher in gestations of 20-27 weeks than those at term (Embree et al, 1980; Kundsin et al, 1984). In our stillbirth studies, 55% of the stillbirths occurred between 20 and 28 weeks of gestation (Quinn, et al, 1985a). Chorioamnionitis was more prevalent in the gestations of 20-28 weeks than in longer gestations (Quinn et al, 1987a).

Recent studies have shown an increased risk of preterm birth (Kimpen et al, 1986) and preterm labour in women colonized with *U. urealyticum* in pregnancy, compared to control groups (Goulet et al, 1987; Rudd et al, 1984; Hillier et al, 1986). Hillier et al (1986) observed that in women colonized with *U. urealyticum* in the vagina or in the placental membrane, there was a higher prevalence of preterm births. Increased vaginal concentrations of *U. urealyticum* and other microorganisms associated with bacterial vaginosis may be associated with premature rupture of membranes, preterm labour and amniotic fluid infection when demographic and obstetrical variables associated with prematurity were controlled in a linear logistic regression model (Gravett and Eschenbach, 1986).

In a study examining the significance of C-reactive protein, an indicator of infection, *U. urealyticum* was isolated from maternal urine more often when C-reactive protein was elevated in the cord blood (Kimpen et al, 1986). A significant relationship was also observed between isolation of ureaplasmas from the mothers' urine and low gestational age.

A prospective study of women with preterm premature rupture of membranes matched to women without preterm premature rupture of membranes is currently underway. In the preliminary analysis of infectious etiologies, the most significant factors were the isolation of *U. urealyticum* from the maternal vagina and from the placenta in women with preterm premature rupture of membranes compared to the control women (Goulet et al, 1987). The prevalence of group B streptococcus in the genital tract was not significantly different between women with and without preterm premature rupture of membranes. There was also no significant difference in the isolation of other bacteria including anaerobes, *M. hominis*, *C. trachomatis* or viruses. Delineation of the role of demographic and clinical factors in this study will add to our understanding of the significance of preterm premature rupture of membranes.

One concept put forward in terms of the role of infection as the cause of premature delivery relates to the phospholipase activity of microorganisms in the placenta. It has been demonstrated that certain bacteria, particularly perinatal pathogens, have elevated phospholipase levels compared to other types of bacteria (Dennis, 1983). It is proposed that the activity of microbial phopholipases would produce exogenous arachadonic acid which could initiate the prostaglandin cascade leading to premature onset of labour (Bejar et al, 1981). Ureaplasmas have significant amounts of phospholipids (Smith, 1971) and we have demonstrated the presence of phospholipase activities (DeSilva and Quinn, 1986). Phospholipase A2 activity in *U. urealyticum* was ten fold higher than phospholipase A1 and phospholipase C, and was comparable to the higher activities observed in bacteria associated with perinatal infections. Furthermore, phospholipase A2 activity was three times higher in serotype 8, compared to serotypes 3 and 4. This was of special interest since serotype 8 and not serotype 3 was found in the case of fatal ureaplasma pneumonia, despite the mother being colonized with both serotypes. Enzyme activities such as phospholipase may be of special importance in mycoplasmas because of their unique morphology. Since they do not have a cell wall, membrane-associated enzymes have ready access to substrates in the external environment. In ureaplasmas, the phospholipase activity was shown to be present in the membrane fraction (DeSilva and Quinn, 1986). Thus the production of arachadonic acid could occur outside the control of normal prostaglandin biosynthesis in the placenta. Phospholipases are also considered to be toxins in other microbial-host systems.

It is now well documented that premature delivery and stillbirth is associated with the isolation of *U. urealyticum* from the placenta. This fact may be very important in the use of tocolytic agents to prevent premature delivery (Hameed et al, 1984). Is it in the best interest of the fetus to prolong the pregnancy if the presence of intrauterine infection is compromising lung function or fetal well being? It is also possible that certain cases, refractory to the use of tocolytic agents may be related to placental infection.

These observations suggest that in some way *U. urealyticum* alone or in combination with other microorganisms is associated with premature delivery. Genital tract colonization may or may not be an indicator of risk depending on the population. Epidemiological studies are now required to assess specific risk factors such as bacterial vaginosis and determine the prevalence of intrauterine ureaplasma infection in premature birth. Once such women can be identified, the efficacy of antibiotic therapy to prevent prematurity could be evaluated. Trials on women known to be mycoplasma positive in the lower genital tract as the only inclusion criterion will be confounded by the inclusion of a large proportion of normal women colonized, yet not at risk.

NEONATAL RESPIRATORY DISEASE

Mycoplasma species are associated with respiratory disease in a wide spectrum of animals and poultry. Respiratory infections in humans and animals and the pathogenic mechanisms are reviewed by Cassell et al, (1985). *U. urealyticum* may be associated with neonatal respiratory disease from two perspectives. Ureaplasmas could infect the placenta and indirectly initiate premature labour, resulting in the birth of a neonate with respiratory disease due to immature lungs. On the other hand, the mycoplasmas could pass through the membranes or the placenta into the amniotic fluid (Cassell et al, 1983a) and gain direct access to the lung *in utero* (Brunell et al, 1969; Dische et al, 1979; Romano et al, 1971; Tafari et al, 1976) leading to infection and damage of lung function. The severity of this neonatal lung disease may be dependent on the duration of the infection *in utero*. It is becoming apparent that neonates born under 32 weeks or of ≤1500 grams tend to develop chronic lung disease in association with U. urealyticum (Cassell et al, 1974;

Wang et al, 1987). Neonates born closer to term tend to have severe pneumonia which is fatal despite antibiotic therapy (Quinn et al, 1985a, 1985b; unpublished observations).

In many of the reports on the isolation of mycoplasmas in pregnancy failures, *U. urealyticum* and *M. hominis* were isolated in association with an inflammatory response in the lungs of stillborns and neonates who died of respiratory failure (Jones 1967; Caspi et al, 1971; Somplinsky et al, 1975; Tafari et al, 1976; Naeye et al, 1977; Dische et al, 1979; Christensen et al, 1982; Quinn et al, 1985a). Evidence of infection and isolation of mycoplasmas were often not found in other organs of the fetuses and neonates autopsied, except where overall sepsis occurred. Alterations in the ciliated epithelium of the trachea observed by scanning electron microscopy have also been reported in a very premature neonate who died of respiratory failure. (Dische et al, 1979). There was clumping and disorganization of the cilia, sloughing of ciliated cells and large patches of tracheal epithelium with no cilia present, which was not due to intubation or autolysis as the autopsy was done within a few hours of death.

Subsequent experiments were done in which the isolate from this case was used to infect human fetal tracheal organ cultures. This ureaplasma strain was shown to induce the same type of pathogenic effects within 8 hours post-infection, which were not found in control cultures inoculated with mycoplasma medium (Quinn et al, 1979). The same cytopathogenic effects were observed by scanning electron microscopy despite the fact that ciliary activity as observed by light microscopy appeared to be normal. These observations suggest that *U. urealyticum* has a toxic effect on the ciliated epithelium of the human respiratory tract. This effect is not unusual in that it has been documented with other mycoplasma species in ciliated tracheal cultures (Collier, 1979) and in fallopian tube cultures (Baldetorp et al, 1983; Stalheim et al, 1976).

In field and experimental studies of stillborn and premature calves with respiratory disease, *U. diversum* was isolated from the lung at autopsy but not from the other organs (Miller et al, 1983; Ruhnke et al, 1984). Experimental inoculation of amniotic fluid proved that *U. diversum* could cause inflammation in the lung in stillborn and premature calves and cause respiratory disease. There is also evidence from other animal models eg. rats and mice, that mycoplasmas such as *M. pulmonis* cause infection in pregnancy and are associated with respiratory disease (Cassell, 1982; Taylor-Robinson and Furr, 1985). Ureaplasma infection of the mucous membranes in the respiratory and genital tract are also found in large domestic animals and in poultry (Howard, 1984).

In 1980, we first reported on a case of a term neonate who was in respiratory distress within 15 minutes of delivery, developed acute pneumonia and died following an episode of bradycardia (Quinn et al, 1985b). The parents who had been infertile, were colonized with *U. urealyticum* during the pregnancy but it was not isolated from the neonate's nasopharynx. However at autopsy, it was the only organism isolated from the lung. The lung exhibited localized areas of inflammation with the development of fibrin strands particularly in the alveoli. In some respects it resembled "patchy" hyaline membrane disease.

The mother had been colonized with serotype 3 and 8; the father with serotype 8 and the lung isolate was serotype 8. The neonate had an antibody titre of 1:64 to serotype 8 which was 1:128 at autopsy; a titre of 1:16 to serotype 3 and was negative for the other serotypes. The antibody was indirectly shown to be Ig M specific. The mother had a titre of 1:16 to serotype 3 and no detectable antibody response to serotype 8, nor did she mount one postpartum.

Immunofluorescent staining of the lung tissue was positive for *U. urealyticum* serotype 8 and negative for the 7 other serotypes. The control lungs from cases including bacterial pneumonia and respiratory distress syndrome were negative. The fluorescent staining localized the organism on the surface of the alveoli and bronchus. Mycoplasma-like particles were observed along the epithelium of the bronchus by electron microscopy.

Cases of ureaplasma pneumonia in neonates associated with persistent pulmonary hypertension has recently been reported (Waites et al, 1988b).

The observations from these cases, from the human and bovine stillbirths, and bovine calf respiratory disease indicate that the focus of *U. urealyticum* is the lower respiratory tract, particularly in the alveoli. This fact is important for the diagnosis of neonatal respiratory disease associated with ureaplasmas. Since neonates do not cough, cultures must be taken from the lower respiratory tract to isolate organisms associated with respiratory disease. This would explain why studies based on neonatal colonization of the nasopharynx do not show a correlation between the isolation of genital mycoplasmas and neonatal respiratory disease (Taylor-Robinson and McCormack, 1979; Taylor-Robinson et al, 1984). Preliminary evidence from a recent study suggested a correlation between the isolation of mycoplasmas from tracheal aspirates but not nasopharyngeal specimens and an increased incidence of neonatal death or chronic lung disease (Cassell et al, 1987).

On the premise that there was an association between intrauterine exposure to *U. urealyticum* and fetal-neonatal lung disease, we examined the antibody response to *U. urealyticum* as a means of differentiating which neonates might be truly infected among those born colonized.

In 1983 we first reported that 55.6% of 21 neonates with respiratory disease (RD) and 28.6% of their mothers had at least one titre ≥1:32 to the *U. urealyticum* serotypes compared to 4.2% of 24 normal neonates and 0% of their mothers (Quinn et al, 1983c). The sera were drawn up to 21 days of age and none of the neonates were on erythromycin therapy at the time. These antibody responses were not likely due to development of normal antibody in colonized neonates since even in normal colonized women, the background prevalence of titres ≥1:32 is only 8%. Since neonates could acquire this antibody from the mother, the incidence of titres four-fold higher in the neonate above the maternal level were assessed. Among the RD neonates 52.4% versus 0% in controls had a higher titre which suggested the antibody was of neonatal origin and not due to passive transfer from the mother. Furthermore the mortality rate was 40% among RD neonates with four-fold higher titres compared to 16.6% of RD neonates with titres equal or less than their mothers. These antibody titres suggested that a significant proportion of neonates had been exposed to *U. urealyticum.*

Significance of the antibody response to *U. urealyticum* was then assessed in a larger cohort of 259 neonates with respiratory disease compared to 22 stillborns and 46 normal term neonates and their mothers whose sera were drawn shortly after delivery (Quinn, 1986). An elevated antibody response of ≥1:32 to at least one serotype was found in 58.3% of the neonates with respiratory disease compared to 77.3% of stillbirths and only 6.5% of normal term neonates. Within the respiratory disease group of neonates, 69.3% of the neonates who died and 80.4% of the term neonates had elevated antibody responses resembling the incidence in stillbirths. A titre four-fold higher than their mother was observed in 56.5% of RD neonates compared to 2.2% of the normal term neonates; in 72.7% of those who died and in 73.3% of the term RD neonates who most closely matched the control group. Since these percentages were similar to the overall presence of elevated antibody titres, the data confirms that most of the antibody response is neonatal in origin, not due to passive transfer from the mother. The mounting of an antibody response is indicative of infection, but does not establish a causal role.

Upon further analysis, 80.4% of term neonates compared to 52.2% of premature neonates had elevated ureaplasma antibody titres. It is possible that with ongoing exposure *in utero*, the term fetus experiencing a longer period of infection has more time to mount an antibody response. Of particular concern was the fact that 69.3% of the neonates who died under 28 days of age had an elevated antibody response which was significantly higher statistically than the 53.8% observed in neonates who survived. When all cases were combined, the mortality rate was 61.3% among the fetus-neonate with a titre ≥1:32 compared to 27.1% for the fetus-neonate who had a titre of ≤1:16. These observations suggested that neonates who mounted an antibody response to *U. urealyticum* had a higher rate of mortality and morbidity associated with respiratory disease than neonates who did not.

Based on our serological studies and our experience in a Neonatal Intensive Care Unit, I proposed in 1986 that two patterns of respiratory disease associated with *U. urealyticum* were becoming apparent (Quinn, 1986). First there was the pattern of severe congenital pneumonia presenting with acute respiratory failure immediately after birth. These neonates often died quickly or remained oxygen dependent for prolonged periods of which a high proportion die within 6 months of other nosocomial infections (Quinn et al, 1985b). The second pattern included neonates presenting with classic "wet lung" which failed to clear. The neonates required increasing concentrations of oxygen in the first weeks of life and developed a chronic pattern of respiratory disease.

A third possibility is also emerging. The neonate acquires *U. urealyticum in utero* or at birth and develops a less severe pattern of chronic respiratory problems with subsequent infections due to other respiratory pathogens such as respiratory syncitial virus, adenovirus, cytomegalovirus etc. in the first year of life (Stagno et al, 1981, unpublished observations). The severity of these respiratory infections appears to be increased and may be fatal when combined with *U. urealyticum.* Ureaplasmas have been isolated at autopsy in conjunction with elevated ureaplasma antibody responses from infants with these other infections. In one case, a seven month old infant who had recurrent bronchiolectasis and died of respiratory failure, was found to have respiratory syncitial virus and *U. urealyticum* in his lungs at autopsy. He also had an elevated antibody response to *U. urealyticum* in serum collected at birth which declined at 5 months of age and rose four-fold by seven months of age.

For many, the hypothesis that *U. urealyticum* was associated with neonatal respiratory disease was untenable in the early eighties, despite the reports from a limited series of cases and serological studies indicating an association worth investigating. This attitude unfortunately limited collaboration and funding for properly controlled studies. However, preliminary reports from two current studies on the infectious etiology of chronic lung disease of the neonate, confirm an association with *U. urealyticum.* Isolation of *U. urealyticum* from the lower respiratory tract of premature neonates was significantly associated with increased mortality and chronic lung disease in neonates under 1500 gm (Cassell et al, 1987). In the second study, neonates with and without chronic lung disease were cultured for all microorganisms at 28 days of age. In the analysis, after an increased requirement for oxygen, isolation of *U. urealyticum* from tracheal aspirates was the most significant factor (Wang et al, 1987). There was no correlation with the isolation of bacteria, viruses or chlamydia in either study. In the first study, isolation of Group B streptococcus was significant for increased mortality and sepsis but not respiratory disease.

The evidence from human studies strongly supports the hypothesis that *U. urealyticum* is associated with lung disease in the fetus and neonate. Experimental evidence from studies in the bovine model demonstrates that U. diversum causes lung disease in utero and respiratory disease in calves. The demonstration of lung infection in the newborn mouse model with *U. urealyticum* from humans points towards causality in neonatal respiratory disease.

INCREASED MORBIDITY AND MORTALITY BETWEEN 20 AND 32 WEEKS OF GESTATION ASSOCIATED WITH *U. UREALYTICUM* INFECTION

Among the many reports published on the isolation of genital mycoplasma in poor pregnancy outcome, there is a clustering of stillbirths or premature births between 20 and 32 weeks of gestation. In the study of Embree and colleagues (1980), genital mycoplasmas were isolated from 34% of placentas in high risk cases with birth weights ≥2500 gm compared to 9% of those with birthweights <2500 gm. When assessed by gestational age, 32% of births at less than 38 weeks had mycoplasma positive placentas compared to 9% of gestations greater than 38 weeks. The incidence rose to 50% for gestations of 26-30 weeks.

In the study of Kundsin et al (1985) genital mycoplasmas were isolated from the placenta in 25% of perinatal deaths of birth weight <999 gm and of 1000-1500 gm compared to 10% of birth weight >2500 gm. The incidence was 34% for neonates born at less than 1000 gm requiring intensive care and 20% for those 1000-1500 gm. In our study, 54.8% of the perinatal deaths occurred between 18 and 27 weeks of gestation with 15.1% at 28-31 weeks, 19.4% between 32-37 weeks and 9.7% at term (Quinn et al, 1985a). When the data were assessed in terms of placental infection, chorioamnionitis was present in 73.7% of gestations between 20-27 weeks and 80% of fetuses-neonates weighing ≤1000 gm compared to 4.3% of term gestations and 8% of neonates weighing ≥2500 gm. These studies point to the fact that the major focus of *U. urealyticum* infection in the pregnancy is associated with loss or premature delivery around 20-28 weeks of gestation or birthweights less than 1500 gm. However, in cases delivered after 32 weeks and even at term, chorioamnionitis and evidence of lung disease were observed in a smaller proportion. In one of the recent studies on chronic lung disease of the newborn, isolation of mycoplasmas from the trachea, was more associated with the development of chronic lung disease or death in neonates born under 1000 grams than neonates born over 2500 grams (Cassell et al, 1987). The correlation was less significant for those born between 1000 and 1500 grams.

These observations suggest that the genital mycoplasmas, particularly *U. urealyticum* are associated with intrauterine infection leading to stillbirth and premature delivery mainly between 20 to 28 weeks of gestation.

DEVELOPMENT OF ANTIBIOTIC TREATMENT REGIMENS IN PREGNANCY

In the development of antibiotic therapies to prevent pregnancy loss associated with intrauterine *U. urealyticum* infection, this pattern of increased loss at 20-28 weeks warrants consideration. Antibiotic therapy must begin sufficiently early to prevent the development of infection by 20 weeks of gestation by which time mycoplasmas may already be present in the amniotic fluid (Cassell et al, 1983a). Antibiotic treatment should also be based on the concept that one is treating the placenta and fetus and not aiming solely for the eradication of the organism from the lower genital tract. In one woman treated to clear prior to conception, the ureaplasma recurred in her genital tract and was isolated from the neonate and placenta in her sixth and seventh pregnancies (unpublished observations). The couple was treated to clear with doxycycline and she was administered erythromycin from the first month of gestation in the eighth pregnancy and used barrier contraception until admitted to the hospital at five months. The ureaplasmas recurred in her vagina at 2 months of gestation and persisted, but were not isolated from the neonate, amniotic fluid or placenta at delivery. This is a single case but highlights what may actually happen in the treatment of such patients.

In our experience, antibiotic therapy prior to conception or during pregnancy does not eliminate colonization or recurrence in the lower genital tract of most women. It was observed that in couples treated to clear with doxycycline prior to conception, the mycoplasmas were re-isolated from 45% of the women between the second and fourth months of gestation (Quinn et al, 1981). Treatment with erythromycin (1000 mgm/day) throughout the pregnancy of women who are positive initially or in whom the mycoplasmas recur, indicate that the organisms are usually not eradicated from the lower genital tract. For the few ureaplasma isolates we tested, this lack of eradication does not appear to be related to antibiotic resistance in the ureaplasma strains (unpublished observations). However, strain resistance has been suggested by other authors (Robertson et al, 1981; Spaepen and Kundsin, 1977). The effects of coexistence of *M. hominis* with other vaginal flora including *U. urealyticum* may be a factor in antibiotic effectiveness (Quinn et al, 1982; Koutsky et al, 1983). Since the antibiotic concentrations achieved in the placenta are higher than in the genital tract, the antibiotics may still be efficacious. Further work will be required to delineate what factors are involved.

To date, three approaches to the prevention of poor pregnancy outcomes using antibiotic therapy have been tested: the use of antibiotic therapy prior to conception to eradicate the mycoplasmas (Quinn et al, 1983a; Taylor-Robinson and McCormack, 1979); the use of 6 weeks of therapy after 30 weeks of gestation to reduce the prevalence of low birth weight (Elder et al, 1971), McCormack et al,1977); and the use of therapy throughout the pregnancy to prevent spontaneous abortion, stillbirth and perhaps prematurity and neonatal morbidity (Quinn et al, 1983a). The latter two concepts are currently undergoing evaluation in blind trials. In our preliminary studies to develop an effective treatment regimen for evaluation, we found that treatment prior to conception appeared to reduce the abortion rate among mycoplasma-positive women with a history of three or more losses under 12 weeks gestation but not for women with a history of later losses (Quinn et al, 1983a). Treatment with erythromycin during the pregnancy held more promise for the women with late losses. This approach may be more appropriate since we do not know when the fetus becomes infected.

MYCOPLASMA HOMINIS INFECTIONS

For many years, discussions on infections associated with genital mycoplasmas have grouped *U. urealyticum* and *M. hominis* together. However, the spectrum of infections with these organisms is diverging. Evidence suggests that *U. urealyticum* is more associated with early infection in pregnancy leading to abortion, stillbirth, and fetal-neonatal lung disease as discussed. *M. hominis* on the other hand, is more frequently associated with intra-amniotic infection late in pregnancy (Gibbs et al, 1983, 1986), postpartum fever, endometritis and salpingitis (Taylor-Robinson and McCormack, 1979, Moller, 1983), as well as with neonatal infections including respiratory disease (Brunell et al, 1969; Mufson, 1983), central nervous system infections (Mardh, 1983; Waites et al, 1988a), conjunctivitis (Jones and Tobin, 1968), abscesses (Sacker et al, 1970) and septicemia (Harwick et al, 1967; Unsworth et al, 1985).

M. hominis has been isolated from the placenta and fetal tissues in stillbirths and poor pregnancy outcomes but appears to be less common than *U. urealyticum* (Brunell et al, 1969; Embree et al, 1983; Jones, 1967; Quinn et al,1985a). In studies of infection in pregnancy, seroconversion to *U. urealyticum* was associated with low birth weight but a similar effect was not noted with *M. hominis* (Kass et al, 1981). In individual cases, *M. hominis* was isolated from amniotic fluid and the placenta in association with chorioamnionitis and funisitis alone and in combination with *U. urealyticum* (Embree et al, 1980, Cassell et al, 1983a). Thus the clinical significance of intrauterine M. hominis is not clear. Although an association between the isolation of *U. urealyticum* and chorioamnionitis has been reported, no significant correlation was found with *M. hominis* in large scale studies, perhaps because of the lower prevalence.

Two factors may play a role in these observations. First, in the population at large, the prevalence of *M. hominis* in women is lower, ranging up to 20% compared to 40-80% for *U. urealyticum* (Lamey et al, 1974; Taylor-Robinson and McCormack, 1979; Quinn et al, 1983b). Secondly, there may be distinct differences in the pathogenic mechanisms of the two species.

Since *M. hominis* is found in the genital tract of women, it could be transmitted to the fetus, as is *U. urealyticum,* by intrauterine infection, by aspiration of organisms during the birth process or by infection at a later stage due to organisms acquired at birth. In cases with intrauterine infection late in gestation, *M. hominis* is isolated more often from the amniotic fluid removed by uterine catheter compared to asymptomatic controls (Gibbs et al, 1983). However, it is also found in association with other highly virulent bacteria. Many of these women proceed to postpartum fever or endometritis. A rise in *M. hominis* antibody occurred more frequently in women with intra-amniotic infection and isolation of *M. hominis* from the amniotic fluid than from women without clinical evidence of intra-amniotic infection or from control women in whom the organism was not isolated (Gibbs et al, 1986).

In a number of case reports, *M. hominis* has been associated with neonatal respiratory disease and chorioamnionitis (Brunell et al, 1969; Dische et al, 1979). *M. hominis* can occur in both premature and term neonates with respiratory disease (Mufson, 1983). We have documented a few cases of chronic respiratory disease in which only *M. hominis* was isolated from the tracheal aspirates of the neonates (unpublished observations).

M. hominis has been recovered from extragenital sites in newborns such as in infections of the eyes, abscesses, joints and blood. A number of reports indicate that *M. hominis* may be involved in central nervous system infections of the newborn such as meningitis, meningoencephalitis, and meningoceles (Mardh, 1983; Waites et al, 1988a). However, M. hominis has also been isolated from cerebrospinal fluid of neonates who had no evidence of clinical infection (Waites et al, 1988b). Thus there exists a spectrum of extragenital infections which could be due to intrauterine infection or transmission of genital mycoplasmas at delivery.

TREATMENT OF NEONATAL MYCOPLASMA INFECTIONS

It is generally assumed that antibiotic treatment regimens appropriate for bacteria are suitable for mycoplasmas. However, that may not hold true. Recurrence of urethritis in males after 7 days of doxycycline (200 mgm/day) is more frequent for those with *U. urealyticum* than chlamydia (Fong et al, 1987). In couples with reproductive failure, treated for 4 weeks with doxycycline (100 mgm/day), 100% of those with *M. hominis* cleared of the organism, 89% of those with *U. urealyticum* but only 66% of those with *U. urealyticum* and *M. hominis* (Quinn et al, 1982). Koutsky et al (1983) reviewed the effect of other factors on the susceptibility of *M. hominis*. These observations suggest that the duration of therapy and the presence of both mycoplasmas and bacteria in the genital flora may influence the efficacy of antibiotic therapy. Controlled trials are essential to determine appropriate treatment regimens for genital mycoplasma infections.

In pregnancy and neonates, the drug of choice for treating *U. urealyticum* infections is erythromycin. However, controlled trials on the efficacy of treating ureaplasma infection in neonates have not yet been done. Most strains of U. urealyticum are sensitive to erythromycin but resistant strains do exist (Spaepen and Kundsin, 1977; Robertson et al, 1981; Taylor-Robinson and Furr, 1986).

In the treatment of the newborn with *M. hominis* infections, care must be given to the selection of proper antibiotics (Myhre and Mardh, 1983). In general, *M. hominis* is not sensitive to erythromycin (Bygdeman and Mardh, 1983). Thus the drugs which are available include lincomycin, clindamycin, tetracyclines, and chloramphenicol with the drug of choice being tetracycline. The life threatening nature of central nervous system infections and severe respiratory failure may warrant the use of tetracycline despite the side effects. However, tetracycline resistant strains of *M. hominis* are increasing in prevalence in the Seattle area, for example (Koutsky et al, 1983; Roberts et al, 1985). For neonates with chronic respiratory disease, clindamycin is an alternative to tetracycline and can be given to neonates. We have successfully treated with clindamycin a few neonates who had chronic lung disease associated with only *M. hominis*. However, one must be mindful that *Clostridium difficle*-associated colitis is a serious if rare side effect. *M. hominis* strains also exhibit a moderate sensitivity to chloramphenicol.

MODEL OF MYCOPLASMA INFECTION IN PREGNANCY

The evidence from human and bovine studies confirms that ureaplasmas cause infection in pregnancy leading to stillbirth, neonatal lung disease and death in certain cases. On the other hand many patients are colonized with ureaplasmas with no apparent signs of infection.

Since mycoplasmas are very host specific, it has been difficult to establish animal models of disease to study pathogenicity. However, Koch's postulate has been fulfilled with the demonstration that inoculation of *U. diversum* into the amniotic fluid of pregnant heifers causes spontaneous abortion, premature delivery and fetal-neonatal lung disease (Miller et al, 1983). Inoculation of *U. urealyticum* into the lung of newborn mice also supports the concept that human ureaplasmas are pathogenic for the neonatal lung (Rudd et al, 1986). In humans, the fetus has now been shown to develop an inflammatory response in the placenta and fetal lung in association with mycoplasmas, and mount an antibody response to *U. urealyticum in utero*. Both are indicative of a response to the presence of an infecting organism.

It is therefore important to study the virulence factors, adherence factors, pathogenic mechanisms of different strains and the influence of host responses to further our understanding of *U. urealyticum* infection in pregnancy and in the neonate.

The time has come to set aside the concept that genital mycoplasmas cannot cause disease because so many people have them. As with many microorganisms, certain strains or serotypes may be more pathogenic than others under certain circumstances. One approach is that there may be differences among the now 16 serotypes of *U. urealyticum* and 7 serotypes of *M. hominis* (Robertson and Stemke, 1982; Lin, 1985). In our studies, 80% of patients in our local population whether fertile or with a history of reproductive failure, carried serotype 3 whereas couples who were infertile for no known reason also had a higher prevalence of serotype 8 (Quinn and Arshoff, 1986). Yet when we examined the serotype specific antibody response in various populations, there was not a significantly elevated mean titre to serotype 3 in normal women, in women with a history of pregnancy loss (Quinn et al, 1983b), or in neonates with respiratory disease, or their mothers (Quinn et al, 1983c).

A difference in pathogenic potential for specific serotypes is suggested in our case of congenital ureaplasma pneumonia (Quinn et al, 1985b). The father of the child carried serotype 8 and the mother serotypes 3 and 8 in her genital tract. The lung isolate was identified as *U. urealyticum* serotype 8. The neonate had an elevated Ig M antibody response to serotype 8 but not to the other serotypes. Serotype 8 was identified in the lung tissue by immunofluorescent staining but the lung was negative for serotype 3 and the other specific serotypes. Penetration studies (Busolo and Zanchetta, 1985a,b), serotypes 4,6 and 8 demonstrated an inhibition of sperm penetration whereas serotype 1 was comparable to the control group. In studies of patient isolates, a predominance of serotype 4 was found in males with non-specific urethritis (Shepard and Lunceford, 1978).

In other studies contrary to our findings, an increased incidence of serotype 3 was found in infertile compared to fertile couples (Lefevre et al, 1986) and no difference was found in patients with spontaneous abortion versus therapeutic abortions, or with and without non-specific urethritis (Robertson et al, 1986). In the experience of Lin (1985), neither the serotypes of *U. urealyticum* nor *M. hominis* appears to be associated with a specific disease entity. At this time serotyping studies have been done by a variety of methods often on selected colonies or subcultures. Since couples carry a mixture of serotypes (Lin, 1985; Quinn and Arshoff, 1986) and the serotypes grow at different rates, the results may not reflect the serotypes actually present in the primary specimen.

In bovines the majority of serotypes isolated from the fetuses are of Group B, and Group A strains are found in other parts of the genital tract. However, the experimental studies in pregnant heifers were done with a Group A strain. This argues against an association between serotypes and specific disease entities.

A model of infection in pregnancy is proposed in Figure 1 to stimulate studies on the pathogenesis of *U. urealyticum* in reproductive failure. Studies have been done with many pathogenic animal mycoplasmas (Cassell, 1982; Levisohn, 1984) and *M. pneumonia* (Gabridge et al, 1985, 1974) which suggest directions for studies of human genital mycoplasmas. There are many aspects of pathogenicity worth investigating such as: adherence factors and receptor sites (Kahane et al,1982; Razin, 1985; Gabridge et al, 1985; Geary and Gabridge, 1987); the lypoglycans and external polysaccharide coat of *U. urealyticum* (Robertson and Smook, 1976; Smith, 1984; 1987); the specific and non-specific stimulation of the immune system (Biberfeld, 1985; Taylor-Robinson and Furr, 1985; Simecka et al, 1987) and the interaction of *U. urealyticum* and *M. hominis* with lymphocytes as reported for other mycoplasma species (Cole et al, 1985; Naot et al, 1977; Makhoul et al, 1987). Other possible virulence factors in ureaplasmas which could be examined include hemolysis (Minion, 1987), hemadsorption (Baseman et al, 1984; 1987) and enzyme activities (Pollack, 1986; Robertson, 1986) including immunoglobulin A1 protease (Kilian et al, 1984; Robertson et al, 1984), and phospholipases (DeSilva and Quinn, 1986) which are considered to be toxins in certain systems.

There is also evidence that in women with recurrent pregnancy loss there is an alteration in their immune system which is reflected in increased levels of autoantibodies(Lafer et al,1981, Branch et al, 1985) or decreased immunological responsiveness (Johnson et al, 1984). We have also observed an increased level of anti-complementary activity in the serum of such women (Quinn and Petric, 1988). These alterations could be idiopathic or could be due to infection. *M. pneumoniae* is known to non-specifically stimulate B cells, and certain patients develop anti-phospholipid and anti-cardiolipin antibodies (Biberfeld, 1985). Since *U. urealyticum* is implicated as a cause of intrauterine infection and 73% of women experiencing late pregnancy loss are colonized, it is

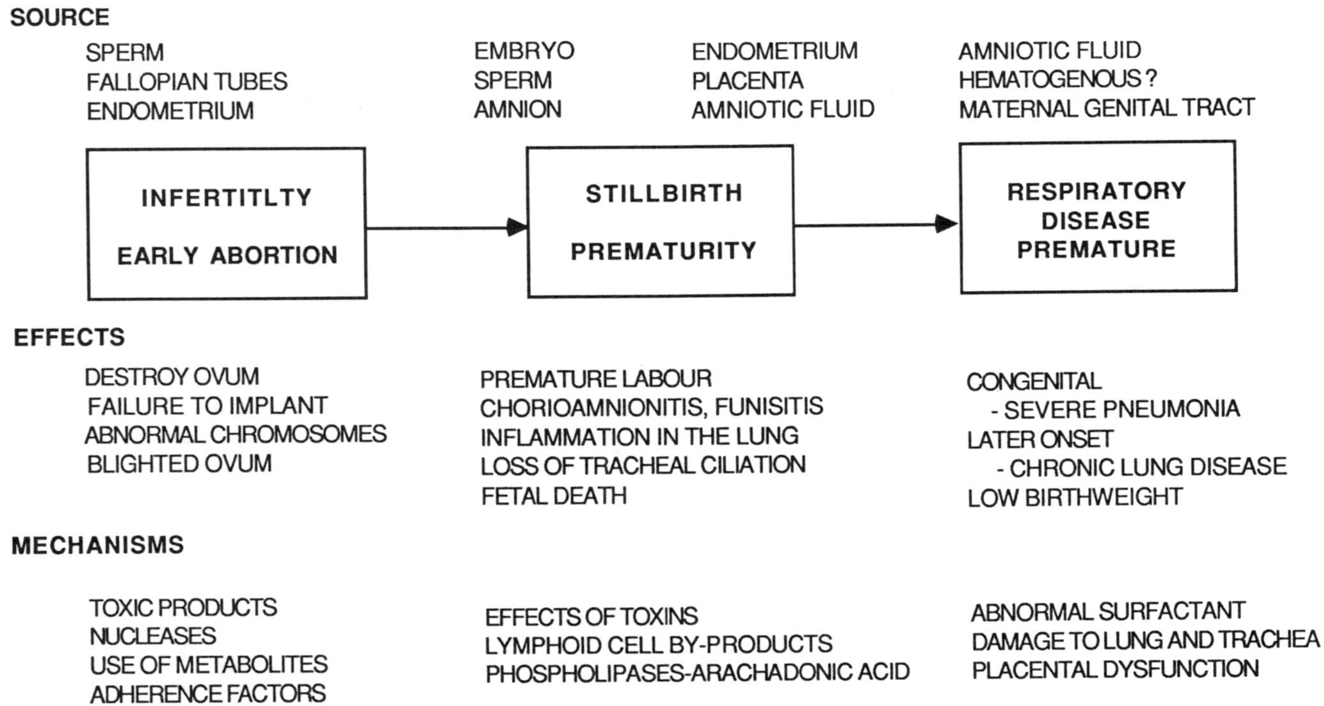

FIGURE 1. MODEL OF INTRAUTERINE INFECTION WITH UREAPLASMA UREALYTICUM

important that studies of immunological causes of pregnancy loss interface with studies of intrauterine infection.

WHY THE CONTROVERSY

The concept that *U. urealyticum* is a cause of intrauterine infection leading to stillbirth and neonatal morbidity and mortality remains controversial for a number of reasons. One prevalent notion is that mycoplasmas are secondary invaders gaining access to the fetus and placenta after death. There is no direct evidence to confirm this concept and inadequate technologies have made it difficult to disprove. However it has been demonstrated that dead tissues and cells are toxic to mycoplasmas and inhibit their growth (Taylor-Robinson and Chen, 1983). In the laboratory, one frequently observes that the first or second ten-fold dilution of tissue, semen and urine specimens are negative for mycoplasmas while higher dilutions turn positive. One explanation is that lysolecithins released from damaged cells are toxic to mycoplasmas which have about 30% lipid in their membranes.

In the investigation of stillbirths and early neonatal deaths, frequently the placenta is not examined. If the main focus of infection is chorioamnionitis, this could easily be missed. A second problem is that the placenta is not appropriately cultured for mycoplasmas, anaerobic bacteria and viruses. A swab submitted for routine bacteriology culture is considered negative for all organisms rather than negative for the bacteria specifically isolated in the culture system used. It is also possible that microorganisms involved in the perinatal death are found only in the placenta thereby being missed in cultures done only on the fetus. If the fetus died from a toxic by-product associated with the presence of organisms in the placenta, the organisms may not need to gain access to the fetus. In cases of prolonged fetal death, the placental tissue may also provide some measure of protection allowing for isolation of significant organisms. It is therefore important that the placenta be properly examined. In our perinatal death studies evidence of chorioamnionitis occurred in 71% of deaths of unknown cause compared to 5% of normal placentas. In addition, mycoplasmas can be isolated from the placenta and fetal lung but not from extensive cultures of the parents post delivery (unpublished observations). Thus culturing the parents after the fact is not of value in such cases.

Another argument which counters the notion that mycoplasmas infect the dead fetus, is that the fetus must be alive to mount both an antibody and inflammatory response to the invading organism (Quinn et al, 1985a; Quinn, 1986). Serological studies have demonstrated not only the presence of antibody in the fetus but levels four fold higher than maternal levels (Quinn et al, 1983c; Quinn, 1986) and of Ig M specificity (Quinn et al, 1985b). On the other hand, genital mycoplasmas might well be a co-factor in causing the death of a fetus already compromised in some unknown way.

Conflicting evidence on the role of mycoplasmas in pregnancy loss comes from studies based on genital tract colonization of the mother. Past studies have indicated that there was no correlation between genital tract colonization and increased risk of bad perinatal outcome (Harrison et al, 1983; Rudd et al, 1986). This observation may be valid but does not lead to the conclusion that there is no association between intrauterine genital mycoplasma infection and poor pregnancy outcome. The studies which do demonstrate an association are based on direct isolation of mycoplasmas from the placenta (Somplinsky et al, 1975; Embree et al, 1980; Kundsin et al, 1984; Quinn et al, 1985a) and fetal-neonatal or rising maternal antibody responses (Lin, 1985; Quinn , 1986). These latter observations are more indicative of infection than mere colonization.

Developments in the field are hindered by the attitude that because so many patients are colonized with genital mycoplasmas, these organisms do not cause disease. This attitude has stymied research into human disease associated with the genital mycoplasmas. There are many situations where high colonization rates exist such as with *E. coli* in the gastrointestinal tract. But diarrhoeal disease is associated with specific strains which produce a virulence factor such as verotoxin. This attitude is reflected in the fact that review articles and book chapters discussing pregnancy loss often fail to mention infectious causes in general and in association with mycoplasmas. References on the role of mycoplasmas are often outdated such that publications in the late 1980's are citing references from the early 1970's with no mention of the recent literature (Gold and Josimovich, 1985). No doubt infection-related issues fall outside the expertise of many of these authors but the current evidence indicates that infectious causes of perinatal death should be recognized.

The quality of research studies on genital mycoplasmas has been lacking in some respects in the past. Part of the reason is that studies relating to human infections are frequently undertaken by physicians in other specialties who are not familiar with the complex nature of mycoplasmas, or do not have access to, or recognize the need for quality methodologies in working with mycoplasmas. Since the role of mycoplasmas is very controversial, it has been difficult to raise research funding. Thus many studies have been done with limited resources and could rarely afford extensive statistical and epidemiological input. As the importance of the role of perinatal mycoplasma gains acceptance, well controlled studies are now being funded which have as a base the preliminary data gained by the pioneers in the field.

Since mycoplasmas are very host specific, acceptance that they cause infection has suffered because animal models were not available to study pathogenicity. Natural models of ureaplasma genital tract infection in sheep and cattle have contributed to our knowledge as experimental models and will continue to do so. Human mycoplasmas have now been shown to infect certain primates (Taylor-Robinson et al, 1985). However, such models are very expensive and the study groups are limited. Studies of organotypic cultures of lung, trachea and fallopian tubes and more recently the neonatal mouse lung model for U. urealyticum hold much promise in the study of virulence factors.

FUTURE DIRECTIONS

The fundamental problem at this time is that we cannot identify women who are at risk or who have intrauterine mycoplasma infection in pregnancy. The infection undoubtedly occurs in some women but many others are colonized with no ill effect. Antibiotic treatments are being evaluated which could be used to treat or prevent this infection. In our perinatal death study, the pregnancy studied was the first pregnancy with a poor outcome or the first pregnancy in 52% of women. These women had no identifiable factors of risk. Among the other 48%, they had a previous loss which could identify them as being at risk. Yet, many of these women would not be classified as at risk if the previous pregnancy resulted in a first trimester abortion or even a premature infant. Thus a very high proportion of the women experiencing perinatal death would not be identified as being at risk.

One promising direction lies with the identification of an elevated or rising antibody response. It has been shown that women who seroconvert in pregnancy have a higher risk of low birthweight infants (Lin, 1985). In our serological studies, 54.7% of the mothers of neonates with respiratory disease and 43% who had a history of prior spontaneous loss had elevated antibody responses to *U. urealyticum* compared to 8.5% of control women (Quinn et al, 1983a). In the perinatal death study 26.3% of mothers had titres ≥1:64 compared to 0% of control mothers. This antibody was detected only in mothers of stillbirths of unknown cause and not in those with a possible cause of death. Since these blood samples were drawn after the neonate was admitted to the Intensive Care Unit or the women had delivered, it is not known when the mothers developed the antibody response. In a few cases we have documented a four-fold rise in maternal titre after delivery of the neonate.

There are a number of explanations. Women may mount the antibody response after the delivery of a currently infected neonate. Secondly, this antibody response may develop during the pregnancy while carrying the infected fetus (Lin, 1985). Thirdly, the antibody may be due to a residual response from previous exposure to *U. urealyticum*, since many of these women had experienced previous poor pregnancy outcomes. Studies are now required to confirm the prevalence of women who mount an antibody response and whether the presence of antibody could be diagnostic in identifying women at risk for silent chronic intrauterine ureaplasma infection. A new approach from the bovine studies which holds promise, is the detection of Ig A antibody in vaginal secretions (Kreplin et al, 1987). Development of rapid serological assays for *U. urealyticum* are essential. Many assays which are rapid and sensitive for M. hominis antibody responses, for example, do not work well for the detection of ureaplasma antibody.

There is also the possibility that certain serotypes of *U. urealyticum* or *M. hominis* have greater potential to cause intrauterine infection than other serotypes. There is evidence both for and against this hypothesis but comprehensive studies with a sensitive serotyping method on primary isolates will be required to evaluate the concept.

Both these approaches have their limitations. Truly innovative studies are needed to determine the nature of virulence factors in genital mycoplasmas. The actual diagnosis of women at risk may rest with a combination of host factors such as immune status plus specific characteristics of virulence among the strains of *U. urealyticum* and *M. hominis*.

Once we have a means of identifying women at risk, epidemiological studies will be required to determine what proportion of women are at risk for spontaneous abortion, stillbirth, prematurity, neonatal mortality and morbidity associated with intrauterine mycoplasma infection. Antibiotic trials can then be evaluated in women at risk who could most benefit from the prevention of intrauterine infection.

ACKNOWLEDGEMENTS

The author acknowledges the collaboration of many colleagues over the years and the significant contribution of A. Nurkkala and A. McArthur in this manuscript.

REFERENCES

Baldetorp BO, Mardh PA, Westrom L (1983). Mucociliary wave activity in organ cultures of human fallopian tubes challenged with Mycoplasma hominis. Sex Transm Dis 10:363.

Ball HJ, McCaughey WJ (1982). Experimental production of vulvitis in ewes with a ureaplasma isolate. Vet Rec 114:271.

Baseman JB, Daly KL, Trevino LB et al (1984). Distinctions among pathogenic human mycoplasmas. Isr J Med Sci 20:866.

Baseman JB, Morrison-Plummer J, Drouillard D et al (1987). Identification of a 32-kilodalton protein of Mycoplasma pneumoniae associated with hemadsorption. Isr J Med Sci 23:474

Bejar R, Curbelo V, Dairs C et al (1981). Premature labour. Bacterial sources of phospholipase. Obstet Gynaecol 57:47.

Biberfeld G (1985). Infection sequelae and autoimmune reactions in Mycoplasma pneumoniae infection. In Razin S, Barile MF (eds): "The Mycoplasmas IV," New York: Academic Press, p 293.

Blanc WA (1980). Infection. In: Ciba Foundation Symposium on Perinatal Infections. Amsterdam: Excerpta Medica 77:17.

Branch DW, Scott JR, Kochenour NK et al (1985). Obstetric complications associated with the lupus anticoagulant. N Engl J Med 313:1322.

Braun P, Lee Y-H, Lein JO et al (1971). Birthweight and genital mycoplasmas in pregnancy. N Engl J Med 284:167.

Britton AP, Ruhnke HL, Miller RB et al (1987). In vitro exposure of bovine morulae to Ureaplasma diversum. Can J Vet Res 51:198.

Brunnell PA, Dische MR, Walker MB (1969). Mycoplasma, amnionitis and respiratory distress syndrome. J Am Med Assoc 207:2097.

Busolo F, Zanchetta R (1985a). Do mycoplasmas inhibit the human sperm fertilizing ability in vitro? Isr J Med Sci 20:902.

Busolo F, Zanchetta R (1985b). The effect of Mycoplasma hominis and Ureaplasma urealyticum on hamster egg in vitro

penetration by human spermatozoa. Fertil Steril 43:110.
Bygdeman SM, Mardh PA (1983). Antimicrobial susceptibility and susceptibility testing of Mycoplasma hominis. (A Review). Sex Trans Dis 10:366.
Caspi E, Herezeg E, Solomon F et al (1971). Amnionitis and T-strain mycoplasmemia. Am J Obstet Gynecol 111:1102.
Caspi E, Solomon L, Langer R et al (1976). Isolation of mycoplasma from the placenta after cesarean section. Obstet Gynecol 48:682.
Caspi E, Solomon F, Somplinsky D (1972). Early abortion and mycoplasma infection. Isr J Med Sci 8:122.
Cassell GH (1982). Pathogenic potential of mycoplasmas: Mycoplasma pulmonis as a model. Rev Infect Dis 4:S18.
Cassell GH, Clyde WA, Davis JK (1985). Mycoplasmal respiratory infections. In Razin S, Barile MF (eds): "The Mycoplasmas IV," New York: Academic Press, p 65.
Cassell GH, Davis RO, Waites KB et al (1983a). Isolation of Mycoplasma hominis and Ureaplasma urealyticum from amniotic fluid at 16-20 weeks gestation: potential effect on outcome of pregnancy. Sex Transm Dis 10:294.
Cassell GH, Lamey JR, Foy HM et al (1974). Infection with Mycoplasma hominis and T-strain in the female genital tract. Obstet Gynecol 44:703.
Cassell GH, Waites KB, Gibbs RS et al (1986). Role of Ureaplasma urealyticum in amnionitis. Pediatr Infect Dis 5:S247.
Cassell GH, Waites KB, Rudd PT et al (1987). Ureaplasma urealyticum is associated with development of chronic lung disease in preterm infants. 27th Interscience Conference on Antimicrobial Agents and Chemotherapy. October 4-7, New York. Abstract No. 533.
Cassell GH, Younger JB, Blackwell RE et al (1983b). Microbiologic study of infertile women at the time of diagnostic laparoscopy: association of Ureaplasma urealyticum with a defined subpopulation. N Engl J Med 308:502.
Christensen KK, Hagerstrand I, Mardh PA (1982). Late spontaneous abortion associated with Mycoplasma hominis infection of the fetus. Scand J Infect Dis 14:73.
Cole BC, Naot Y, Stanbridge EJ et al (1985). Interactions of mycoplasmas and their products with lymphoid cells in vitro. In Razin S, Barile MF (eds): "The Mycoplasmas IV," New York: Academic Press, p 203.
Collier AM (1979). Mycoplasmas in organ culture. In Tully JG, Whitcomb RF (eds): "The Mycoplasmas II," New York: Academic Press, p 475.

Comhaire FH, Rowe PJ, Farley TMN (1986). The effect of doxycycline in infertile couples with male accessory gland infection: a double blind prospective study. Int J Androl 9:91.

Dennis EA (1983). Phospholipases. In Boyer PD (ed): "Enzymes: XVI," New York: Academic Press, p 307.

DeSilva N, Quinn PA (1986). Endogenous activity of phospholipases A and C in Ureaplasma urealyticum. J Clin Microbiol 23:354.

Dische MR, Quinn PA, Czegledy-Nagy N et al (1979). Genital mycoplasma infection. Intrauterine infection: pathologic study of the fetus and placenta. Am J Clin Pathol 72:167.

Doig PA, Ruhnke HL (1977). Isolation of ureaplasmas from sheep with granular vulvitis. Vet Rec 100:179-80.

Doig PA, Ruhnke HL (1984). Effects of ureaplasma infection on bovine reproduction. Current Therapy in Theriogenology II. p 282.

Doig PA, Ruhnke HL, Mackay AL, Palmer NC (1979). Bovine granular vulvitis associated with ureaplasma infection. Can Vet J 20:89-94.

Doig PA, Ruhnke HL, Mackay AL, Palmer NC (1980a). Experimental bovine genital ureaplasmosis I. Granular vulvitis following vulvar inoculation. Can J Comp Med 44:252.

Doig PA, Ruhnke, HL, Palmer NC (1980b). Experimental bovine genital ureaplasmosis II. Granular vulvitis, endometritis and salpingitis following uterine inoculation. Can J Comp Med 44:259.

Doig PA, Ruhnke HL, Waelchli-Suter R et al (1981). The role of ureaplasma infection in bovine reproductive disease. In: Compendium on Continuing Education for the Practicing Veterinarian. Princeton: Veterinary Learning Systems, 3:S324.

Driscoll SG, Kundsin RB, Horne HW et al (1969). Infections and first trimester losses: possible role of mycoplasmas. Fertil Steril 20:1017.

Elder HA, Santamarina BAG, Smith S et al (1971). The natural history of asymptomatic bacteriuria during pregnancy: the effect of tetracycline on the clinical course and the outcome of pregnancy. Am J Obstet Gynecol 111:441.

Embree JE, Krause VW, Embil JA et al (1980). Placental infection with Mycoplasma hominis and Ureaplasma urealyticum: clinical correlation. Obstet Gynecol 56:475.

Embree JE, Krause VW, Embil JA (1983). Mycoplasma hominis: a placental pathogen? Sex Transm Dis 10:307.

Fong IW, Linton W, Simbul M et al (1987). Treatment of nongonococcal urethritis with ciprofloxacin. Am J Med 82:311.
Fowlkes DM, Dooher GB, O'Leary WM (1975a). Evidence by scanning electron microscopy for an association between spermatozoa and T-mycoplasmas in men of infertile marriage. Fertil Steril 26:1203.
Fowlkes DM, MacLeod J, O'Leary WM (1975b). T-mycoplasmas and human infertility: correlation of infection with alterations in seminal parameters. Fertil Steril 26:1212.
Fraser LR, Taylor-Robinson D (1977). The effect of Mycoplasma pulmonis on fertilization and preimplantation development in vitro of mouse eggs. Fertil Steril 28:488.
Gabridge MG, Chandler KF, Daniels MJ (1985). Pathogenicity factors in mycoplasmas and spiroplasmas. In Razin S, Barile MF (eds): "The Mycoplasmas IV," New York: Academic Press, p 313.
Gabridge MG, Johnson CK, Cameron AM (1974). Cytotoxicity of Mycoplasma pneumoniae membranes. Infect Immun 10:112.
Geary SJ, Gabridge MG (1987). Characterization of a human lung fibroblast receptor site for Mycoplasma pneumoniae. Isr J Med Sci 23:462.
Gibbs RS, Blanco JD, St. Clair PJ et al (1983). Mycoplasma hominis and intrauterine infection in late pregnancy. Sex Transm Dis 10:303.
Gibbs RS, Cassell G, Davis J et al (1986). Further studies on genital mycoplasmas in intra-amniotic infection: blood cultures and serologic response. Am J Obstet Gynecol 154:717.
Gold JJ, Josimovich JB (1985). "Gynecologic Endocrinology." Hagerstown: Harper and Row.
Goulet C, Ritchie KW, Quinn PA et al (1987). A case-control study to assess the role of infection in preterm premature rupture of membranes. 27th Interscience Conference of Antimicrobial Agents and Chemotherapy. October 4-7, New York. Abstract No. 37.
Gravett MG, Eschenbach DA (1986). Possible role of Ureaplasma urealyticum in preterm premature rupture of the fetal membranes. Pediatr Infect Dis 5:S253.
Gump DW, Gibson MG, Ashicaga T (1984). Lack of association between genital mycoplasmas and infertility. N Engl J Med 310:937.
Hameed C, Tejani N, Verma UL, Archbald F (1984). Silent chorioamnionitis as a cause of preterm labor refractory to tocolytic therapy. Am J Obstet Gynecol 149:726.

Harrison RH, Boyce WT, Haffner WHJ et al (1983). The prevalence of genital Chlamydia trachomatis and mycoplasmal infections during pregnancy in an American Indian population. Sex Transm Dis 10:184.

Harwick HJ, Luppa JB, Purcell RH et al (1967). Mycoplasma hominis septicemia associated with abortion. Am J Obstet Gynecol 99:725.

Hillier SL, Krohn MJ, Kiviat N et al (1986). The association of Ureaplasma urealyticum with preterm birth, chorioamnionitis, postpartum fever, intrapartum fever and bacterial vaginosis. Pediatr Infect Dis 5:S348.

Hinton RA, Egdell LM, Andrews BE et al (1979). A double-blind cross-over study of the effect of doxycycline on mycoplasma infection and infertility. Br J Obstet Gynaecol 86:37.

Horne HW, Hertig AT, Kundsin RB et al (1973). Subclinical endometrial inflammation and T-mycoplasma: a possible cause of human reproductive failure. Int J Fertil 18:226.

Howard CJ (1984). Animal ureaplasmas: their ecological niche and role in disease. Isr J Med Sci 20:954.

Johnson PM, Barnes RMR, Hart CA et al (1984). Determinants of immunological responsiveness in recurrent spontaneous abortion. Transplantation 38:280.

Jones DM (1967). Mycoplasma hominis in abortion. Brit Med J 1:338.

Jones DM, Tobin B (1968). Neonatal eye infection due to Mycoplasma hominis. Brit Med J 2:467.

Jurmanova K, Sterbova J (1977). Correlation between impaired spermatozoan motility and mycoplasma findings in bull semen. Vet Rec 100:157.

Kahane I, Banai M, Razin S et al (1982). Attachment of mycoplasmas to host cell membranes. Rev Infect Dis 4:S185.

Kass EH, Lin J-S, McCormack WM (1986). Low birth weight and maternal colonization with genital mycoplasmas. Pediatr Infect Dis 5:S279.

Kass EH, McCormack WM, Lin J-S et al (1981). Genital mycoplasmas as a cause of excess premature delivery. Trans Assoc Am Physicians 94:26.

Kaufman M, Goldberg R, Quinn PA (1985). Genital mycoplasma in adolescence. Proceed 54th Ann Mtg Royal College of Physicians and Surgeons and Canadian Paediatric Society. September 9-11, Vancouver.

Kilian M, Brown MB, Brown TA et al (1984). Immunoglobulin Al protease activity in strains of Ureaplasma urealyticum. Acta Pathol Microbiol Scand Sect B 92:61.

Kimpen J, Bosmans E, Janssen J et al (1986). Screening for

Ureaplasma urealyticum infections in the neonate and the association with prematurity. Eur J Obstet Gynecol Reprod Biol 22:53.
Koutsky LA, Stamm WE, Brunham RC et al (1983). Persistence of Mycoplasma hominis after therapy: importance of tetracycline resistance and of coexisting vaginal flora. Sex Transm Dis 10:374.
Kreplin CMA, Ruhnke HL, Miller RB et al (1987). The effect of intrauterine inoculation with Ureaplasma diversum on bovine fertility. Can J Vet Res 51:440.
Kundsin RB, Ampola M, Streeter X, Neurath P (1971). Chromosomal aberrations induced by T-strain mycoplasmas. J Med Gen 8:181.
Kundsin RB, Driscoll SG, Ming P-ML (1967). Strain of mycoplasma associated with human reproductive failure. Science 157:1573.
Kundsin RB, Driscoll SG, Monson RR et al (1984). Association of Ureaplasma urealyticum in the placenta with perinatal morbidity and mortality. N Engl J Med 310:94.
Lafer EM, Rauch J, Andrezejewski C et al (1981). Polyspecific monoclonal lupus autoantibodies reactive with both polynucleotides and phospholipids. J Exp Med 153:897.
Lamey JR, Foy HM, Kenny GE (1974). Infection with Mycoplasma hominis and T-strains in the female genital tract. Obstet Gynecol 44:703.
Leader A, Mortimer D, Bryan LE et al (1987). Influence of Ureaplasma urealyticum infection on semen characteristics of suspected infertile men. 43rd Ann Mtg Society of Obstetricians and Gynaecologists of Canada. June 24-27. Abstract No. 3.
Lefevre J, Granger L, St. Michel P et al (1986). Serotype distribution of Ureaplasma urealyticum in infertile and pregnant women. Pediatr Infect Dis 5:S348.
Levisohn S (1984). Early stages in the interaction between Mycoplasma gallisepticum and the chick trachea, as related to pathogenicity and immunogenicity. Isr J Med Sci 20:982.
Lin J-SL (1985). Human mycoplasmal infections: serologic observations. Rev Infect Dis 7:216.
Lindsey JR, Cassell GH (1973). Experimental Mycoplasma pulmonis infection in pathogen-free mice. Models for studying mycoplasmosis of the respiratory tract. Am J Pathol 72:63.
Makhoul N, Merchav S, Tatarsky I et al (1987). Mycoplasma-induced in vitro production of interleukin-2 and colony stimulating activity. Isr J Med Sci 23:480.
Mardh PA (1983). Mycoplasma hominis infection of the

central nervous system in newborn infants. Sex Transm Dis 10:331.

McCormack WM, George H, Donner A et al (1977). Hepatotoxicity of erythromycin estolate during pregnancy. Antimicrob Agents Chemother 12:630.

Miller RB, Ruhnke HL, Doig BF et al (1983). The effects of Ureaplasma diversum inoculated into the amniotic cavity in cows. Theriogenology 20:367.

Minion CF (1987). Correlation of Mycoplasma pulmonis-mediated hemolysis with translocation of a fluorescent cholesterol probe. Isr J Med Sci 23:458.

Moller BR (1983). The role of mycoplasmas in the upper genital tract of women. Sex Transm Dis 10:281.

Morrison I (1985). Perinatal mortality: basic considerations. Seminars in Perinatol 9:144.

Mueller RF, Sybert VP, Johnson J et al (1983). Evaluation of a protocol for post-mortem examination of stillbirths. N Engl J Med 309:585.

Mufson MA (1983). Mycoplasma hominis: a review of its role as a respiratory tract pathogen of humans. Sex Transm Dis 10:335.

Myhre EB, Mardh PA (1983). Treatment of extragenital infections caused by Mycoplasma hominis. Sex Transm Dis 10:382.

Naessens A, Foulon W, Debrucker P et al (1986). Recovery of microorganisms in semen and relationship to semen evaluation. Fertil Steril 45:101.

Naeye RL (1983). The investigation of perinatal deaths. N Engl J Med 309:611.

Naeye RL, Maisel MJ, Lorenz RP et al (1983). The clinical significance of placental villous edema. Pediatrics 71:588.

Naeye RL, Tafari N, Judge D et al (1977). Amniotic fluid infections in an African city. J Pediatr 90:965.

Naot Y, Tully JG, Ginsburg H (1977). Lymphocyte activation by various mycoplasma strains and species. Infect Immun 8:310.

Ontario. Registrar General (1983). Vital statistics for 1981. Toronto: Government of Ontario, p 52.

Ornoy A, Solomon-Arnon J, Ben-Zui Z et al (1981). Placental findings in spontaneous abortions and stillbirths. Teratology 24:243.

Paavonen J, Critchlow CW, DeRouen T et al (1986). Ureaplasma urealyticum associated with mucopurulent cervicitis. Pediatr Infect Dis 5:S354.

Pankuch GA, Applebaum PC, Lorenz RP, et al (1984).

Placental microbiology and histology and the pathogenesis of chorioamnionitis. Obstet Gynecol 64:802.
Piot P (1976). Distribution of eight serotypes of Ureaplasma urealyticum in cases of non-gonococcal urethritis and gonorrhea and in healthy persons. Br J Vener Dis 52:266.
Pollack JD (1986). Metabolic distinctiveness of ureaplasmas. Pediatr Infect Dis 5:S305.
Porter IH, Hook EB (1980). Terminological Conventions, Methodological Considerations, Temporal Trends, Specific Genes, Environmental Hazards and some other Factors Pertaining to Embryonic and Fetal Death. New York: Academic Press, p 1-17.
Quinn PA (1986). Evidence of an immune response to Ureaplasma urealyticum in perinatal morbidity and mortality. Pediatr Infect Dis 5:S282.
Quinn PA, Arshoff LU (1986). Serotypes of Ureaplasma urealyticum found in fertile and infertile couples. Pediatr Infect Dis 5:S352.
Quinn PA, Butany J, Chipman M et al (1985a). A prospective study of microbial infection in stillbirths and early neonatal death. Am J Obstet Gynecol 151:238.
Quinn PA, Butany J, Taylor J et al (1987a). Chorioamnionitis: its association with pregnancy outcome and microbial infection. Am J Obstet Gynecol 156:379.
Quinn PA, Czegledy-Nagy E, Dische MR et al (1979). Mycoplasma infection in human fetal trachea. Proceed 79th Meeting, American Society for Microbiology p 86.
Quinn PA, Gillan J, Markestad T et al (1985b). Intrauterine infection with Ureaplasma urealyticum as a cause of fatal neonatal pneumonia. Pediatr Infect Dis 4:538.
Quinn PA, Gysler M, Chipman ML et al (1987c). Incidence of late loss and Ureaplasma urealyticum in women with recurrent pregnancy loss. 27th Interscience Conference on Antimicrobial Agents and Chemotherapy. October 4-7, New York. Abstract No. 431.
Quinn PA, Petric M (1988). Anticomplementary activity in serum of women with a history of recurrent pregnancy loss. Am J Obstet Gynecol 158:368.
Quinn PA, Petric M, Barkin M et al (1987b). Prevalence of antibody to Chlamydia trachomatis in spontaneous abortion and infertility. Am J Obstet Gynecol 156:291.
Quinn PA, Rubin S, Nocilla DM et al (1983c). Serological evidence of Ureaplasma urealyticum infection in neonatal respiratory disease. Yale J Biol Med 56:565.
Quinn PA, Rudd NL (1974). T-strain mycoplasma infection in

amniotic fluid cell cultures. Can J Public Health 65:61.
Quinn PA, Shewchuck AB, Lie K et al (1982). The efficacy of doxycycline in the eradication of mycoplasmas from the urogenital tract in couples with reproductive failure. Proceed. 58th Annual Meeting of Society of Obstetricians and Gynaecologists of Canada. June 15-19, Toronto.
Quinn PA, Shewchuck AB, Shuber J et al (1981). Recurrence of genital mycoplasma infection in pregnancy. Proceed 49th Conjoint Meeting on Infectious Diseases. November 25-27, Ottawa. p 5.
Quinn PA, Shewchuck AB, Shuber J et al (1983a). Efficacy of antibiotic therapy in preventing spontaneous pregnancy loss among couples colonized with genital mycoplasmas. Am J Obstet Gynecol 145:239.
Quinn PA, Shewchuck AB, Shuber J et al (1983b). Serological evidence of Ureaplasma urealyticum infection in women with spontaneous pregnancy loss. Am J Obstet Gynecol 145:245-52.
Razin S (1985). Mycoplasma adherence. In Razin S, Barile MF (eds): "The Mycoplasmas IV," New York: Academic Press, p 161.
Roberts MC, Koutsky LA, Holmes KK et al (1985). Tetracycline resistant Mycoplasma hominis strains contain streptococcal tetM sequences. Antimicrob Agents Chemother 28:141.
Robertson JA (1986). Potential virulence factors of Ureaplasma urealyticum. Pediatr Infect Dis 5:S322.
Robertson JA, Coppola JE, Heisler OR (1981). Standardized method for determining antimicrobial susceptibility of strains of Ureaplasma urealyticum and their response to tetracycline, erythromycin and rosaramicin. Antimicrob Agents Chemother 20:53.
Robertson JA, Honore LH, Stemke GW (1986). Serotypes of Ureaplasma urealyticum in spontaneous abortion. Pediatr Infect Dis 5:S270.
Robertson JA, Smook E (1976). Cytochemical evidence of extramembranous carbohydrates on Ureaplasma urealyticum (T-strain mycoplasmas). J Bacteriol 128:658.
Robertson JA, Stemke GW (1982). Expanded serotyping scheme for Ureaplasma urealyticum strains isolated from humans. J Clin Microbiol 15:873.
Robertson JA, Stemler ME, Stemke GW (1984). Immunoglobulin A protease activity of Ureaplasma urealyticum. J Clin Microbiol 19:255.
Romano N, Romano F, Carollo P (1971). T-strain of mycoplasma in bronchopneumonic lungs of an aborted fetus. N Engl J Med 285:950.

Rudd PT, Brown MB, Cassell GH (1984). A prospective study of mycoplasma infection in the preterm infant. Isr J Med Sci 20:899.
Rudd NL, Quinn PA (1973). Potential causative agent in amniotic fluid culture mosaicism. Mammalian Chromosome Newsletter 14:76.
Rudd PT, Waites KB, Duffy LB et al (1986). Ureaplasma urealyticum and its possible role in pneumonia during the neonatal period and infancy. Pediatr Infect Dis 5S288.
Ruhnke HL, Doig PA, MacKay AL et al (1977). Isolation of ureaplasma from bovine granular vulvitis. Can J Comp Med 42:151.
Ruhnke HL, Palmer NC, Doig PA et al (1984). Bovine abortion and neonatal death associated with Ureaplasma diversum. Theriogenology 21:367.
Sacker T, Walker M, Brunell PA (1970). Abscess in a newborn infant caused by mycoplasmas. Pediatrics 46:303.
Shepard MC, Lunceford CD (1978). Serological typing of Ureaplasma urealyticum isolates from urethritis patients by an agar growth inhibition method. J Clin Microbiol 8:566.
Shurin PA, Alpert S, Rosner B et al (1975). Chorioamnionitis and colonization of the newborn infant with genital mycoplasma. N Engl J Med 293:5.
Simecka JW, Davis JK, Cassell GH (1987). Specific vs nonspecific immune responses in murine respiratory mycoplasmosis. Isr J Med Sci 23:485.
Smith PF (1971). "Biology of Mycoplasmas." New York: Academic Press, p 114.
Smith PF (1984). Lipoglycans in mycoplasmas. CRC Crit Rev Microbiol 11:157.
Smith PF (1987). Antigenic character of membrane lipoglycans from Mollicutes - a review. Isr J Med Sci 23:448.
Somplinsky D, Solomon D, Elkina L et al (1975). Infections with mycoplasma and bacteria in induced mid-trimester abortion and fetal loss. Am J Obstet Gynecol 121:610.
Spaepen MS, Kundsin RB (1977). Simple direct broth disc method for antibiotic susceptibility testing of Ureaplasma urealyticum. Antimicrob Agents Chemother 11:267.
Stagno S, Brasfield DM, Brown MB et al (1981). Infant pneumonitis associated with cytomegalovirus, chlamydia, pneumocystis, and ureaplasma: a prospective study. Pediatrics 68:322.
Stalheim OHV, Proctor SJ, Gallagher JE (1976). Growth and effects of ureaplasmas (T-mycoplasmas) in bovine oviductal

organ cultures. Infect Immun 13:915.
Stray-Pedersen B, Eng J, Reikvan TM (1978). Uterine T-mycoplasma colonization in reproductive failure. Am J Obstet Gynecol 130:301.
Strobino BR, Kline J, Shrout P et al (1980). Recurrent spontaneous abortion: definition of a syndrome. In Porter IH, Hook EB (eds): "Human Embryonic and Fetal Death," New York: Academic Press, p 315.
Svensson L, Ingemarsson I, Mardh PA (1986). Chorioamnionitis and the isolation of microorganisms from the placenta. Obstet Gynecol 67:403.
Swenson CE (1982). Effect of Mycoplasma pulmonis on in vivo fertilization in the mouse. J Reprod Fertil 65:257.
Swenson CE, Toth A, O'Leary (1979). Ureaplasma urealyticum and human infertility; the effect of antibiotic therapy on semen quality. Fertil Steril 31:660.
Tafari N, Ross S, Naeye RL et al (1976). Mycoplasma T-strains and perinatal death. Lancet 1:108.
Taylor-Robinson D (1986). Evaluation of the role of Ureaplasma urealyticum in infertility. Pediatr Infect Dis 5:S262.
Taylor-Robinson D, Chen TA (1983). Growth inhibitory factors in animal and plant tissues. In Razin S, Tully JG (eds): "Methods in Mycoplasmology I," New York: Academic Press, p 109.
Taylor-Robinson D, Furr PM (1985). The interplay of host and organism factors in infection of the mouse genital tract by Mycoplasma pulmonis. J Hyg (Lond) 95:7.
Taylor-Robinson D, Furr PM (1986). Clinical antibiotic resistance of Ureaplasma urealyticum. Pediatr Infect Dis 5:S335.
Taylor-Robinson D, Furr PM, Liberman MM (1984). The occurrence of genital mycoplasmas in babies with and without respiratory distress. Acta Pediatr Scand 73:383.
Taylor-Robinson D, McCormack W (1979). Mycoplasmas in human genitourinary infections. In Tully JG, Whitcomb RF (eds): New York: Academic Press, p 30.
Taylor-Robinson D, Tully JG, Barile MF (1985). Urethral infection in male chimpanzees produced experimentally by Mycoplasma genitalium. Br J Exp Pathol 66:95.
Unsworth PF, Taylor-Robinson D, Shoo EE et al (1985). Neonatal mycoplasmaemia: Mycoplasma hominis as significant cause of disease? J Infect 10:163.
Waites KB, Crouse DT, Philips JB et al (1988b). Persistent pulmonary hypertension in neonates with ureaplasmal pneumonia. Pediatrics (In Press).

Waites KB, Rudd PT, Crouse DT et al (1988a). Chronic Ureaplasma urealyticum and Mycoplasma hominis infections of central nervous system in preterm infants. Lancet 1:17.

Wang E, Frayha H, Wilson J et al (1987). Genital mycoplasmas, Chlamydia trachomatis and viruses, and chronic lung disease of prematurity. 27th Interscience Conference on Antimicrobial Agents and Chemotherapy. October 4-7, New York. Abstract No. 532.

DISCUSSION

DR. NAEYE: Do the various mycoplasmas destroy surfactant?

DR. QUINN: Based on our research, I have put forward the hypothesis that ureaplasmas are associated with neonatal respiratory disease. One of the target organs in an infected pregnancy is the fetal lung in both human and bovine infections. Ureaplasmas are isolated from the lung and placenta but not from other organs, and an inflammatory response is seen in the lung. Neonatal respiratory disease is associated with abnormal surfactant function. In the immature lung, lack of development is a major confounding factor. But in more mature gestations, I ask why is the surfactant abnormal, particularly in term neonates?

My hypothesis is that ureaplasmas either directly alter surfactant composition and therefore function, or they indirectly affect the biosynthetic system by affecting the alveolar type II cells which produce surfactant. This hypothesis is supported by the fact that we have demonstrated the presence of phospholipases in human ureaplasmas. The specific activity of phospholipase A_2 is 100 fold higher than phospholipase A_1 or C. Phospholipase A_2 activity in some serotypes is 10 times higher than phospholipase A reported in bacterial pathogens of neonates. Since ureaplasmas have no cell wall and the phospholipase activity is associated with the membrane, these enzymes may play a role in the development of surfactant dysfunction.

DR. NAEYE: Almost every newborn infant with the respiratory distress syndrome received 2 or more antibiotics. Are these antibiotics usually ineffective against mycoplasma?

DR. QUINN: Ampicillin and gentamicin are used extensively in treating "infected" neonates. However these antibiotics are not particularly effective against ureaplasmas or mycoplasmas. Antibiotics which warrant consideration for the treatment of neonatal respiratory disease include erythromycin and chloramphenicol for ureaplasmas and clindamycin for M. hominis positive cases. We have had some success in treating neonates with chronic lung disease. The use of antibiotics is of lesser value in treating neonates with severe congenital ureaplasma pneumonia.

DR. LAMMER: You showed a slide which seemed to indicate that there was no difference in the percentage of mycoplasmas present in cervical cultures from women who previously had normal outcomes and those with aborted fetuses. And, yet, one of your recommendations for screening was that it might be worthwhile to screen women who have had a previous stillbirth. I would assume that the screening would be done by culturing the cervices of these women. It is unclear how these culture results could be interpreted.

DR. QUINN: From our perspective, pregnancy loss is associated with intrauterine ureaplasma infection. Unfortunately, we cannot culture specimens from the pregnancy. We, therefore, culture the lower genital tracts of the couple. However, we are mindful that 50-80% of women with normal pregnancies carry these organisms. In our new studies, 45% of women with normal pregnancies are colonized, as are 48% of women with a history of pregnancy loss under 20 weeks and 73% of women with a history of pregnancy loss after 20 weeks.

For this reason we looked for a second factor which would subset the ureaplasma positive population into those more at risk. We chose the following: a history of 2 or more pregnancy losses or 1 stillbirth known to be positive for genital mycoplasma. The best means of identifying such women at this time is to carry out proper mycoplasma cultures on the placenta, fetal lung and liver of all stillbirths, and the lung in neonatal deaths.

At this time we do not have the technology to identify women at risk of intrauterine ureaplasma infection in a given pregnancy. The development of such techniques is an important direction for future research. Concepts being proposed are that some of the 14 ureaplasma serotypes may be more pathogenic than others or have a propensity to infect the placenta and fetus. Another is that women who actually are infected would develop a significant immune response to ureaplasma which would not be present in women who are only surface colonized.

DR. V. ANDERSON: I think it might be important to know the duration from the time of intrauterine demise and the actual delivery of the baby, as well as the time span between ruptured membranes and parturition. Is there any possibility that mycoplasma may be an opportunistic infection that could have occurred after the demise of the fetus?

DR. QUINN: I am cognizant of that concept. I think there are two factors that argue against it. First, there is the presence of the inflammatory response. The fetus has to be alive to develop an inflammatory response, particularly in its lung. Second, it would have to be living to mount an antibody response. These facts argue against the idea that the infection is initiated after the fetus has died. In addition, we isolate mycoplasmas from the placenta and lung. Dead tissues are toxic to mycoplasmas so it is unlikely the organisms would grow in dead tissues. In some placentas, ureaplasma concentrations are as high as 10^7 to 10^9 colour changing units/gm of tissues.

DR. V. ANDERSON: IgM antibody?

DR. QUINN: In the few cases that we have been able to examine, we have fractionated the serum and run the assays on each fraction. We have been able to demonstrate the presence of IgM specific antibody in the neonates. We also find titers in the fetuses and neonates which are 4 fold greater than those in the serum of the mothers.

Transplacental Effects on Fetal Health, pages 153–164

SARCOCYSTIS INDUCED ABORTION AND FETAL DEATH

R. Fayer and J.P. Dubey

Animal Parasitology Institute
Agricultural Research Service
U.S. Department of Agriculture
Beltsville, Maryland 20705

INTRODUCTION

Protozoan parasites of the genus *Sarcocystis* share similar life cycle patterns and morphological features with their better known relatives, the organisms that cause malaria and toxoplasmosis. Infectious units (oocysts) of *Sarcocystis* species are distributed throughout the environment when a carnivorous definitive host disperses the egg-like stage in its feces. Spread mechanically by people, animals, tools, wind and water, oocysts contaminate vegetation and water supplies. When ingested by a susceptible intermediate host, motile banana-shaped sporozoites leave the oocyst, penetrate the intestinal wall and eventually enter endothelial cells lining small arteries or arterioles. Here each sporozoite undergoes nuclear multiplication to produce a cluster of merozoites which, like the sporozoites before them, enter endothelial cells lining blood vessels (usually capillaries) throughout the body and produce a cluster of second generation merozoites. The clusters are called schizonts. At the time or shortly after second generation merozoites leave the schizont, acute sarcocystosis can develop in those hosts harboring sufficient numbers of a pathogenic *Sarcocystis*. Acute sarcocystosis may be concurrent with abortion in pregnant hosts, or inapparent infection may lead to premature parturition or fetal death. Those events and possible mechanisms will be reviewed.

GENERAL CLINICOPAHTIC FINDINGS

In general, the most prominent signs of acute sarcocystosis include fever, anemia, clotting disorder, anorexia, weight loss, weakness, prostration or even death (for review see Fayer, Dubey 1986). Lactating animals may decrease or cease milk production. Pregnant animals may prematurely terminate gestation. In the laboratory, erythrocyte and hemoglobin values may be greatly depressed during the period of anemic crisis. Hemolysis, hemorrhage and removal of circulating erthyrocytes in the spleen all account for the 50 to 70% loss of erythrocytes. At this time, serum bilirubin, BUN, CPK, LDH, AAT and SBDH levels are elevated. Prothrombin time is much longer than normal but other parameters of clotting remain normal except for platelet dysfunction and Factor VII deficiency in some individuals. Histological examination shows hemorrhage and inflammation characterized by moderate to severe mononuclear cell infiltration in the perivascular and interstitial tissues of many organs with some accompanying areas of parenchymal necrosis. The most commmonly observed inflammatory cells are lymphocytes and macrophages.

PREMATURE PARTURITION

Abortion and fetal death have resulted when animals became infected with pathogenic species of Sarcocystis during pregnancy. Most cattle, sheep, goats, roe deer, and pigs that developed clinical signs of sarcocystosis from experimental infections induced mid to late in gestation underwent abortion (Barnett et al 1977; Dubey 1981; Erber et al 1978 a,b; Fayer et al 1976; Leek, Fayer 1978; Proctor et al 1976; Stalheim et al 1976; Vickers, Brooks 1983) whereas infected animals that did not have signs of infection usually carried their fetus to term (Dubey 1981; Munday 1981). Lesions were not found in any fetal tissues examined from any of these experimentally infected host species with the exception of one lamb. Parasites (only 2) were found in only 2 (Barnett et al 1977) of 18 bovine fetuses and only 4 schizonts were found in fetal membranes of 3 sheep (Leek, Fayer 1978). In contrast, both parasites and lesions were found in the maternal placentome of cattle, sheep, and goats (Barnett et al 1977; Dubey 1981; Leek, Fayer 1978). One might conclude from these experimentally infected animals that although Sarcocystis is present in the maternal placenta, it rarely crosses the fetal placenta to infect the fetus or fetal membranes. Unlike experimentally infected animals, those cattle with naturally acquired infections have had either parasites or lesions or both observed in fetuses by numerous investigators (Dubey, Bergeron 1982; Hong et al 1982; Jerrett et al 1984; Jolley et al 1983; Kunde et al 1980; McCausland et al 1984; Munday, Black 1976; Schmitz, Wolf 1977). And unlike experimentally infected cattle, parasites as well as lesions were found in the placenta from several natural infections (Corner et al 1963; Dubey, Bergeron 1982; Munday, Black 1976). Furthermore, some naturally infected cows showed no clinical signs of infection although organisms were detected in the fetus or placenta (Dubey, Bergeron 1982). Confirmation that the natural infections and the experimental infections were due to the same species is not possible although parasites were morphologically similar, were located in the same type of host cells, and in some cases responded serologically to the same antigen. Thus, some question remains as to whether differences observed between experimentally infected animals and naturally infected animals may be due to different species or strains of the parasite.

FETAL INFECTION AND LESIONS

Parasites in naturally infected bovine fetuses were found in virtually all organs examined but were most often described from the brain. Immature and mature schizonts as well as free merozoites were found, usually within endothelial cells of capillaries but occasionally free in the lumen of a vessel or in neural tissue (Hong et al 1982; Jerrett et al 1984; Jolley et al 1983; Kunde et al 1980; McCausland et al 1984; Munday, Black 1976).. A composite description of the lesions in the brain would include nonsuppurative encephalitis or meningitis with small foci, composed of glial cells surrounding a central necrotic area, throughout the gray and white matter of the cerebrum, cerebellum or brainstem with some perivascular mononuclear cell infiltration and occasional microthrombi in vessels. Other affected organs appear similar to those of infected postnatal animals with nonsuppurative myocarditis, pneumonitis, hepatitis, and glomerulitis accompanied by focal necrosis and hemorrhage.

Apart from one premature lamb born to an experimentally infected ewe, no significant lesions or organisms were found in any experimentally infected sheep (Munday 1981). That lamb had cerebral congestion and edema as well as areas of leucoencephalomalacia in the cerebrum and midbrain. Another lamb, from a naturally infected ewe, was found with encephalitis characterized by mononuclear cell infiltration and gliosis (Dubey, Towle 1986).

PLACENTAL INFECTION AND LESIONS

Free merozoites and schizonts, often associated with lesions, have been observed in maternal or fetal placentas of some cattle, sheep and goats. Immunofluorescent staining of placentomes from 6 experimentally infected cows revealed numerous merozoites and schizonts only in maternal caruncles but none in fetal cotyledons (Barnett et al 1977). Caruncles from all 6 cows were atrophied. Carnucles from naturally infected aborting cows were also found to contain numerous parasites but were hemorrhagic and necrotic with calcification of epithelial cells and of the fibrous connective tissue (Corner et al 1963). In other natural infections resulting in abortion, fetal placental lesions ranged from mild to severe with accompanying mononuclear cell infiltration (Dubey, Bergeron 1982; Munday, Black 1976). In 11 experimentally infected sheep, only 4 schizonts were found in fetal membranes from three ewes (Leek, Fayer 1978). Neither organisms nor lesions were found in any placenta or uterine tissues from any of these sheep.

In experimentally infected goats, schizonts were found in the maternal placentome and endometrium but not in the fetal membranes (Dubey 1981). Lesions also were confined to the maternal placentome and endometrium where there was heavy mononuclear cell infiltration and some focal necrosis.

POSSIBLE MECHANISMS RESULTING IN PREMATURE PARTURITION

Hypoxia

Based on the foregoing observations there appear to be several possible ways in which sarcocystosis might initiate abortion or fetal death (Figure 1).

In the intensely studied ovine model, one hypothetical sequence of events leading to the onset of labor begins at

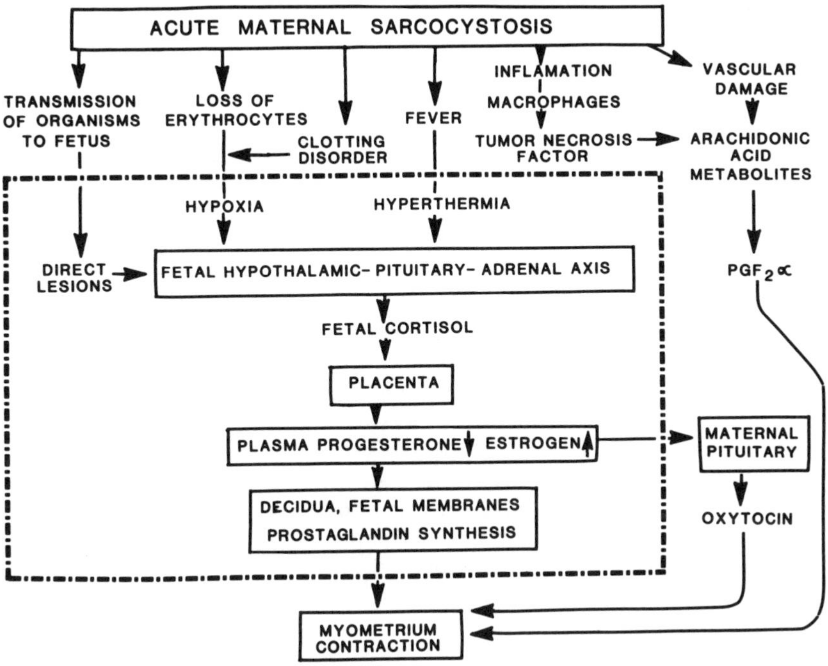

Figure 1. A hypothetical diagrammatic presentation of Sarcocystis-induced pathologic changes in the maternal host that may initiate hormonal events leading to parturition. Fetal hormonal events are shown within the area marked by dotted lines. Both fetal and maternal events induce myometrial gap junctions increasing free ionized calcium leading to myometrium contraction and expulsion of the fetus.

the level of the fetal brain in the hypothalamus and is transmitted via the pituitary to the fetal adrenal where cortisol provides the fetal trigger to maternal endocrine changes (Challis, Lye 1986). These in turn are followed by release of steroids and prostaglandins from the placenta, the decidua, and the fetal membranes which stimulate the myometrium to contract and the cervix to dilate. This concept that the sheep fetus initiated parturition is based in part on the following experimental evidence (for review see Challis, Lye 1986; Challis, Mitchell 1983). Fetal hypophysectomy or bilateral adenalectomy prolonged pregnancy whereas administration of ACTH or glucocorticoid hormone into the *in utero* fetus resulted in premature parturition. Maternal hypophysectomy or administration of ACTH or synthetic glucocorticoids at similar doses did not affect parturition. Under normal conditions it is thought that there is a rise in the concentration of plasma cortisol secreted from the fetal adrenal as it grows and develops with the highest concentrations during the last 2 or 3 days of fetal life (Challis, Lye 1986). What mechanisms might act to stimulate high ACTH or cortisol concentrations in the fetus leading to premature parturition or abortion? One possible sequence of events might begin with anemia in the dam which could result in hypoxia in the fetus. Hypoxia could also result from insufficient blood flow through the maternal placentome due to occlusion of capillaries by schizonts, localized hemorrhage or disseminated intravascular coagulation. Evidence of hypoxia comes from the finding of leukoencephalomalacia in some fetuses. Vasopressin is known to stimulate ACTH release in fetal sheep and although circulating concentrations of vasopressin are very low in fetal sheep they rise several fold with the approach of spontaneous parturition and in response to hypoxia (Challis, Lye 1986). Although hypoxia has been shown to raise the concentration of immunoreactive ACTH in fetal plasma at all times during gestation when it was studied, only after day 139 of the usual 148 day gestation period was the increase in ACTH associated with a large increase in plasma glucocorticoid concentration. Isolated fetal adrenal cells appeared to be responsive and secreted large amounts of cortisol in response to ACTH, a form of GTP, or dibutyrylcyclic AMP as early as day 50 of gestation and at term but not at day 100 (Challis, Lye 1986).

Endothelial Damage and Immune Responses

To determine if vascular damage associated with sarcocystosis in the dam might lead to changes in concentration of hormones associated with the maintenance of gestation, the plasma concentration of progesterone, E_1, E_2, PGFM, and alpha-fetoprotein was monitored in pregnant cows experimentally infected with *Sarcocystis* (Baetz et al 1980, 1981; Lowe et al 1982).

Progesterone production after day 50 of gestation in sheep is primarily in the placenta; ovariectomy at this time will not induce abortion (Challis, Lye 1986). Progesterone acts through suppressing potentials in the myometrium by maintaining it refractory to stimulation by oxytocin or PGF_{2alpha}. Decrease in placental progesterone at term, based on measurement of plasma progesterone concentration, follows and is caused by a rise in fetal cortisol levels. Progesterone withdrawal initiates increased PGF_{2alpha} secretion and parturition in sheep.

During late pregnancy, estrogens promote uterine contractility in most species, increase the responsiveness of the uterus to agonists such as oxytocin and PGF_{2alpha}, inhibit progesterone production, and stimulate prostaglandin synthesis and release. Maternal estrogen in prepartum sheep increases in response to fetal adrenal activity. Both the major source of estrogen and the site of action for fetal cortisol is in the placenta. Although parturition is associated with an increased concentration of maternal estrogen, it is not a prerequisite.

Unfortunately, changes recorded in progesterone, E_1 and E_2 concentration in the experimentally infected cows by Lowe et al (1982) and Baetz et al (1980, 1981) could not be categorized as cause or effect. Although preceded or concurrent with abortion, similar changes were documented at the time of normal parturition.

Four lines of evidence suggest the prostaglandins initiate labor by stimulating myometrial contractions and by softening the cervix: (1) an increased concentration of prostaglandins is found in amniotic fluid and maternal serum in late pregnancy; (2) prostaglandin cyclooxygenase inhibitors such as aspirin and indomethocin suppress uterine activity and prolong gestation; (3) some myometrium (especially primate) is very sensitive to stimulation by exogenous prostaglandins; and (4) intracervical administration of PGE_2 to sheep caused localized softening and distention of the cervix (Challis, Lye, 1986). Two specific lines of observation suggest that events in acute sarcocystosis might result in increased concentration of prostaglandins in the general peripheral circulation of the dam or specifically in the maternal placentome and fetal placenta. First, the release of second generation merozoites is associated with damage of capillary endothelium, an event known to trigger the arachidonic acid cascade leading to PGF_{2alpha} release. Parasite disruption of cell membranes as well as the action of inflammatory cells may stimulate platelet activity including the release of PGF_{2alpha} by platelets and by damaged endothelium. Second, at the time second generation merozoites mature, numerous mononuclear inflammatory cells are found perivascularly throughout the body and in the placenta. Many of these cells are macrophages. Recent *in vitro* studies suggest that macrophages can be stimulated by *Sarcocystis* lysates to release tumor necrosis factor (TNF) (Fayer, 1987). One of the many activities of TNF is its ability to trigger the arachidonic acid cascade leading to PGF_{2alpha} release. Because the findings of Lowe et al (1982) were inconclusive with respect to the sequence of events leading to high maternal plasma PGF_{2alpha} concentration preceeding bovine abortion, studies with appropriate controls need to be conducted to clarify the relationship between sarcocystosis and those events.

Fever

Although fever has been associated with premature parturition and perhaps regarded as the cause, it is not clear if fever itself is a cause or an effect of some other action. Pyrogens from infectious agents such as bacteria or protozoa or pyrogens released from degenerating body tissues cause fever during disease. Pyrogens may act directly on the hypothalamus to raise the set-point of its thermostatic control or may act indirectly by stimulating leukocytes to produce endogenous pyrogen. Endogenous pyrogen is thought to cause fever by first inducing prostaglandin E_1 formation which in turn elicits the fever reaction. Thus, it is not clear if fever itself directly affects the fetus or if the initiators of fever, in this case *Sarcocystis* pyrogens or prostaglandins, induce pathological changes.

Direct Parasitism of Fetus

In addition to the foregoing possibilities leading indirectly to death or premature parturition of the fetus, invasion of fetal tissues by the parasite might result in specific lesions with similar end results. Distribution of parasites throughout the brain with associated lesions might stimulate the fetal hypothalamic-pituitary-adrenal axis or destroy significant brain tissue leading to death. Evidence of fetal myocarditis, pneumonitis, and hepatitis suggest other possible avenues leading directly to fetal death.

SUMMARY

There are many unanswered questions and observations that appear contradictory within the subject of how sarcocystosis affects fetal health. Some fetuses are infected and have lesions, others are unaffected. Some fetal placentas are infected and have lesions, others are unaffected. Some maternal placentomes are infected and have lesions, others are unaffected. Most pregnant animals have overt clinical illness at the time the fetus is affected, others do not. Several possible mechanisms have been hypothesized by which sarcocystosis may directly or indirectly affect fetal health.

REFERENCES

Baetz AL, Barnett D, Bryner JH, Cysewski SJ (1980). Plasma progesterone concentration in the bovine before abortion or parturtion in pregnant animals exposed to Sarcocystis cruzi, Campylobacter fetus, or Aspergillus fumigatus. Am J Vet Res 41:1767-1768.

Baetz AL, Crandell SE, Schmerr MJF, Barnett D, Bryner JH (1981). Plasma alpha-fetoprotein concentrations in pregnant cows exposed to Sarcocystis cruzi, Campylobacter fetus, or Aspergillus fumigatus. Am J Vet Res 42:2146-2148.

Barnett D, Carter BA, Hughes DE, Baetz AL, Fayer R. (1977). Practicable diagnosis of acute bovine sarcocystosis causally related to bovine abortion. Am Assoc Vet Lab Diag 20 Ann Proc:131-138.

Challis JRG, Lye SJ (1986). Parturition. In Clarke JR (ed): "Oxford reviews of reproductive biology," Volume 8, Oxford: Clarendon Press, pp. 61-112.

Challis JRG, Mitchell BF (1983). Endocrinology of pregnancy and parturition. In Warshaw JB (ed): "The Biological Basis of Reproductive and Developmental Medicine," New York: Elsevier Biomedical, pp. 105-139.

Corner AH, Mitchell D, Meads EB, Taylor PA (1963). Dalmeny disease. An infection of cattle presumed to be caused by an unidentified protozoon. Can Vet J 4:252-264.

Dubey JP (1981). Abortion and death in goats inoculated with _Sarcocystis_ sporocysts from coyote feces. J Am Vet Med Assoc 178:700-703.

Dubey JP, Bergeron JA (1982). _Sarcocystis_ as a cause of placentitis and abortion in cattle. Vet Pathol 19:315-318.

Dubey JP, Towle A (1986). Toxoplasmosis in sheep: A review and annotated bibliography. Miscellaneous publication No. 10 of the Commonwealth Institute of Parasitology, London. 1-152.

Erber M, Boch J, Barth D (1978a). Drei Sarkosporidienarten des Rehwildes. Berl Munch Tierarztl Wochenschr 91:482-486

Erber M, Meyer J, Boch J (1978b). Aborte beim Schwein durch Sarkosporidien (_Sarcocystis suicanis_). Berl Munch Tierarztl Wochenschr 91:393-395.

Fayer R (1987). Influence of parasitism on growth of cattle possibly mediated through tumor necrosis factor. Proc XII Beltsville Symp (in press).

Fayer R, Dubey JP (1986). Bovine sarcocystosis. Compend Contin Educ Pract Vet 8:F130-142.

Fayer R, Johnson AJ, Lunde M (1976). Abortion and other signs of disease in cows experimentally infected with _Sarcocystis fusiformis_ from dogs. J Inf Dis 134:624-628.

Hong CB, Giles RC, Newman LE, Fayer R. (1982). Sarcocystosis in an aborted bovine fetus. J Am Vet Med Assoc 181:585-588.

Jerrett IV, McOrist S, Waddington J, Browning JW, Malecki JC, McCausland IP (1984). Diagnostic studies of the fetus, placenta and maternal blood form 265 bovine abortions. Cornell Vet 74:8-20.

Jolley WR, Jensen R, Hancock HA, Swift BL (1983). Encephalitic sarcocystosis in a newborn calf. Am J Vet Res 44:1908-1911.

Kunde JM, Jones LP, Craig TM (1980). Protozoal encephalitis in a bovine fetus. Southwest Vet 33:231-232.

Leek RG, Fayer R. (1978). Sheep experimentally infected with Sarcocystis from dogs II. Abortion and disease in ewes. Cornell Vet 68:108-123.

Lowe KJ, Williams WF, Fayer R, Gross TS (1982). Reproductive hormone and prostaglandin metabolite profiles of pregnant cows infected with the abortifacient Sarcocystis cruzi. Am Dairy Sci Assoc 77 Ann Meet:198.

McCausland IP, Badman RT, Hides S, Slee KJ (1984). Multiple apparent Sarcocystis abortion in four bovine herds. Cornell Vet 74:146-154.

Munday BL, Black H (1976). Suspected Sarcocystis infections of the bovine placenta and foetus. Z Parasitenk 51:129-132.

Munday BL (1981). Premature parturition in ewes inoculated with Sarcocystis ovicanis. Vet Parasitol 9:17-26.

Proctor SJ, Barnett D, Stalheim OHV, Fayer R (1976). Pathology of Sarcocystis fusiformis in cattle. Am Assoc Vet Lab Pract 19 Ann Meet:329-336.

Stalheim OH, Proctor SJ, Fayer R, Lunde M (1976). Death and abortion in cows experimentally infected with Sarcocystis from dogs. Am Assoc Vet Lab Diag 19 Ann Meet:317-328.

Schmitz JA, Wolf WW (1977). Spontaneous fatal sarcocystosis in a calf. Vet Pathol 14:527-531.

Vickers MC, Brooks HV (1983). Suspected Sarcocystis infection in an aborted bovine foetus. NZ Vet J 31:166

DISCUSSION

DR. OSBURN: I was wondering about the aborted fetal calf you showed. It looked like it had alopecia. Is there any specific reason for that?

DR. FAYER: I really can't explain that. Out of 18 bovine fetuses that we have examined, that was the only calf with alopecia.

DR. WAHL: Have you found any instances where one calf was clearly affected with *Sarcocystis* infection and the other ones seemed to be normal?

DR. FAYER: As far as experimental animals are concerned, every animal has appeared normal. There have been only two fetuses in which organisms were identified. So there have not been any specific lesions or anomalies that we have seen.

DR. ALDERINK: You said there was about a 100% infection rate in cattle. Approximately what is the incidence of clinical cases of *Sarcocystis* infection?

DR. FAYER: I really can't tell you because clinical sarcocystosis is very difficult to diagnose. Basically, what we see in the field are anemic, feverish, and unthrifty animals. There also are abortions and a dramatic decrease in milk production. We receive very few referrals, and these usually are from veterinarians who have tried to rule out other causes of disease. We have dealt with dairy herds and feedlots in which many animals were affected, but the incidence of infection in cattle has not been determined.

DR. POHLENZ: Are there any interactions between different types of *Sarcocystis*, either *S. bovihominis* or *S. bovicanis* or others, in which the one excludes the other?

DR. FAYER: We have conducted some experimental studies in which we have tried to produce a protective immunity in animals to two times an LD_{50} from *S. cruzi*. *Sarcocystis cruzi* is the species that we have used to challenge cattle. The cat-derived species (*S. hirsuta*), which is generally a nonpathogen, was not protective.

Transplacental Effects on Fetal Health, pages 165–173

ANTENATAL MALARIAL INFECTIONS

Richard L. Naeye

Department of Pathology, Pennsylvania State University College of Medicine Hershey, Pennsylvania 17033

INTRODUCTION

With a few exceptions the same disorders of pregnancy are encountered in every population group in the world. One of the exceptions is malaria, whose influence is usually limited to low altitude tropical and subtropical areas. Since malaria has such an important effect on human health it might be assumed that plentiful information is available about its effects on pregnancy and the fetus. Much information is available but gaps remain. Most of these gaps relate to the fact that malaria often exists in an environment where multiple other factors adversely affect pregnancy outcome. This makes it necessary to separate out possible effects due to the malaria from the effects that are caused by other factors. For example, the gravidas who are most often affected by malaria are young, poorly nourished and receive little or no antenatal medical care. It is thus difficult to determine in some malarial areas how many of the frequent unfavorable pregnancy outcomes are due to malaria and how many to other influences in the community.

Endemic Malaria

The differing effects of malaria on immune and non-immune populations must be understood to understand the role of malaria in pregnancy. In communities where malaria is endemic the majority of residents probably receive several sporozoite inoculations each year (McGregor, 1984 and 1987; McGregor and Smith, 1952). Most newborns in this setting have antibodies that passed the placenta from their mothers with the result that they are partially immune for several months after birth. Their first malarial attacks are usually mild and sometimes asymptomatic (McGregor et al., 1956). The next attacks are usually more severe and reach their peak between 1-3 years of age. These more severe attacks are often accompanied by anemia and by a slowing of body growth or even a loss of body weight (McGregor, 1984 and 1987). All of this occurs after the children have lost their passively acquired immunity and have not yet developed effective active immunity. By three years of age many children in this setting are immune and are able to tolerate dense levels of parasitemia without symptoms or further growth retardation (McGregor and Smith, 1952; McGregor et al., 1956). Studies have shown that such older children have little or no benefit from chemotherapeutic malarial prophylaxis in terms of better growth or fewer days of illness each year (Archibald and Bruce-Chwatt, 1956).

Taking the aforementioned facts into consideration, it is somewhat surprising that there are many reports in the literature that pregnancy enhances the severity of malarial infections (McGregor, 1984; McGregor and Smith, 1952; McGregor et al., 1956; Covell, 1950). These reports are largely based on the fact that pregnant women usually have more plasmodial parasites in their blood than nonpregnant women. This is somewhat of a paradox because most pregnant women in malarial endemic areas have a high level of active immunity against the parasite and both they and their fetuses have few if any clinical evidences of a malarial infection. The fact that gravidas with enhanced parasitemia die no more frequently than nonpregnant women in populations where the infection is endemic is additional evidence that the increased parasitemia is not a reactivation of an old infection or an increased response to a new one (McGregor, 1984).

The fact that malarial parasitemia is both more prevalent and heavier during pregnancy has led to speculation that pregnancy in some way depresses pre-existing acquired immunity (McGregor, 1984 and 1987; McGregor and Smith, 1952; Reinhardt, 1980). This speculation has been encouraged by the discoveries that corticosteroid production increases during pregnancy and that serum from pregnant women can inhibit the phagocytic activity and chemotactic responsiveness of phagocytes (McGregor, 1984; Bjorksten, 1980). However, as McGregor has pointed out, these findings have not been matched by any clear demonstration that pregnant women are more susceptible to malarial or to other infections than the non-pregnant (McGregor, 1984).

If pregnant women are not more susceptible to infection than the non-pregnant, what is the cause of their enhanced parasitemia? A full explanation is not available but some partial answers can be suggested. It has been observed that parasite prevalence, density and maternal gestational anemia are greatest in primigravidas (McGregor, 1984 and 1987; Reinhardt, 1978). Primigravidas have a somewhat different intrauterine environment than multigravidas, particularly in the third world, and these differences may contribute to the enhancement of parasitemia during first pregnancies. Third world primigravidas are often unmarried, have less to eat and receive less antenatal medical care than multigravidas who are usually married. The nutrition of primigravidas is further compromised by the fact that they are usually young enough to be still growing so that their growth needs compete with the growth needs of their fetuses for available nutrients (Naeye, 1981). Resulting undernutrition predisposes to both infection and to low uteroplacental blood flow (Naeye et al., 1983; Naeye 1983). It is thus possible that this undernutrition and the low blood flow predispose to the enhanced parasitemia

The older literature has many claims that the enhanced parasitemia of pregnancy predisposes to low birth weights without explaining if the low birth weights are due to more frequent preterm deliveries or to fetal growth retardation. McGregor's finding that birth weights increased in the Gambia with increasing parity, with or without the presence of placental parasites, casts doubt on the possibility that parasitemia causes low birth weights (McGregor, 1984). Reinhardt found in a malarial population he studied that maternal anemia would explain only about 1% of birth weight variance (Reinhardt, 1980). Since anemia is a marker for malaria in such a population, his findings are strong evidence against the possibility that malarial parasitemia causes fetal growth retardation. Thus, there are many reasons to doubt that malaria has much effect on pregnancy outcome in communities where the infection is endemic.

Epidemic Malaria and Pregnancy Outcome

Epidemic malaria has a very different effect on pregnancy and its outcome than does endemic malaria. Poor pregnancy outcomes are particularly frequent with epidemics of *P. falciparum*. Epidemic malaria develops when a poorly immune or non-immune population is suddenly exposed to the parasite (McGregor, 1984). In this situation the infection leads to high fever, rapid hemolysis and severe anemia. This combination presumably accounts for the maternal deaths, high rates of abortion, stillbirth and preterm delivery that occur in malarial epidemics (Wickramasuriya, 1937; Le Van Hung, 1951; Menon, 1972). It needs to be determined if maternal metabolic acidosis contributes to these poor outcomes. Such acidosis can develop with any type of acute maternal infection during pregnancy (Naeye, 1981). Both the fever and the fasting that often accompany these infections predispose to the metabolic acidosis, which can develop within 24 hours of the time that gravidas stop eating (Naeye, 1983; Felig and Lynch, 1970). This acidosis could be a major contributor to the increase in fetal and neonatal deaths associated with such infections (Naeye, 1981). Acidosis is particularly lethal to fetuses when gravidas are undernourished, a common situation for unmarried primigravidas in the third world (Naeye, 1979).

Malaria in the Fetus and Newborn

Fetal infection has been reported with each of the four species of plasmodia that infect man (Covell, 1950). Transplacental transmission of the parasite to the fetus appears to be common but clinical infection is rare in the neonate. In a study conducted in the Ivory Coast Reinhardt reported that 55% of the newborns of infected mothers had parasites in their blood, suggesting that transplacental passage of the parasites had been frequent (Reinhardt, 1980). Only a few of the infected neonates had an elevated blood level of IgM, so the parasite presumably reached the fetus only a few days before birth. Despite this frequent transplacental transmission, symptomatic congenitally acquired malarial infections are rare. The few reported cases have presented as pyrexial illness within 24 hours of birth in non-immune and partially immune newborns (Menon, 1972). It needs to be noted that not every study that has found heavy parasitemia in maternal and placental blood has found parasites in the blood of the associated newborns (McGregor, 1984) (Table 1).

TABLE 1 - Malarial parasites/ul of blood in Gambian women

	Primigravidas	Multigravidas
Placental blood	32,846	11,477
Peripheral blood	5,137	1,767
Newborn blood	0	0

-modified from McGregor (1984)

If malarial parasites are frequently transmitted to the fetus but rarely produce neonatal illness, what happens to the parasites? McGregor and his associates have found that in Gambia the prevalence of placental malaria shows little change from the dry, low transmission season to the wet, high transmission season, suggesting that the chances of transplacental fetal infection are as great in the dry as in the wet months (McGregor, 1984) (Table 2). However, detectable parasitemia at several months of age was much more frequent in the wet months. This suggests that transplacentally transferred parasites were destroyed in the circulation of fetuses and neonates whereas parasites acquired several months after birth persisted after transplacentally transferred antibodies against the parasites had largely disappeared. This is strong evidence that fetal and neonatal defense mechanisms, in conjunction with transplacentally transferred antibodies, constitute a potent fetal defense against the parasite. Logie et al have reported that pregnant women are strongly immunoresponsive to plasmodial infection (Logie et al., 1973). Those that have many parasites in their placental circulation have high plasma concentrations of IgG.

TABLE 2 - Prevalence of malarial parasites in placentas and subsequently in the peripheral blood of children less than 3 months of age in rural Gambia.

	Prevalence During	
	Dry Season	Wet Season
Placenta	27%	28%
Peripheral blood	1%	12%

-modified from McGregor (1984)

The density of plasmodial parasites is usually greater in placental than in maternal peripheral blood (McGregor, 1984) (Table 1). This has led McGregor to argue that the placenta constitutes an environment that shields the parasite from destruction by extrauterine immune effector mechanisms (McGregor, 1984). These extrauterine immune mechanisms are apparently least effective in primigravidas because primigravidas have a higher density of plasmodial parasites in their placentas than multigravidas.

In summary, it appears that malaria rarely affects pregnancy outcome in populations where the parasite is endemic, whereas the effects of the infection on pregnancy outcome can be great in partially immune and non-immune populations. Maternal deaths and high rates of abortions and stillbirths in these unprotected populations remain a major health problem. Such non-immune women can of course be protected by anti-malarial drugs, but the use of such drugs is far from universal and will probably never be fully employed. It therefore seems important to learn more about how the damaging mechanisms that develop during acute infections in non-immune gravidas exert their effects on the fetus. Are all of the effects due to rapid hemolysis? Are some due to maternal metabolic acidosis and rapid fall in utero-placental blood flow? Answers to these questions might provide information that would help improve pregnancy outcomes when malaria appears in partially immune and non-immune populations.

Finally, there are many recent reports that severe, symptomatic malaria has reappeared in previously immune individuals who have become immunoincompetent as the result of developing the acquired immune deficiency syndrome (AIDS). It remains to be determined how much of a role malaria will play in the management and outcome of the current AIDS epidemic in Africa and elsewhere.

REFERENCES

Archibald HM, Bruce-Chwatt LJ (1956). Suppression of malaria with pyrimethamine in Nigerian school-children. Bull WHO 15:775-784.

Bjorksten B (1980). Phagocyte function in pregnancy. Immunol Today 1:55-56.

Covell G (1950). Congenital malaria. Trop Dis Bull 47:1147.

Felig P, Lynch V (1970). Starvation in human pregnancy,

hypoglycemia, hypoinsulinemia and hyperketonemia. Science 170:990.
Le Van Hung (1951). Paludisme et grossesse a Saigon. Rev Paludisme Med Trop 83:75-112.
Logie DE, McGregor IA, Rowe DS, Billewicz WZ (1973). Plasma immunoglobulin concentrations in mothers and newborn children in Africa and Europe with special reference to malaria. Studies in the Gambia, Nigeria and Switzerland. Bull WHO 49:547-554.
McGregor IA (1984). Epidemiology, malaria and pregnancy. Am J Trop Med Hyg 33:517-525.
McGregor IA (1987). The significance of parasitic infections in terms of clinical disease: a personal view. Parasitology 94:S159-S178.
McGregor IA, Gilles HM, Walters JH, Davies AH and Pearson FA (1956). Effects of heavy and repeated malarial infections on Gambian infants and children; effects of erythrocytic parasitization. Br Med J 2:686-692.
McGregor IA, Smith DA (1952). A health nutrition and parasitology survey in a rural village, Keneba, in West Kiang, The Gambia. Trans R Soc Trop Med Hyg 62:341-352.
Menon R (1972). Pregnancy and malaria. Med J Malaysia 27:115-119.
Naeye RL (1983). Effects of maternal nutrition on fetal and neonatal survival. Birth 10:109-113.
Naeye RL (1981). Nutritional/nonnutritional interactions that affect the outcome of pregnancy. Am J Clin Nutr 34:727-731.
Naeye RL (1979). Weight gain and the outcome of pregnancy. Am J Obstet Gynecol 135:3.
Naeye RL, Tafari N (1983). Risk Factors in Pregnancy and Diseases of the Fetus and Newborn. Baltimore: Williams & Wilkins.
Reinhardt MC (1980). The African newborn in Abidjan, maternal and environmental factors influencing the outcome of pregnancy. In Abei H, Whitehead R: "Maternal Nutrition During Pregnancy and Lactation," Bern: Hans Huber Publ, pp 132.
Reinhardt MC, Ambroise-Thomas P, Cavallo-Serra R, Meylan C and Gautier R (1978). Malaria at delivery in Abidjan. Helv Paediatr Acta 33 (suppl 41):65-84.
Wickramasuriya GA (1937). Clincal features of malaria in pregnancy. In GAW Wickramasuriya (ed): Malaria and Ancylostomiasis in the Pregnant Women. London: Oxford University Press, pp 5-90.

DISCUSSION

DR. ROSA: There have been several trials of antimalarial drugs in pregnancy and I wonder if you could evaluate them?

DR. NAEYE: Antimalarial drugs have been shown to be effective in protecting pregnant women in malaria susceptible populations.

DR. QUINN: You have shown an increase in stillbirths from parity one to parity two and subsequently. Do you think this could be more associated with genital tract infections?

DR. NAEYE: It is only indirectly related to other infections. In the rural areas of many African nations, a woman's nutritional status decreases with each successive pregnancy because the amount of food available to the family doesn't increase and therefore has to be divided into progressively smaller per capita shares as family size increases. This predisposes to a number of disorders that produce poor pregnancy outcomes, including acute bacterial chorioamnionitis.

DR. QUINN: I believe it is an important factor. There is no sense in treating malaria in pregnant women if they actually are aborting because of infection with normal flora or with sexually transmitted disease microorganisms.

DR. NAEYE: To my knowledge gonorrhea is not a cause of fetal or neonatal death in these settings. Congenital syphilis is an important disorder but it causes only a small percentage of the unfavorable pregnancy outcomes in the malarial populations with which I am familiar.

DR. V. ANDERSON: I have reviewed 500 cases from Zaire and there was no difference in the incidence of malaria in the HIV positive and the HIV negative mothers. However, we don't know about clinical AIDS yet. So, until the disease expresses itself, we can't really know if patients with malaria develop clinical AIDS at the same rate as nonparasitized individuals.

DR. NAEYE: I agree. In an endemic population the number of malarial parasites in a placenta has very little clinical significance.

DR. V. ANDERSON: I use this information regarding malaria and HIV infections for public health purposes because everyone wants to know whether or not mosquitoes transmit HIV infection.

DR. NAEYE: The evidence seems very strong that HIV is not carried by mosquitoes. This is shown by the fact that HIV is almost absent in children between about 5-15 years of age in HIV endemic areas. Children in this age group were born before HIV became endemic and have not yet become sexually active. If mosquitoes were a vector for HIV, the infection should be frequent in them.

DR. FAYER: I would like to suggest the possible importance of tumor necrosis factor (TNF). In Lancet a couple of months ago, Scuderi and colleagues reported examining sera from a number of people with chronic infections which included some viruses, bacteria, and parasites. It is of interest that in individuals with plasmodium and trypanosome infection they found elevated levels of TNF, which in turn raised PGF_{2alpha} levels.

III. METABOLIC, DRUG, AND CHEMICAL TERATOGENS

Transplacental Effects on Fetal Health, pages 177–191

HUMAN TERATOGENS: DELINEATING THE PHENOTYPIC EFFECTS, THE PERIOD OF GREATEST SENSITIVITY, THE DOSE-RESPONSE RELATIONSHIP AND MECHANISMS OF ACTION

Lewis B. Holmes

Embryology-Teratology Unit, Children's Service, Massachusetts General Hospital and Department of Pediatrics, Harvard Medical School, Boston, MA 02114

The number of recognized human teratogens is short (Table 1), shorter than most doctors and patients expect it to be. "New" human teratogens continue to be recognized, with two exposures with a high risk of serious damage, the anticonvulsant valproic acid and the medication used to treat cystic acne, isotretinoin, being added to the list in 1982.

We have learned valuable lessons from the experience to date. Current and future studies can build on this experience to provide more precise information as to the teratogenic effects in exposed human pregnancies. Several aspects of this experience are relevant to the metabolic, drug and chemical teratogens being discussed at this conference.

RECOGNIZING THE SPECTRUM OF PHENOTYPIC EFFECTS

The potential effects of an intrauterine exposure to a teratogen include:

- spontaneous abortion
- growth retardation
- microcephaly
- major and minor malformations
- metabolic dysfunction
- cognitive dysfunction or mental deficiency
- altered social behavior
- malignancy

TABLE 1. Recognized Human Teratogens

1. Drugs
   - Aminopterin/amethopterin
   - Androgenic hormones
   - Busulfan
   - Chlorobiphenyls
   - Cyclophosphamide
   - Diethylstilbestrol
   - Heroin/methadone
   - Iodide
   - Isotretinoin (13-cis-retinoic acid)
   - Lithium
   - Phenytoin
   - Propylthiouracil
   - Tetracycline
   - Trimethadione
   - Valproic Acid
   - Warfarin

2. Heavy Metals
   - Lead
   - Mercury

3. Radiation
   - Cancer therapy

4. Maternal Conditions
   - Alcoholism
   - Insulin-dependent diabetes mellitus
   - Maternal phenylketonuria
   - Myasthenia gravis
   - Myotonic dystrophy
   - Smoking
   - Systemic lupus erythematosus

5. Intrauterine Infections
   - Cytomeglovirus
   - Herpes Simplex
   - Rubella
   - Syphilis
   - Toxoplasmosis
   - Varicella
   - Venezuelan equine encephalitis virus

This wide spectrum of phenotypic effects emphasizes the need for studies of exposed fetuses that will start early enough to identify events before the expected birth, such as spontaneous abortion and stillbirth, and continue long enough to identify late effects, such as the increased frequency of insulin-dependent diabetes mellitus among individuals with congenital rubella syndrome and the decreased rate of marriage among individuals exposed to diethylstilbestrol _in utero_ (Beral and Colwell, 1981).

The experience to date with several teratogenic drugs has shown that the affected infant has a recognizable pattern of malformations. Some of these patterns involve multiple major malformations. For example, infants exposed to thalidomide may have: microtia, bilateral preaxial arm malformations (e.g. absent or finger-like thumb), (Figure 1) and shortened long bones, abnormal shoulder joint, preaxial polydactyly of the first toes (Figure 2) and absence of the tibia. Experience in Sweden showed that the epidemic produced by thalidomide could only be identified if the infants with the rare bilateral anomalies amelia, phocomelia or bilateral preaxial forearm deficiencies (e.g. radius and/or thumb aplasia) were tabulated (Kallen et al., 1984). By contrast, the tabulation of "limb reduction defects", a category which includes a wide variety of unilateral limb malformations, did not identify the "epidemic".

In general, drugs which have a high risk of damaging the exposed fetus, like thalidomide, aminopterin, isotretinoin, and valproic acid, produce multiple major malformations. This makes it easier for these correlations to be confirmed in large data bases, such as national malformations surveillance programs. The first successful use of these programs was in the delineation of the teratogenicity of valproic acid because of its association with the occurrence of spina bifida (Robert and Guibaud, 1982).

The creation of these large-scale malformation surveillance programs was a sequel to the tragic occurrence of the thalidomide epidemic. However, these programs are only effective in identifying strong teratogens which produce an increase in the occurrence of one or more major malformations that are readily detected and when there is a widespread exposure among pregnant women (Khoury and Holtzman, 1987).

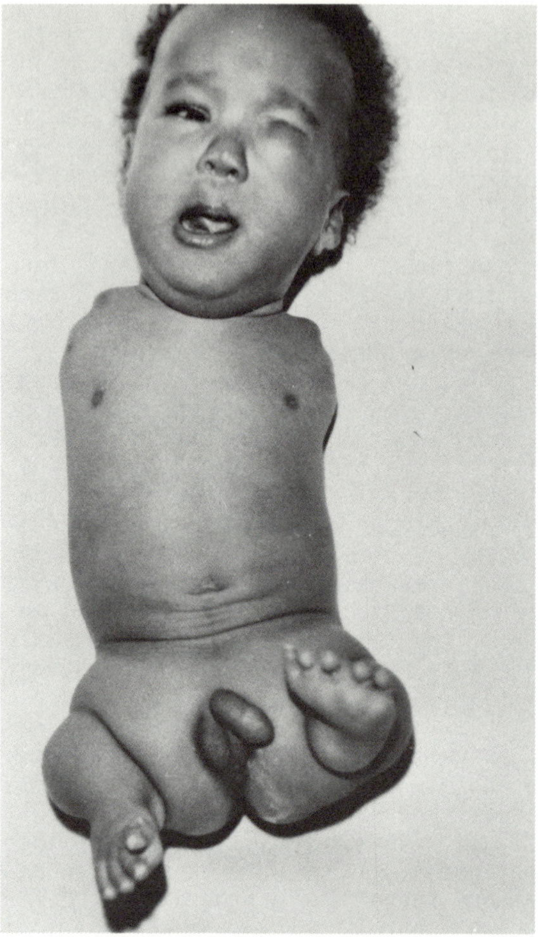

Figure 1. An English boy exposed to thalidomide *in utero* who was born with absence of the left eye, facial nevus, amelia of both arms and phocomelia of both legs (Courtesy of Dr. CGH Newman, London, England).

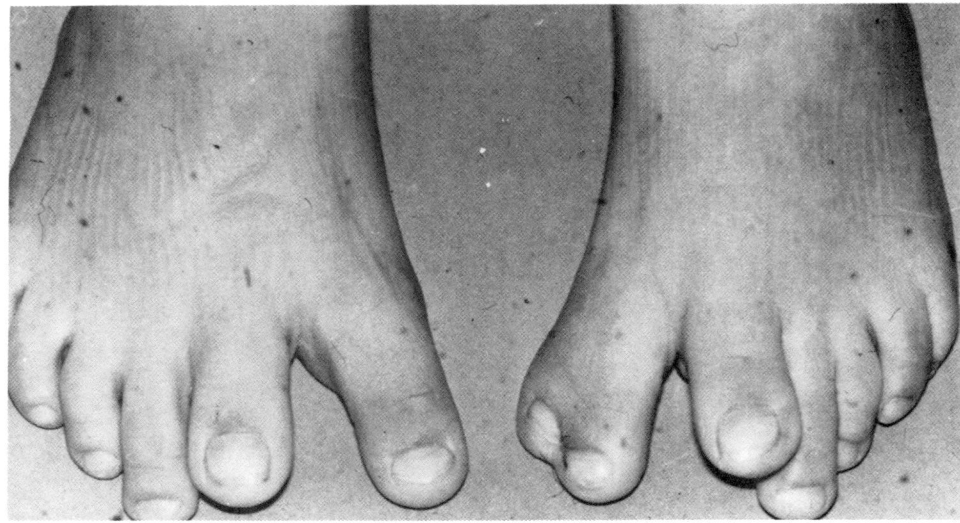

Figure 2. Shows preaxial polydactyly of the first toe caused by exposure to thalidomide during pregnancy (Courtesy of Dr. CGH Newman, London, England).

By contrast, drugs like phenytoin and warfarin, produce distinctive patterns of abnormalities that may not be coded on hospital discharge summaries, a source of information in some epidemiologic studies. More intensive examinations of exposed individuals are required to identify the phenotypic features (Figures 3 and 4). The difficulty in identifying the phenotypic effects of phenytoin was illustrated emphatically by the different findings in the evaluations of the same group of exposed infants in the National Collaborative Perinatal Project (Hanson et al., 1976; Hanson and Smith, 1977; Shapiro et al., 1976; Shapiro et al., 1977). An epidemiologic approach was to tabulate the frequency of "all identified malformations" (Shapiro et al., 1976). These investigators concluded that the fetal damage might be due to the epilepsy itself. By contrast, clinicians who reviewed personally the findings in the examination forms of the same exposed and matched control infants concluded that

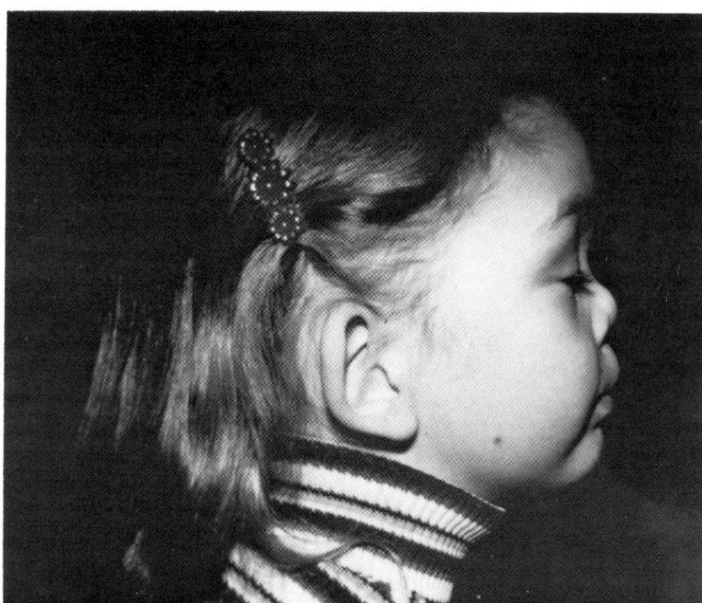

Figure 3. Shows the marked nose hypoplasia that is a common and distinctive effect of exposure to warfarin.

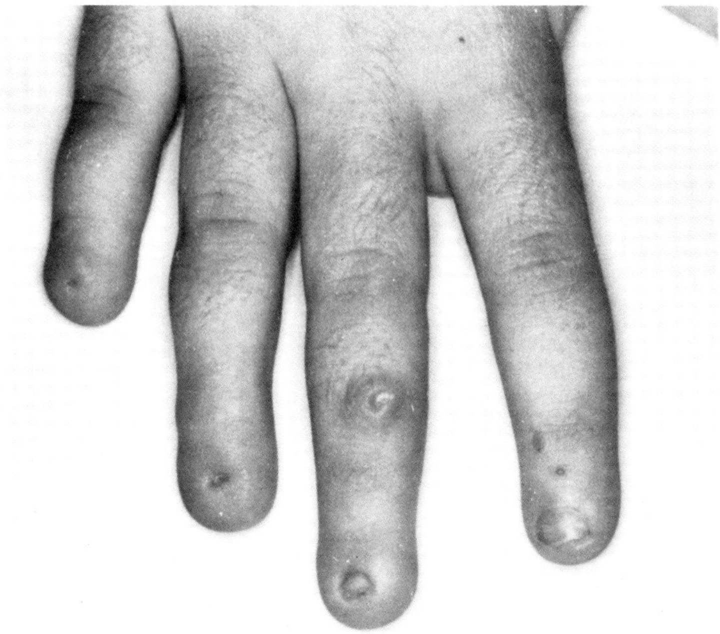

Figure 4. Shows the symphalangism of the distal interphalangeal joints and severe nail hypoplasia due to exposure to phenytoin.

prenatal exposure to phenytoin caused a distinctive pattern of growth retardation and major and minor malformations (Hanson et al., 1976). Each group defended its approach (Hanson and Smith, 1977; Shapiro et al., 1977). We know now that exposure to phenytoin and other anticonvulsants in pregnancy does produce an increased occurrence of growth retardation, certain major malformations and a pattern of subtle craniofacial abnormalities and other minor anomalies such as nail hypoplasia. However, the increase in major malformations is only slight--about two-fold. Therefore, it is not surprising that a large-scale epidemiologic study which tabulated only major malformations would not identify this more subtle, but specific, phenotypic effect.

The experience with teratogens with a relative risk of damage of 2 or 3 which produce more subtle patterns of growth retardation and anomalies emphasizes the need to use more sophisticated approaches to delineate teratogens. Components of this approach include using examination protocols with definitions of the features being looked for, making objective measurements whenever possible, having the examiner unaware of the exposure status (e.g. exposed or control) of the infant being examined and an assessment of the reproducibility of the findings by two examiners of the same infant. Since the phenotypic features can be subtle in the newborn infant, long-term follow-up may be needed to identify abnormal physical features in older children and evidence of cognitive dysfunction.

DETERMINING THE PERIOD OF GREATEST SENSITIVITY

Many of the drugs that are teratogenic are administered for long periods of time during pregnancy, thus obviating the possibility of determining the period of time when the fetus is most vulnerable to damage. It is assumed that exposure in the first trimester must occur to produce malformations and that exposure in the second and third trimesters can produce other phenotypic effects such as growth retardations, microcephaly and cognitive dysfunction. Only for thalidomide has a specific period of greatest sensitivity been postulated. Lenz (1971) proposed that this period was days 34 to 50 after the last menstrual period. He suggested that the exposure within this period had different effects: days 34 to 39 correlated with the occurrence of ear anomalies and cranial nerve palsies; days 39 to 43 with severe defects of the arms; days 42 to 46 with severe defects of the legs and days 47 to 50 with mild malformations of the thumbs. Hopefully those exposures, which can be for only a few days during pregnancy, like isotretinoin, tetracycline, and warfarin, will be evaluated to determine more precisely the period of greatest sensitivity and the risks from exposures at specific periods of gestation.

DETERMINING THE DOSE-RESPONSE RELATIONSHIP

Theoretically the greater the exposure the greater the risk of damage to the unborn fetus. There is some limited evidence to support this. Clarren and his associates (1987) found that infants exposed to over four ounces of pure alcohol a day during pregnancy were likely to have a recognizable pattern of craniofacial abnormalities, whereas infants exposed to lower amounts did not. The likelihood of major malformations correlated with the blood level of phenytoin during pregnancy, although few levels were available for the first trimester of pregnancy (Dansky et al., 1982). Differences in social behavior of adults who had been exposed to diethylstilbestrol *in utero* correlated with the period and the dose of the exposure (Beral and Colwell, 1981).

DETERMINING THE UNDERLYING MECHANISM OF TERATOGENICITY

Several mechanisms of action have been postulated:

Iodide: excessive intake by the mother produces fetal thyroid inhibition with secondary compensatory hypertrophy.

Propylthiouracil: inhibits thyroid hormone synthesis.

Tetracycline: deposits in areas of active mineralization in the organic matrix of newly proliferating bone.

Warfarin: a vitamin K antagonist that prevents the formation of calcium-binding amino acids that alter the effect of growth factors (osteocalcin) essential for normal chondrogenesis (Pauli et al., 1987).

Phenytoin: lowered levels of epoxide hydratase and/or an altered ability to detoxify the arene oxide of phenytoin makes the fetus more vulnerable to damage (Buehler, 1985; Strickler et al., 1985).

Valproic acid: a weakly acidic drug that increases the intracellular pH in the early embryo (Nau and Scott, 1986).

The information available on each of the postulated mechanisms is quite limited. Warfarin has been studied extensively in experimental animals and only recently have any correlations in humans been made (Pauli et al., 1987). Studies of children exposed to the anticonvulsant phenytoin *in utero* have suggested that these children may inherit an abnormality in the metabolism of the drug to its arene oxide metabolite which predisposes them to the teratogenic effects (Buehler, 1985; Strickler et al., 1985). However, it has also been noted that other anticonvulsant drugs with different chemical structure, including phenobarbital (Krauss et al., 1984) and ethotoin (Finnell and DiLiberti, 1983), produce the same phenotypic effects. This raises the question as to whether it is the arene oxide metabolites that are teratogenic or instead some factor common to several types of anticonvulsants.

One can hope that continued progress will be made in delineating the mechanism of action of human teratogens. This would make it possible to screen women in the child-bearing age group to identify those with an increased risk of having a child damaged by an exposure, such as an anticonvulsant, during pregnancy.

REFERENCES

Beral V, Colwell L (1981). Randomized trial of high doses of stilbestrol and ethisterone therapy in pregnancy: long-term follow-up of the children. J Epidemiol Community Health 35:155.

Buehler BA (1985). Epoxide hydralase and the fetal hydantoin syndrome. Am J Hum Genet 37 Suppl:A7.

Clarren SK, Sampson PD, Larsen J, Donnell DJ, Barr HM, Bookstein FL, Martin DC, Streissguth AP (1987). Facial effects of fetal alcohol exposure: assessment by photographs and morphometric analysis. Am J Med Gen 26:651.

Dansky L, Andermann E, Andermann F, Sherwin AL, Kinch RA (1982). Maternal epilepsy and congenital malformations: correlation with maternal plasma anticonvulsant levels. In Janz D et al (eds): "Epilepsy, Pregnancy, and the Child", New York: Raven Press, p 251.

Finnell RH, DiLiberti JH (1983). Hydantoin-induced teratogenesis: are arene oxide intermediates really responsible? Helv Paediatr Acta 38:171.

Hanson JW, Myrianthopoulos NC, Harvey MAS, Smith DW (1976). Risk to the offspring of women treated with hydantoin anticonvulsants, with emphasis on the fetal hydantoin syndrome. J Pediatr 89:662.

Hanson JW, Smith DW (1977). Reply. J Pediatr 90:674.

Kallen B, Rahmani T M-Z, Winberg J (1984). Infants with congenital limb reduction registered in the Swedish Register

of Congenital Malformations. Teratology 29:73.
Khoury MJ, Holtzman NA (1987). On the ability of birth defects monitoring to detect new teratogens. Am J Epidemiol 126:136.
Krauss CM, Holmes LB, VanLang QN, Keith DA (1984). Four siblings with similar malformations after exposure to phenytoin and primidone. J Pediatr 105:750.
Lenz W (1971). How can the teratogenic action of a factor be established in man? South Med J Suppl 64:41.
Nau H, Scott WJ Jr (1986). Weak acids may act as teratogens by accumulating in the basic milieu of the early mammalian embryo. Nature 323:276.
Pauli RM, Lian JB, Mosher DF, Suttie JW (1987). Association of congenital deficiency of multiple vitamin K dependent coagulation factors and the phenotype of the warfarin embryopathy: clues to the mechanism of teratogenicity of coumarin derivatives. Am J Hum Genet 41:566.
Robert E, Guibaud P (1982). Maternal valproic acid and congenital neural tube defects. Lancet 1:937.
Shapiro S, Slone D, Hartz SC, Rosenberg L, Siskind V, Monson RR, Mitchell AA, Heinonen OP, Idanpaan-Heikkila J, Haro S, Saxen L (1976). Anticonvulsants and parental epilepsy in the development of birth defects. Lancet 1:272.
Shapiro S, Slone D, Hartz SC, Rosenberg L, Siskind V, Monson RR, Mitchell AA, Heinonen OP (1977). Are hydantoins (phenytoins) human teratogens? J Pediatr 90:673.
Strickler SM, Dansky LV, Miller MA, Seni M-H, Andermann E, Spielberg S (1985). Genetic predisposition to phenytoin-induced birth defects. Lancet 2:746.

DISCUSSION

DR. MARNOY: You mentioned that in the fetal alcohol syndrome the abnormal facial characteristics develop when exposure is at the 4 ounce level. What is the threshold dose below which there is no effect on the fetus?

DR. HOLMES: The slide I showed on the effects of prenatal exposure to alcohol is from a study by Ann Streissguth and her associates in Seattle. To my knowledge she has not published information on the effect of lower doses of exposure on morphologic effects such as head size, height, and weight. The paper to which I referred by Clarren et al concerned only the facial features among alcohol-exposed children at age 7 years.

DR. NAEYE: Do the phenytoin-exposed neonates have small heads and, if so, how small?

DR. HOLMES: We define microcephaly as a head circumference that is over two standard deviations below the mean value for infants of the same gestational age, sex, and race. We do not know in our own study what the frequency of microcephaly among phenytoin-exposed infants is as compared to controls, since this is currently underway. However, our pilot studies showed the risk of microcephaly is greater in infants exposed to multiple anticonvulsant drugs than in those infants exposed to phenytoin alone.

DR. LEVY: It is interesting that valproic acid produces embryopathy because valproic acid has certain rather interesting metabolic effects in the individual. First, it elevates the blood ammonia level of those individuals who are taking rather large doses. Second, it elevates the blood glycine concentration. Third, it can produce at least a mild metabolic acidosis, which, of course, would relate to the theory that lowering of the intracellular pH might be the reason for the embryopathy. But it raises the question in my mind as to whether women with inborn errors of metabolism that are associated with high ammonia levels or with hyperglycinemia are going to have children with embryopathic effects.

DR. HOLMES: That was the reason why I referred to the recent paper by Pauli et al in my presentation. Do you believe exposure to valproic acid produces a deficiency of carnitine?

DR. LEVY: I think it results from valproic acid ingestion and it could be directly related to the effects of valproic acid.

DR. QUINN: There are a number of ongoing studies investigating the efficacy of erythromycin therapy in the prevention of poor pregnancy outcome. What advice do you have regarding neonatal assessment of teratogenic effects in these exposed neonates? I am most concerned about studies in which patients are treated for eight months of gestation.

DR. HOLMES: I would suggest checking the data from the National Collaborative Perinatal Project published by Heinonen et al on the therapeutic use of erythromycin in pregnancy. However, I would predict they do not have information on exposure for eight months of pregnancy.

DR. QUINN: In our erythromycin study, one of the caveats required was that we follow these children to six years of age. We had great difficulty designing a comprehensive neonatal follow-up that would be subtle enough to pick up teratogenic effects when we don't know what we are looking for.

DR. HOLMES: Clinical follow-up studies are labor-intensive, but will provide some reassurance. I suggest these be kept simple and focused on birth weight, length, head-size, the presence/absence of major malformations and a minimal number of minor physical features. An examination protocol should be used employing a small number of examiners who should be kept blind as to whether the child under examination was an exposed one or a control.

DR. SCARPELLI: Are any of the metabolites of phenytoin capable of binding to DNA?

DR. HOLMES: I am not aware that anyone has studied that.

DR. NAEYE: There is a greater than expected number of children with cerebral palsy and lesser neurologic abnormalities whose mothers had seizure disorders. Could you speculate on whether these neurologic abnormalities are due to drugs used to control the seizures, fetal asphyxia during the maternal seizures or to genetic disorders that can express both as seizures and as other neurologic abnormalities?

DR. HOLMES: I am not aware of any study that shows a harmful effect from having seizures during pregnancy. In our ongoing study we are comparing the phenotypic features of three groups of infants--infants exposed to epilepsy medication, infants whose mothers have had epilepsy in the past, and unexposed control infants. At this point in the study there appears to be an effect only in the first group. We will not know unless we follow the children for several years how many in each group are considered to have "cerebral palsy". Furthermore, our sample size may not be large enough.

DR. SEVER: Let me reaffirm the importance and difficulty of making epidemiologic associations. In the Collaborative Study, which was conducted between 1960 and 1966, we were able to study the rubella epidemic which occurred in 1964. During that year we had 6,000 pregnant women in the study and were able to identify with certainty 135 women who had rubella. When we looked at specific defects, such as eye damage, heart defects and so forth, we could not find an association with rubella. When we combined the defects of the congenital rubella syndrome, however, we did find the association with rubella. It is really very difficult to make an epidemiologic association if defects are considered individually.

DR. HOLMES: I agree. In evaluating "mild teratogens", like phenytoin, some phenotypic effects can be identified at birth while others are identifiable only when the child is old enough to have developmental assessments and more sophisticated examinations, such as evaluation of craniofacial development.

DR. V. ANDERSON: Are there any clues in the mothers themselves?

DR. HOLMES: We are looking into the issue of family resemblance by assessing facial features in frontal and lateral views in photographs of the infants and both parents in all three groups of infants. We have not found any other correlations in the mothers of infants with the phenytoin embryopathy, such as a higher frequency of gum hyperplasia. We plan to carry out studies of phenytoin metabolism to look for markers of greater genetic susceptibility in certain families.

DR. SMITH: I was wondering about your examination of the retina.

DR. HOLMES: That was listed as a general slide outlining the types of evaluations that could be done in follow-up studies. We are not doing that in children who have been exposed to phenytoin *in utero*.

DR. SMITH: Studies with mice exposed to a very low dose of a DNA alkylating agent such as MNU during pregnancy have shown the late onset of retinal degeneration in their offspring.

DR. HOLMES: I believe follow-up studies are necessary on all human teratogens with an evaluation that is sufficiently thorough to uncover new correlations. Tomorrow we will hear, I suspect, about the effects of DES on adult social behavior, a good example of the importance of long-term follow-up.

Transplacental Effects on Fetal Health, pages 193–202

DEVELOPMENTAL TOXICITY OF SYNTHETIC RETINOIDS IN HUMANS

Edward J. Lammer

California Birth Defects Monitoring Program,
Berkeley, California 94703

INTRODUCTION

Synthetic derivatives of retinol (vitamin A) have been exploited for their potential benefits in the treatment of chronic skin disorders and cancers, and as potential chemopreventive agents for cancers. Only two of these agents have been approved for marketing in the United States. Isotretinoin (13-cis-retinoic acid) was approved for treatment of severe cystic acne in September 1982. Etretinate was approved for treatment of severe recalcitrant psoriasis in November 1986 (FDA 1986). At the time of their initial marketings, it was known that both of these compounds were teratogenic in experimental animals. Both drugs were labelled as "contraindicated for use during pregnancy". Concerns about the potential for human teratogenicity were not unfounded. Clinical and epidemiologic studies have provided substantial evidence for isotretinoin teratogenicity (Lammer et al 1985). A number of case reports from Europe of malformed fetuses and infants exposed to etretinate have recently appeared, suggesting that it is probably a human teratogen also (Happle et al 1984; Grote et al 1985).

To learn more about the risks of adverse outcomes following retinoid use, we began Phase I of the Longitudinal Study of Infants Exposed to Isotretinoin in Utero in May 1985. The purposes of the study were to improve the quantitative measures of risk for major malformation, to define the range of major malformations caused by isotretinoin, and to quantitate and define the risks of minor malformation, sensory deficits, hormonal deficiencies, and early growth problems. The exposed pregnancies were identified by contacts made with the manufacturer, the Food and Drug Administration, or a member of our research group. We have studied two populations of fetuses/infants whose mothers used isotretinoin in utero: 1) a prospectively ascertained cohort of exposed infants; and 2) a retrospectively ascertained case series of malformed, exposed fetuses/infants. The first group was composed of fetuses/infants born to mothers whose use of isotretinoin was reported to a member of the research group during the pregnancy itself. At the time that the exposed pregnancy was reported, there was no knowledge of the fetal outcome. The outcomes of the prospectively ascertained cohort of exposed pregnancies represent an unbiased spectrum of possible adverse effects associated with isotretinoin exposure. The retrospective group was composed of malformed infants who were identified after birth when the history of isotretinoin use during pregnancy was obtained. In general, these infants represent the severe end of the spectrum of possible outcomes.

RESULTS

Phase I of the study was completed in July 1987. Only a small part of the data analysis has been completed at this time. We reported on two of the adverse outcomes, abortion and major malformation, among the prospective cohort of exposed pregnancies at the annual meeting of the Teratology Society in May 1987 (Lammer et al 1987a). Among 57 exposed pregnancies, there were 9 spontaneous abortions, 1 malformed stillbirth, 10 malformed livebirths and 37 livebirths with no major malformations. The pattern of major malformation involved the embryogenesis of 4 structures: face and cranium, heart, thymus, and brain. Brain and craniofacial malformations occurred more frequently than cardiac or thymic defects. The specific types of major malformations have been described in more detail elsewhere (Lammer et al 1985; Lammer 1987). Among the craniofacial malformations, dysgenesis of the external ear and canal were most common. Micrognathia and midfacial underdevelopment were also common. Cleft palate was uncommon and was only found among retrospectively reported cases. Lammer et al (1987b) have also reported on the frequent occurrence of facial asymmetry among infants exposed to isotretinoin. The pattern of facial asymmetry differed from that described in oculoauriculo-vertebral dysplasia (Goldenhar syndrome) and similar disorders. Among exposed infants who had congenital heart defects, the defects were categorized into 2 main mechanistic categories: abnormalities of aorticopulmonary septation and branchial arch mesenchymal tissue defects (Lammer et al 1985). We have found 5 different types of aorticopulmonary septation abnormalities: double outlet right ventricle, D-transposition of the great vessels, tetralogy of Fallot, truncus arteriosus communis, and supracristal ventricular septal defects. We have also found thymic dysmorphogenesis (ectopia, hypoplasia, aplasia) among exposed infants with or without congenital heart defects. The central nervous system malformations cover a wide spectrum of problems: hydrocephaly, microcephaly, macro- and micro-dysgenesis of the cerebellum, and cranial nerve deficits. In general, cerebellar development appears to be much more susceptible to the adverse effects of isotretinoin than does the cerebral cortex. At least 4 types of hydrocephalus have been found (Lammer et al 1985). Cranial nerve deficits have involved cranial nerves 2, 3, 4, 7, and 8.

In general, the types of malformations found among infants exposed to isotretinoin resembled those induced by retinoids in a number of different experimental animal species (Kochhar 1967; Shenefelt 1972; Geelen 1979; Wilhite et al 1986). Although retinoids have been used to induce neural tube and limb reduction defects in experimental animals, no infants have been born with limb reduction defects following isotretinoin exposure recently. One child with spina bifida has been identified (personal communication, JF Atkin). In contrast, both neural tube and limb reduction defects have been reported following etretinate exposure during or before pregnancy (Happle et al 1984; Grote et al 1985). The similarity between the patterns of malformation among human cases and the experimental animal models suggested that the pathogenetic mechanisms were likely to be similar. It was hypothesized that the craniofacial, cardiac and thymic malformations resulted from adverse effects on cranial neural crest cells (Lammer et al 1985). This hypothesis was supported by experimental studies (Webster et al 1986; Goulding and Pratt 1986) that showed a direct interference with development of cranial neural crest cells. Deficiency of crest cell-derived mesenchyme and abnormal crest cell interactions with other cell populations (inductive activities) explain most of the non-CNS malformations induced by isotretinoin. Sulik et al (1987) have also hypothesized that isotretinoin adversely affects epibranchial placodal cells and that some of the craniofacial malformations may result from abnormalities of that cell population. A direct effect on that cell population, however, was not demonstrated in their study and it remains unclear whether the excess cell death in the region of the placodes involved neural crest-derived cells or placodal-derived cells.

It is possible, and probable, that cell populations other than cranial neural crest are susceptible to isotretinoin. However, neuroectodermally derived cells, especially from the rhombencephalic area of the neural tube, appear to be particularly susceptible to retinoids during embryogenesis. The factors that determine susceptibility remain unknown but they may be related to properties of cell populations with migratory activity. In addition, the distribution and concentration of cellular retinoic acid binding protein (RABP) or retinoid receptors may be important in determining susceptibility.

DISCUSSION

Fetal exposure to synthetic retinoids increases the risk for a characteristic pattern of malformation. It does not increase the risk for all malformations. Although a common link between craniofacial, cardiac and thymic malformations may not be obvious, there is a substantial amount of experimental evidence that cranial neural crest cells are involved in the morphogenesis of all three structures. The neural crest contributes mesenchyme and inductively interacts with other cell populations during the morphogenesis of those structures. We know little about which other neuroectodermal cell populations are susceptible to retinoids, but the neuroepithelium from the area of the developing rhombencephalon seems more susceptible than more cephalic areas of the neural tube.

The molecular pathogenesis of the malformations is unclear. There is experimental evidence that retinoids can promote cell differentiation, alter cell migration, affect DNA synthesis and cell proliferation, and alter normal patterns of programmed cell death. Any of these pathogenetic mechanisms might contribute to the induction of structural malformations. Studying the patterns and natural history of retinoid-induced malformations and synthesizing that information with the findings of experimental models should continue to yield more information about normal and abnormal human embryogenesis. For example, a number of human craniofacial syndromes were previously attributed to quantitative deficiencies of cranial neural crest cells. Recently, the work of Sulik et al (1987) concerning the pathogenesis of mandibulofacial dysostosis raised questions about whether that disorder is a primary neurocristopathy. Those authors hypothesized that mandibulofacial dysostosis might result from a primary abnormality of epibranchial placodal cells or their interaction with cranial neural crest cells. In addition, Lammer et al (1987b) emphasized that the facial asymmetry and associated major and minor craniofacial malformations in the human retinoic acid embryopathy do not resemble the pattern reported in oculoauriculo-vertebral dysplasia or Goldenhar syndrome. Assuming that oculoauriculo-vertebral dysplasia and related syndromes result from primary defects of cranial neural crest, this suggests that the underlying crest cell abnormality is different from the effects induced by isotretinoin. The opportunity exists to use the experimental models of retinoid teratogenesis to learn more about the role that vitamin A (retinol) and all-trans-retinoic acid play in normal embryogenesis. Recently, Thaller and Eichele (1987) presented evidence that all-trans-retinoic acid may be a morphogen in the developing limb bud. They found that retinoic acid formed a concentration gradient across the limb anlage, with the highest concentration near the part of the limb bud where the zone of polarizing activity is located. Others (Kwarta et al 1985) have identified CRABP within the mouse limb bud, although it is unknown whether its concentration varies regionally within the limb bud. Dencker et al (1987) reported that radiolabelled retinoic acid specifically accumulated in neurectodermal cells and in presumptive cranial neural crest cells of early mouse embryos, but only during restricted periods of development. The temporal and tissue-specific presence of CRABP and accumulation of retinoic acid within embryos suggest that retinoids play an important role in controlling pattern formation and other aspects of the morphogenesis of many structures of vertebrate embryos. Another interesting recent development is the hypothesis of Nau and Scott (1986) that acidity may be a very important property for teratogenesis. Because the pH of early embryos is higher than the pH of maternal serum, weak acids will accumulate to higher concentrations in the embryo compared to maternal serum. Since isotretinoin is a weak acid, it is possible that this physio-chemical property may contribute to its high teratogenic risk. Kraft et al (1987) have also shown that all-trans-retinoic acid accumulates in mouse embryos whose mothers were exposed to 13-cis-retinoic acid during pregnancy. The importance of the acidic nature of 13-cis-retinoic acid and its maternal-fetal metabolism to human teratogenicity is unknown. All of these areas will be important avenues for future research in retinoid teratogenesis. Continued work in this rapidly developing focus of research should help to elucidate some of the roles of retinoids in normal and abnormal embryogenesis.

REFERENCES

Dencker L, d'Argy R, Danielsson BRG, Ghantous H, Sperber GO (1987). Saturable accumulation of retinoic acid in neural and neural crest derived cells in early embryonic development. Dev Pharmacol Ther 10:212-23.

FDA (1986). Etretinate approved. FDA Drug Bulletin; November:16-17.

Geelen JAG (1979). Hypervitaminosis A induced teratogenesis. CRC Crit Rev Toxicol 6:351-75.

Goulding EH, Pratt RM (1986). Isotretinoin teratogenicity in mouse whole embryo culture. J Craniofacial Genet Dev Biol 6:99-112.

Grote W, Harms D, Janig U, Kietzmann H, Ravens U, Schwarze I (1985). Malformation of fetus conceived 4 months after termination of maternal etretinate treatment. Lancet ii:1276.

Happle R, Traupe H, Bounameaux Y, Fisch T (1984). Teratogene wurkung von etretinat beim menschen. Deutsche Med Wochenschr 109:1476-80.

Kochhar DM (1967). Teratogenic activity of retinoic acid. Acta Pathol Microbiol Scand 70:398-404.

Kraft JC, Kochhar DM, Scott WJ, Nau H (1987). Low teratogenicity of 13-cis-retinoic acid (isotretinoin) in the mouse corresponds to low embryo concentrations during organogenesis: Comparison to the all-transisomer. Toxicol Appl Pharm 87:474-82.

Kwarta RJ Jr., Kimmel CA, Kimmel GL, Slikker W Jr. (1985). Identification of the cellular retinoic acid binding protein (CRABP) within the embryonic mouse (CD-1) limb bud. Teratology 32:103-11.

Lammer EJ (1987). Patterns of malformation among fetuses and infants exposed to retinoic acid (isotretinoin). In McLachlan JA, Pratt RM, Markert CL, (eds.): Banbury Report 26. "Developmental Toxicology: Mechanisms and Risk". Cold Spring Harbor Laboratory, pp. 243-55.

Lammer EJ, Chen DT, Hoar RM, Agnish ND, Benke PJ, Braun JT, Curry CJ, Fernhoff PM, Grix AW, Lott IT, Richard JM, Sun SC (1985). Retinoic acid embryopathy. N Engl J Med 313:837-41.

Lammer EJ, Hayes AM, Schunior A, Holmes LB (1987a). Risk for major malformation among human fetuses exposed to isotretinoin (13-cis-retinoic acid). Teratology 35:68A.

Lammer EJ, Hayes AM, Schunior A, Holmes LB (1987b). Facial asymmetry in retinoic acid embryopathy. Presented at the March of Dimes Clinical Genetics Conference on the Neural Crest and Craniofacial Disorders, Minneapolis, July 19-22.

Nau H, Scott WJ (1986). Weak acids may act as teratogens by accumulating in the basic milieu of the early mammalian embryo. Nature 323:276-8.

Shenefelt RE (1972). Morphogenesis of malformations in hamsters caused by retinoic acid: Relation to dose and stage at treatment. Teratology 5:103-18.

Sulik KK, Johnston MC, Smiley SJ, Speight HS, Jarvis BE (1987). Mandibulofacial dysostosis (Treacher Collins syndrome): a new proposal for its pathogenesis. Am J Med Genet 27:359-72.

Thaller C, Eichele G (1987). Identification and spatial distribution of retinoids in the developing chick limb bud. Nature 327:625-8.

Webster WS, Johnston MC, Lammer EJ, Sulik KK (1986). Isotretinoin embryopathy and the cranial neural crest: an in vivo and in vitro study. J Craniofacial Genet Dev Biol 6:211-222.

Wilhite CC, Hill RM, Irving DM (1986). Isotretinoin-induced craniofacial malformations in humans and hamsters. J Craniofacial Genet Dev Biol Suppl 2:193-209.

Acknowledgement: Maureen Torres provided excellent technical assistance with the manuscript.

DISCUSSION

DR. OSBURN: I assume that the major thymic defect is the absence of the epithelial component of the thymus?

DR. LAMMER: Often the thymus is totally absent.

DR. SCARPELLI: We know that vitamin A has important effects on the programming of differentiation. Does the vitamin A have toxic effects or does it actually affect differentiation?

DR. LAMMER: People are actively investigating those ideas now. I think both of those ideas (effects on differentiation and toxic effects) are probably tenable. In the experimental model developed by Kathy Sulik, there are cytoplasmic blebs of many presumptive cranial neural crest cells. That certainly would affect a cell's ability to migrate, since it would not be able to recycle its plasma membrane. The blebbing may be a direct cytotoxic effect of the retinoid on the composition of the cell membrane. Regarding retinoid effects on cell differentiation, we have some evidence from looking at the pattern of ear malformations among isotretinoin-exposed children that the drug may affect pattern formation. That is, isotretinoin alters the positional information of some of the ectomesenchymal cells that are forming the external ear. It alters their positional information in a way that produces duplications of parts of the external ear. Our current speculation is that this process may be similar to the way that retinoids alter cell positional information in regenerating amphibians' limbs and in embryonic chick limb bud cultures that are exposed to these compounds during critical periods of development. We speculate that these ear malformations may result from an alteration of cell position along the axis of the branchial arches.

DR. SCARPELLI: So these are spatial alterations?

DR. LAMMER: Yes, abnormalities of spatial orientation. I would guess that such abnormalities could result from an effect of this drug on cell differentiation.

DR. NAEYE: I wonder what the possibilities are for subtle neurologic abnormalities, particularly those that are first detected long after the neonatal period, often after 1 year of age? Many neurologic abnormalities fit into this category, some caused by antenatal hypoxia and others of unidentified factors that operate in embryonic life.

DR. LAMMER: Your comment is appropriate. A drug that causes major malformations of the brain should certainly be suspected of causing abnormalities that are more subtle. The data that I presented are only a small part of the data that we have accumulated. Basically, I presented only the outcomes of spontaneous abortion and of major malformations. We are still analyzing our data with regard to risks for minor birth defects, hormone deficiencies, growth problems, etc. We have planned a second phase of the study that would assess intellectual function, behavior problems, attention deficit disorders, and similar kinds of problems.

Isotretinoin was first released for human use in late 1982. So, exposed children are still very young. Many of the intelligence and behavioral assessments will be much more predictive of future function if we wait and apply them at age 4-5. In Phase I of this study, the participants were different ages, between 6 months and 3 years when we examined them. It would be very difficult to assess more subtle behavioral outcomes over this age range.

DR. NAEYE: It might also be useful to look for possible relationships between drugs used in pregnancy and the sudden infant death syndrome (SIDS) because the evidence is mounting that SIDS has its roots in brain stem injury during fetal life.

DR. LAMMER: We are currently reviewing the microscopic neuropathology findings from about 16 of these isotretinoin-exposed children who have died. There are a number of abnormalities in the brain stem. We hope to present those results within the next year.

DR. OSTER-GRANITE: I suggest that the common cerebellar malformations and neural crest malformations may share a common developmental mechanism that produces the phenotype.

DR. LAMMER: Yes, that is a good point. Another idea that attempts to explain why cerebellar development and cranial neural crest cells are so susceptible to retinoids assumes that both cell populations share some common properties. In fact, the ectodermal cells that will give rise to the cerebellum and the portion of the cranial neural crest that will migrate into the developing branchial arches are contiguous prior to neurulation and the onset of crest cell migration. One idea is that, perhaps, there is some property that is common both to the cells that are destined to be cerebellar and those that are to become ectomesenchymal. One of the provocative ideas at this time involves an intracellular protein called cellular retinoic acid binding protein. Embryonic cells that are susceptible to retinoids may be unique because, at a critical point in development, all of those cells may be synthesizing large amounts of that protein. The protein would concentrate retinoic acids in specific cells. This lead is under active investigation now.

DR. ROSA: I have a question about the normal exposures. Accutane, like Etretinate, was on the market around the world before it was marketed in the U.S. The Food and Drug Administration (FDA) has accumulated birth defects reports on Etretinate from around the world. FDA has accumulated over 100 reports on birth defects and spontaneous abortion caused by Accutane. All of these reports are from the U.S. and Canada, but we have no reports from outside North America. You have twice as much data on the so-called normal outcomes than I have. Have you examined the dosage and the timing of the exposure to see if a lower dose explains normal outcomes?

DR. LAMMER: This is still under study. It is a slow process because we are trying to be very thorough and we are using multiple sources of information about the exposure events so that we can reconstruct precise and accurate exposure windows. One difficulty is obtaining pharmacy data for women who took isotretinoin during pregnancy. It is very difficult to obtain pharmacy records that are several years old. Yet that data is very valuable for confirming isotretinoin dosages and the date on which the mother probably started taking the medication. So, we are still trying to collect these multiple sources of exposure information and will synthesize an exposure interval for each of the exposed pregnancies in the near future.

Transplacental Effects on Fetal Health, pages 203–226

THE DEVELOPMENT OF THE BRAIN AND TERATOGENESIS

Mary Lou Oster-Granite

Developmental Genetics Laboratory, The Johns Hopkins University School of Medicine, 725 N. Wolfe Street, Baltimore, MD 21205

INTRODUCTION

The development of the central nervous system is a protracted process, spanning a considerable portion of gestation and, in some mammals, of postnatal life. In altricial mammals, much brain development occurs postnatally, while in precocial mammals, this development occurs _in utero_. While critical periods of development in specific brain regions are identified readily, the exact timing of these developmental stages relative to postconception age varies among mammalian species. The purpose of this review is to indicate the relative timing of such critical developmental events in mammals, and to indicate some of the mechanisms by which specific metabolic, drug, and chemical teratogens may exert their deleterious effects at those critical developmental stages.

Generally, three critical periods of development may be identified: neurulation, cell proliferation and migration, and cell differentiation and survival. The duration of the latter two critical periods varies within regions of the central nervous system and among specific cell types. During neurulation, the forming central nervous system is isolated from the amniotic cavity and the peripheral nervous system is established. During the period of cell proliferation and migration, principal or output neurons and interneurons or local circuit neuron populations are established and migrate to their final locations within the neuraxis. During the period of cell differentiation and survival, patterns of synaptogenesis are established and programmed cell death eliminates substantial numbers of neurons in specific cell populations.

NEURULATION

During gastrulation, three distinct tissues, the ectoderm, mesoderm, and endoderm are derived from the epiblast; become specified; and initiate interspecific tissue interactions that result in organogenesis. With the appearance of mesodermal cells migrating into the primitive streak, cell position helps to establish separate, distinctive mesodermal cell populations. Most important to the subsequent development of the nervous system is the formation of the notochord and the paraxial mesoderm. The establishment of the notochord creates a central axial core of cells extending from the primitive streak to the bucopharyngeal (stomodeal) membrane. It also establishes the bilateral symmetry of the embryo. When somite formation is initiated in the paraxial mesoderm, the adjacent and overlying ectoderm is induced to neurulate. During neurulation, the nervous system becomes separated and eventually isolated from the surface ectoderm and from the amniotic cavity. In mammals and other species, neurulation occurs in two distinct phases, denoted as primary and secondary neurulation (Gordon, 1985; Lemire et al., 1975; O'Shea, 1986; Schoenwolf, 1982).

Primary neurulation is characterized by the formation of a continuous cylinder of epithelial cells. In this process, the cuboidal ectoderm overlying the notochord and paraxial mesoderm is induced to change its shape and its rate of proliferation. With these changes, the neuroepithelium loses its cobblestone appearance (O'Shea, 1986). Changes in the number and distribution of microtubules are important features of the elongation of the cells, and the appearance of microfilaments in the apical cell cytoplasm is associated with a constriction of the apical surface to produce a wedge-shaped cell (Karfunkel, 1974). Whether these elements produce the change in cell shape or reflect cytoplasmic alterations produced by mesenchymal expansion, increased intercellular adhesion, or alterations in cell volume is still controversial (O'Shea, 1986). Certainly there is evidence in amphibian systems that membranes and intercellular adhesive properties are very important in this shape change process (Jacobson et al., 1986). These changes are characteristic of dynamic epithelial cell surfaces and are sufficient to create and maintain the integrity of the apical seal while permitting much intra- and intercellular movement. Nonetheless, these changes in cell shape indicate induction of the ectoderm to form the neural plate, a pseudostratified columnar or wedge-shaped epithelium.

With constriction of the apical surfaces of the cells in the midline, and possibly the dynamic constriction and movement of cells on the lateral aspect of the neural tube, the neural plate is transformed into a neural groove. With further constriction, the lateral edges of the neural groove become apposed and eventually fuse, creating a neural tube. Closure first occurs at the level of the fourth somite and proceeds cranially and caudally.

The actual cell populations that effect apposition and eventual fusion vary within portions of the central nervous system. Within the developing brain, for example, neuroepithelial cells (forebrain), surface ectoderm (midbrain), or both (hindbrain) may make the first contact. In the trunk region, it is a zone of flattened cells between the neuroepithelium and surface ectoderm that makes first contact (O'Shea, 1986). This process is mediated in part by changes in the carbohydrate and glycosylaminoglycan composition of the cell surfaces (McLone and Knepper, 1985-6). In addition to the elaboration of a thick carbohydrate cell surface coat and the appearance of specific cell adhesion molecules, lamellopodia and filopodia appear on the surface of the appositional cells facilitating their interdigitation (O'Shea, 1986).

This process of cell shape change, apposition and fusion is critical to the formation of major portions of the central nervous system - the brain and the spinal cord through the upper lumbar region. While closure proceeds sequentially, apposition of the neural folds may not be continuous throughout the length of the neural tube. Some regions become apposed more slowly, and others become apposed so tightly that the lumen of the neural tube is obliterated for short periods of time (O'Shea, 1986). In the cranial portion of the neural tube, a marked differentiation of the forebrain (encephalization) begins before closure is completed and alters appositional relationships (Lemire et al., 1975). With the formation of the neural tube, the open ends of the tube are designated as neuropores. The anterior neuropore closes when there are approximately 18-23 somites (day 25 postconception in human beings) and the posterior neuropore closes when there are approximately 24-28 somites (several days later). In mice, this process of primary neurulation occurs over a 36 hour period (stage 15) beginning on day 8 of gestation (day 0 = copulation plug date).

As closure of the anterior neural tube proceeds, a distinctive basal lamina is established that separates the neuroepithelium and underlying mesenchyme. This basal lamina is thought to act as a scaffolding for morphogenetic cell shape changes, as a functional barrier, and as a barrier to cell migration by the neuroepithelium (O'Shea, 1986). This barrier encapsulates the neuroepithelium, except at places of imminent neural crest cell migration. The neural crest arises from a population of ectodermal cells adjacent to the neural tube, which initiate migration between the neural tube and the somite, or in some cases through the somites to establish the pluripotent forerunners of many different peripheral cell types, but most importantly, of the peripheral nervous system.

Formation of the lumbar and sacral regions of the spinal cord utilizes an entirely different morphogenetic process (secondary neurulation) to create a continuous closed tube. In the area caudal to the primitive streak, mesenchymal cells migrate, aggregate, epithelialize, and fuse with the neuroepithelium of the closing posterior neuropore region (O'Shea, 1986; Schoenwolf, 1984). The actual morphogenetic events of epithelialization during secondary neurulation differ between mammalian and avian species. In mammals, solid cores of cells become associated with the posterior neuropore, develop intercellular junctions and form lumina secondarily that are continuous with the neural tube lumen. In avian species, multiple cyst-like cell aggregations form in cells abundantly interconnected by gap junctions and become interconnected as a ventral or secondary neuroepithelium. Mammals appear to lack an overlap between the primary and secondary neuroepithelia, and the addition of cells to the caudal neuroepithelium occurs continuously (Schoenwolf, 1984). Perhaps as a result, closure of the posterior neuropore is essential to the creation of a closed caudal neural tube in mammals.

With completion of the formation of the neural tube through the coccygeal regions, important remodeling occurs in the terminal part of the spinal cord as the tail regresses, a process called retrogression. During retrogression, the distal spinal cord and its meningeal covers are reshaped to create the conus medullaris, the filum terminale, and the cauda equina. This remodeling process, which begins at about 38 days of gestation in human beings, continues until some time after birth (Lemire et al., 1975). After the fifth month of gestation this process also involves differential growth of the vertebral column relative to the spinal cord itself. Differential growth and positional relationships occur to produce a spinal cord that ends at S_{1-2} at birth and that stabilizes at around S_1 during the first postnatal year.

CELL PROLIFERATION AND MIGRATION

To accomplish the events of neurulation, cell proliferation and migration are essential. Once the neural tube is established, however, a second phase of proliferation and migration transforms the initial pseudocolumnar neuroepithelium into a functional stratified epithelium. During this transitional process, three distinct layers are formed in the neuroepithelium: the ventricular zone, adjacent to the lumen of the neural tube; the mantle zone, a cell rich layer just internal to the ventricular zone; and a cell poor, but process rich zone, the marginal layer. The processes involved are discussed in numerous texts, e.g. Purves and Lichtman (1985).

This epithelial transformation is accomplished in large part by the geometric generation of postmitotic daughter cells. One of the daughter cells ceases mitosis, detaches from the luminal cells, and migrates towards the abluminal (or pial) layer. Such detached cells create a new zone, the mantle zone, comprised initially of postmitotic neurons, and later, additionally, of proliferative astrocytes and oligodendrocytes. The neuroblasts begin to differentiate and to elaborate axons and dendrites. Their axons enter the marginal layer to travel cranially and/or caudally into regions of the developing neuraxis, or to exit the neuraxis altogether.

The developing spinal cord retains this simple arrangement in the adult. The ventricular zone becomes the ependymal layer; the mantle zone, the gray matter; and the marginal zone, the white matter. Differential cell division within the spinal cord converts these concentrically arranged layers into the characteristic external white matter and internal butterfly-shaped gray matter of the adult spinal cord. This is accomplished in part by sequential differential proliferation ventrally, then dorsally. Cells proliferating ventrally give rise in part to principal or output neurons whose axons traverse the marginal zone to exit the spinal cord in the ventral rootlets. Proliferative activity in the dorsal portion of the mantle zone creates the neurons and interneurons that mediate transduction of sensory information. Axons of the principal neuron component of these cells ramify to establish synaptic interactions with neurons in the nearby ventral spinal cord and eventually with distant synaptic relay targets.

Portions of the brain, however, rearrange the simple three-layered pattern of the spinal cord. This is brought about in part because additional changes occur in the relative positions of cell groups, in the proportions of dorsal and ventral cells, in portions of the cranial neural tube, and in the size of the lumen associated with specific developing brain regions. Differential cell division, the establishment of extraventricular zones of mitotic activity, and directed cell migration contribute to this process.

While differential mitotic activity generates principal neurons and interneurons in various regions of the brain, not all neurons arise from the ventricular zone. Early in encephalization, though, changes in the luminal size of the central canal of the cranial neural tube arise in part because of differential mitotic activity in the ventral zone. Such size and shape changes permit distinction of first three and then five brain vesicles. The three primitive brain vesicles are the forebrain or prosencephalon, the midbrain or mesencephalon, and the hindbrain or rhombencephalon. Subsequent subdivision of both the prosencephalon and rhombencephalon create the five final brain vesicles: the telencephalon, diencephalon, mesencephalon, metencephalon, and myelencephalon. With rapid cell proliferation and elongation of the cranial neural tube, a thin, straight cylinder is transformed into a flexed structure with characteristic dilations. Within the walls of this externally complex structure, ventricular, mantle, and marginal zones become established.

For encephalization to continue appropriately, secondary replicative zones, subjacent to the ventricular zone, must now develop. Cells in these extraventricular regions may be generated either geometrically or exponentially. Two particularly important extraventricular proliferative zones are the external germinal layer of the cerebellum, derived from the rhombic lip of the metencephalon, and the subventricular zone of the telencephalon.

The rhombic lip represents an expanded germinal zone associated with ventricular neuroepithelium of the dorsal metencephalon. It gives rise to the principal neurons and interneurons of the vestibular, auditory, and cortical relay nuclei of the adult medulla and pons, and all the neurons of the cerebellum. Importantly, the rhombic lip generates a population of motile neuroblasts that retain their proliferative ability after they migrate to the pial surface of the cerebellar anlage. Exponential proliferation of neurons from this external germinal layer is essential to ensure continued development and differentiation of cells in the cerebellar cortex. Once generated, postmitotic granular neurons migrate radially in an outside-in direction to their final location in the internal granular layer of the cerebellar cortex.

The subventricular zone of the telencephalon is a similar secondary proliferative center, but is established adjacent to the ventricular zone. First principal, then interneurons, of various neocortical regions arise from these contiguous germinative zones. The inside-out migration pattern of the postmitotic cells places progressively younger neuron populations nearer to the cortical pial surface. Depending on the location of the cells within the ventricular or subventricular zone, specific cell populations may arise by geometric or exponential generation.

It is important to realize that the generation of cells in the neuraxis differs from that in other tissues in two significant respects. First, the duration of generation for particular neuron populations is highly variable. Principal or output neurons are usually generated over a very short time interval. In mice this may mean a matter of days; in human beings, a matter of weeks. Interneurons, on the other hand, may undergo quite protracted generation. In mice this may mean a matter of weeks; in human beings, months or occasionally years. Second, generation of principal neurons and interneurons in a given region usually occurs sequentially and exponentially; it may also occur sequentially and geometrically, as is the case with the neurons of Ammon's horn and the dentate gyrus in the developing hippocampal formation. Additionally, the number of principal neurons formed may dictate the final number of interneurons of specific types that are generated or persist. Some neuron populations appear to exist as numerically specific functional units whose number is dictated by the number of principal neurons present. Thus, the vulnerability of specific neuron populations to teratogenic agents and the pattern of disruption that results depend upon the timing and duration of the insult itself. Insults occurring in conjunction with principal neuron formation may exert more catastrophic effects than those occurring in conjunction with the formation of interneuron populations.

Once generated, most neurons migrate to a final location within the neuraxis. Usually, such migration is directed radially, either inside-out, or outside-in, in the vicinity of the cell's birthplace in a generative zone (Ramon y Cajal, 1929). For many cell populations, this is accomplished by migration in association with other cells, the so-called radial glia (Levitt and Rakic, 1980; Rakic, 1971). Some cell populations, however, do not use this mechanism of migration and may undergo extensive cranial and caudal migration. Neurons generated by the rhombic lip, for example, may invade the entire expanse of both the pons and medulla. In some of these populations, migration is circumferential and associated with the pial surface; in others, it appears directed, but not radial.

Disruption of migration may result from alterations in the composition of the extracellular milieu, in recognition molecules on the cell surface, or in the timing of expression of specific molecules used for recognition between specific cells. Molecules implicated as particularly important in this process include substrate adhesion molecules, such as fibronectin and laminin; cell adhesion molecules, such as nCAMs and ngCAMs; various glycosylaminoglycans; and in the visual system, glycosyltransferases (Edelman, 1983; Roth et al., 1971; Toole, 1976).

An inability to complete migration successfully may result in cell death, a typical consequence of disrupted migration of external germinal cells, for example (Rakic and Sidman, 1973a,b). Alternatively, the ectopic cells may survive, in clusters called heterotopic rests. Such rests sometimes occur during the development of some principal neuron populations, particularly those which migrate long distances to reach their expected location within the neuraxis. Survival for such ectopic cells may be dictated in part by their ability to differentiate and to recognize and be recognized by appropriate synaptic targets.

CELL DIFFERENTIATION AND SURVIVAL

Once cells have reached their final destination, many portions of the neuraxis undergo a period of initial cell differentiation, when processes are elaborated and specific organelle systems become arranged in their adult configurations within the cell. This maturation period may involve the elaboration of a characteristic 3-dimensional array of dendrites, the elaboration of numerous, but highly localized, dendritic spines, and the development of pre- and postsynaptic specializations before or during synaptogenesis. Although synapse formation may occur appropriately between respective targets, such synaptic contact is not sufficient to ensure survival of neurons during the maturation process (Landmesser and Pilar, 1974).

Several interconnected neuronal systems undergo extensive cell death during the synaptogenetic period. This death may involve as many as half of the neurons of a given subset, and may serve to limit the diversity of synaptic connectivity occurring in a specific neuronal population (Purves and Lichtman, 1985). It may also be modified by the appearance of peptide factors which stimulate growth or differentiation, putative growth factors (Purves and Lichtman, 1985). Additionally, the premature or extensive removal of particular afferent cell populations can predispose certain populations to express novel cell markers or to continue to express markers that normally are expressed for only a short period of time during development (Forloni et al., 1987; Hohmann et al., 1987). Thus, neuronal number in development is not prespecified, but is rather determined by interaction and competition with other cells, modified by growth factors during critical developmental periods (Purves and Lichtman, 1985).

THE EFFECTS OF SPECIFIC TERATOGENIC AGENTS

Many metabolic insults, drugs, and chemical teratogens result in similar phenotypic effects in the central nervous system, i.e., mental retardation, cellular hypoplasia, etc. The actual mechanisms by which these agents affect nervous system development, however, may be quite different, and may serve to illustrate the limited avenues of response to exogenous teratogens that are available to cell populations in the developing embryo in general (Opitz, 1985). Importantly, one must realize that the tissues or cell populations in which particular morphologic changes are observed may not be the site of action of the teratogen. Such a different site was demonstrated elegantly by Johnson et al (1971) in their studies of influenza A virus infection of chickens. Here, the site of viral infection was not localized to the central nervous system, but to other embryonic and extraembryonic tissues. Similarly, the considerable number of studies by Brent and his colleagues (Leung, 1983) have demonstrated that various types of antibodies can interfere with the function of the visceral yolk sac early in mammalian development and thus cause embryonic malformations.

For a given agent to be considered teratogenic, Shepard (1986) suggests that it fulfill the following criteria: the agent must be present during the critical period of development, the agent should produce congenital defects in an experimental animal with a rate statistically higher in the treated group than the control animals receiving the same vehicle or sham procedure, and the agent in an unaltered state acts on the embryo/fetus directly or indirectly through the placenta. While thalidomide does not fit the third criterion, it is a teratogen, nevertheless.

Not all human teratogens have been identified as a result of catastrophic effects in human or test animal populations, although coumarin derivatives were shown to produce congenital warfarin embryopathy in the absence of animal experimentation (Kreber et al., 1968). At least 3 examples now exist of the results of teratogenicity studies in animals identifying human teratogens (Shepard, 1986). Valproic acid was suspected to be a teratogen before neural tube defects were observed in the offspring of epileptics (Robert and Guiband, 1982; Weinbaum et al., 1986). Hyperthermia was a suspected cause of congenital malformations of the central nervous system and eye in rodents as early as 1978 (Layde et al., 1980; Miller et al., 1978). Finally, isotretinoin, a form of retinoic acid or vitamin A, has been associated with craniofacial defects, and heart and hindbrain abnormalities in a variety of species (Lammer et al., 1985; Rosa, 1983).

Shepard (1986) and Schardein (1985) have reviewed the extensive literature on known, putative, and unlikely human teratogens. These agents may be summarized broadly as follows. Known human teratogens include radiation, infections, maternal metabolic imbalance, drugs, and environmental chemicals. Putative teratogens include cigarette smoking, Valium, zinc deficiency, taurine deficiency, excessive vitamin A, and varicella virus. Unlikely teratogens include aspirin, marihuana, LSD, anesthetics, antinauseants (Bendectin), oral contraceptives, rubella vaccine, video-display terminals, and ultrasound. Examples of each of these broad categories of teratogens and their known or suspected etiologic effects will be discussed and compared below.

Radiation

While mental retardation was known to result from x-irradiation as early as 1929 (Murphy, 1929), it was not until the atomic blasts of Hiroshima and Nagasaki that increased interest and research were devoted to its study (Ornoy and Yanai, 1980). Microcephaly, hydrocephalus, and mental retardation are common effects of *in utero* exposure; sensitivity appears greatest in exponentially dividing cell populations at particular developmental time points. In rodents, even low levels of irradiation, considered safe for adult or even the fetus in general, may produce slight structural and functional damage to the central nervous system. By selecting the developmental period of exposure, Altman and colleagues (Altman and Bayer, 1978; Bayer et al., 1973) could obtain selective lesions of specific cell populations in cerebellum or hippocampal formation, and generate specific behavioral sequaelae.

Infection

Among the infections most commonly producing effects within the central nervous system are rubella virus, cytomegalovirus, herpes virus hominis I and II, toxoplasmosis, parvoviruses, bluetongue virus vaccine, mumps virus, equine abortion virus, and Venezuelan equine encephalitis virus (Lemire et al., 1975; Oster-Granite, 1974; Shepard, 1986)). Other viral infections, although more rare, have also been studied extensively and mechanisms of effects ascertained. An excellent and comprehensive review of the effects of viral infections on the developing nervous system can be found in Johnson (1982). While placental infections, principally of syncytiotrophoblast cells, can produce malformations (i.e., cytomegalovirus and equine abortion virus), there is little evidence that exposure of the fetus to virus through the amniotic fluid or fetal circulation is of consequence unless susceptible fetal cells are present. Several specific mechanisms have been identified with respect to specific viruses. These include acute or chronic generalized encephalitis, chromosome alterations, mitotic inhibition, selective infection of specific cells (such as alterations in organogenesis by selective destruction of mitotic or undifferentiated cell populations), and obstructions of cerebrospinal fluid pathways and hydrocephalus. Examples of each of these mechanisms will be presented below.

Rubella virus. The threat of rubella virus epidemics has been almost eliminated by the licensing of the rubella vaccine in 1969. Unfortunately, the risk of fetal infection in non-immunized individuals is still greatest during the first trimester of pregnancy. The neurobiologic effects to the fetus are considerable, including eye defects (cataracts, retinopathy, microphthalmia, glaucoma, chorioretinitis), deafness, microcephaly, psychomotor retardation, and mental retardation. The effects of rubella virus are due to depression of mitotic activity in chronically infected cells (Rawls and Melnick, 1966), leading to organ hypocellularity (Naeye and Blanc, 1965). The principal neuropathologic effects appear to result from inflammatory vascular disease (Johnson, 1982).

Cytomegalovirus. Cytomegalovirus (CMV) is the most common known cause of mental retardation (Johnson, 1982), producing chorioretinitis, microphthalmia, optic atrophy, cerebral calcifications, microcephaly, microgyria, encephalomalacia, cerebral cysts, cerebellar aplasia and deafness (Hanshaw, 1970). While CMV infection may be "silent" at birth, the presence of symptoms in the neonatal period serves as a very strong predictor of neurologic sequaelae (Pass et al., 1980). Since CMV represents the most common form of fetal infection, recognition that CMV could be transmitted to the fetus (through extraembryonic tissues) when maternal infection had occurred more than one year before conception has considerably dampened hopes for an effective vaccine (Pass et al., 1986). Once a woman gives birth to an infant with congenital anomalies caused by CMV, a second such episode is rare (Embil et al., 1970).

Herpesvirus. Microcephaly and seizures, as well as microphthalmia, hypotonia, and periventricular and hippocampal calcifications characterize the alterations present in infants whose mothers were infected by type 1 or type 2 herpesvirus during the first few weeks of pregnancy (Florman et al., 1973; South et al., 1969)

Toxoplasmosis. While maternal infection with the parasite, _Toxoplasma_, may result in fever, transmission of the tissue cyst or oocyst to the fetus may result in hydrocephalus, hydrancephaly or microcephaly, chorioretinitis, convulsions, and cerebral calcifications (Lemire et al., 1975). Active congenital toxoplasmosis results in bilateral chorioretinitis with variable vision loss.

Parvoviruses. Several classes of mitolytic viruses have been identified. Perhaps the best studied are the parvoviruses, the smallest DNA viruses. Depending on the timing of infection in neonatal rodents, a spectrum of defects ranging from granuloprival cerebellar hypoplasia to obstructive hydrocephalus can be observed (Oster-Granite, 1974). The major mechanism of infection is selective destruction of mitotic or undifferentiated cell populations. While infection of forming neurons in the hippocampal formation and subventricular zone occurs with the parvoviruses, its greatest effects are manifest in those neuron populations undergoing exponential generation, such as the cerebellar granule cells. Selectivity is imparted by the gestational age at the time of infection.

Bluetongue Virus. Another example of selective mitolytic effects by viruses is illustrated by the midgestation infection of sheep by bluetongue virus as a live-virus vaccine (Johnson, 1982). In these animals, the subventricular zone of the developing cerebral cortex is particularly vulnerable to infection. Porencephalic cysts as well as neuronal heterotopias and hydrancephaly may result (Narayan and Johnson, 1972). In human beings, such alterations are usually thought to arise from vascular accidents (Johnson, 1982).

Mumps Virus. Infection of ependymal cells by mumps virus infection in animals and human beings may lead to aqueductal atresia and resultant non-communicating hydrocephalus (Johnson, 1982). Unlike the mitolytic viruses discussed above, the phenotype generated by mumps virus infection appears to be indistinguishable, irrespective of time of infection.

Maternal Metabolic Imbalance

Among the maternal metabolic imbalances adversely affecting the outcome of pregnancy are endemic cretinism, diabetes, PKU, virilizing tumors, alcoholism, and hyperthermia (Schardein, 1985; Shepard, 1986). As several of these causes of birth defects are discussed by other speakers at this Symposium, they will not be discussed in further detail here.

Drugs and Environmental Chemicals

Licit and illicit pharmacologic agents, as well as environmental chemicals, produce profound effects on fetal development. Among the best studied of these agents are androgenic hormones, diethylstilbesterol, antithyroid drugs, aminopterin and methylaminopterin, cyclophosphomide, floxuridine, busulfan, thalidomide, chlorobiphenyls, diazepan, barbiturates, diphenylhydantoin and trimethadione, valproic acid, coumarin anticoagulants, nicotine, ethanol, penicillamide, tetracyclines, 13-cis-retinoic acid (Accutane), inhalant anesthetics, and trace metals, such as organic mercury, lead, cadmium, and lithium. An excellent review of the teratogenic effects of many of these compounds appears in Schardein (1985).

Antimetabolites. A number of chemotherapeutic and antimitotic agents act as human teratogens. These include aminopterin and methylaminopterin, cyclophosphamide, floxuridine. Characteristic among the malformations associated with prenatal exposure to these agents include distinctive malformations of the skull that range from a clover-leaf appearance of the head with hydrocephalus to craniosynostosis. Ocular hypertelorism, wide nasal bridge, and malpositioned ears are also common features. Anencephaly, hydrocephalus, meningomyelocoele, and hypoplasia are common neurologic features, and those individuals surviving birth have variable mental skills. While skeletal abnormalities frequently accompany the neurologic defects observed, they are no more distinctive. One major risk with these types of agents is that they should not be administered in the perinatal period or during infancy. Such administration could be directly deleterious to the continued development of the cerebellar cortex, whose external germinal layer continues to proliferate rapidly for 12-18 months postnatally in human beings.

Anticonvulsants. Anticonvulsants such as hydantoin, trimethadione, barbital, primidone, and valproate have been linked with birth defects. Their effects on fetal development are probably related to effects on folate metabolism, through reduction of polyamine levels (Schardein, 1985). Like fetal alcohol syndrome, fetal anticonvulsant syndromes consist of at least three symptom clusters, facial dysmorphogenesis, growth retardation and mental subnormality (Vorhees, 1986). In rodents, those animals surviving to birth exhibit significant hyperactivity, which could not be correlated with enhanced rates of learning. No reduction, however, could be detected in brain protein or in brain weight, and no gross pathological changes were observed (Vorhees, 1986).

Inhalant Anesthetics. Rodier (1986) examined the effects of nitrous oxide and halothane in pre- and postnatal rodents to determine whether selective vulnerability was related to changes in mitotic activity of affected cells. Prenatal exposure to nitrous oxide or halothane did have permanent effects on brain morphology, but these changes were not the result of mitotic arrest. Nitrous oxide treatment causes reduction in Purkinje cells if administered at a period just after they have formed. Postnatal exposure reduces the number of granule cells and produces a granuloprival cortex with normal numbers of Purkinje cells. Lane et al (1980, 1981) found the same pattern of deficits when these anesthetics were compared for their ability to induce malformations during organogenesis. No direct correlation was found between level of anesthesia and teratogenicity. Other studies (Smith, 1974; Barnard, 1966) indicate that halothane and similar drugs produce cell death by inhibiting enzymes in the electron transport chain, while nitrous oxide may generate hyponitrite ion, which combines with ferrihemes to induce DNA damage.

Organic Mercury. The cellular effect of mercury is to alter cell proliferative rate during embryogenesis (Chen et al., 1979). Methylmercury, unlike its inorganic counterparts, is distributed widely in the mammalian body (Mottet, 1981), and readily crosses the placenta. With the revelation that methylmercury was involved as the causative agent in the defects observed in children with Minamata disease (Takeuchi, 1968), teratologists began to research actively the effects of mercury on fetal development. Based on a large number of studies, it now appears that this decreased proliferative rate results from its limitation of energy metabolism in cells; the action of mercurials appears to be on the sulfhydryl groups of enzymes, rather than on specific denaturation of enzymes.

Lead. Lead has no known nutritional value to mammals (Mottet, 1981; de la Cruz and Oster-Granite, 1988), and exposure to toxic levels of lead represents a significant medical risk for children in many inner city areas. Irrespective of the timing of administration, lead salts are deleterious to developing tissues, principally through their effects on mitochondria function (Goyer, 1971). In mammals, lead produces an encephalopathy that results from the direct increase of lead levels in cerebral tissues (Baudin et al., 1975). When administered during critical periods of cerebellar development, increased necrosis of the external germinal layer was observed with delayed maturation of Purkinje cells (Press, 1977).

Cadmium. Like the mercurials, cadmium appears to exert its effect on fetal development through its impact on sulfhydryl containing enzymes, particularly certain zincmetalloenzymes, such as carbonic anhydrase, alkaline phosphatase, and succinic oxidase (Mottet, 1981). While it is not clear whether cadmium's effects are limited strictly to the fetus, or involve the placenta as well, it appears that many of the malformations observed may arise as the result of alterations in the endothelium of vascular beds (Gabbiani, 1974). Depending on the timing of administration, defects observed in rodents varied from gross facial malformations, including malformations of the eye, micro- and anophthalmia, and of the brain, encephalocoele and exencephaly. Later administration produced anophthalmia, dysplastic or absent ears, and attenuated bony wall (Barr, 1972, 1973; Ferm et al., 1969).

Lithium. While lithium has been of considerable therapeutic value in the treatment of manic and certain other depressive disorders since the late 1940s (Cade, 1949), it is usually administered to susceptible women during their most vulnerable period, the childbearing years. Lithium is teratogenic in rodents (Wright et al., 1967) where it affects structures almost exclusively in the eyes, ears, and palate. In human beings, the most striking defects that arise in babies exposed to excessive lithium appear to be associated with the cardiovascular system, rather than the nervous system (Mottet, 1981).

REFERENCES

Altman J, Bayer SA (1978). Prenatal development of the cerebellum in the rat. I. Cytogenetics and histogenesis of the deep nuclei and cortex of the cerebellum. J Comp Neurol 179:23-45.

Barnard RD (1966). The pathodynamics of hemopoiesis suppression by nitrous oxide. Anesth Analg 45:461-466.

Barr MJ (1972). An animal model for the deficient abdominal muscle syndrome. J Pediatr 81:182.

Barr MJ (1973). The teratogenicity of cadmium chloride in two stocks of Wistar rats. Teratology 7:237-242.

Baudin TW, Mushak P, O'Tauma LA, Krigman RM (1975). Blood-brain barrier dysfunction in acute lead encephalopathy. Environ Health Perspect 12:81-88.

Bayer SA, Brunner RL, Hine R, Altman J (1973). Behavioral effects of interference with postnatal acquisition of hippocampal granule cells. Nature 242:222-223.

Cade JFJ (1949). Lithium salts in the treatment of psychotic excitement. Med J Aust 2:349-352.

Chen WJ, Body RL, Mottet NK (1979). Some effects of continuous low dose congenital exposure to methylmercury

on organ growth in the rat fetus. Teratology 20:31-36.
de la Cruz FF, Oster-Granite ML (1988). Neural bases of mental retardation. In Timiras P, Meisami M (eds): "Handbook of Human Biologic Development." Baco Raton: CRC Press, in press.
Edelman GM (1983). Cell adhesion molecules. Science 219:450-457.
Embil JA, Ozere RL, Haldane EV (1970). Congenital cytomegalovirus infection in two siblings from consecutive pregnancies. J Pediatr 77:417-421.
Ferm VH, Hanlon DP, Urban J (1969). The permeability of the hamster placenta to radioactive cadmium. J Embryol Exp Morphol 22:107.
Florman AL, Gershon AA, Blackett PR, Nahmias AJ (1973). Intrauterine infection with herpes simplex virus: resultant congenital defects. J Am Med Assoc 225:129-132.
Forloni GL, Bendotti C, Hohmann CF, Reeves RH, Oster-Granite ML, Gearhart JD, Coyle JT (1987). Immunocytochemical and in situ hybridization studies of somatostatin expression in mouse brain during normal development and after lesions of the basal forebrain. Soc Neurosci Abst 13:1618.
Gabbiani G (1974). Acute cadmium intoxication - early selective lesions of endothelial clefts. Lab Invest 30:686-695.
Gordon R (1985). A review of the theories of vertebrate neurulation and their relationship to the mechanics of neural tube birth defects. J Embryol Exper Morphol 89S:229-255.
Goyer RA (1971). Lead toxicity: a problem in environmental pathology. Am J Pathol 64:167-182.
Hanshaw JB (1970). Developmental abnormalities associated with congenital cytomegalovirus infection. Adv Teratol 4:64-93.
Hohmann CF, Forloni GL, Oster-Granite ML, Coyle JT (1987). Analysis of abnormal cortical morphogenetic events induced by cholinergic basal forebrain lesions in the newborn mouse. Soc Neurosci Abst 13:1618.
Jacobson AG, Oster GF, Odell GM, Cheng LY (1986). Neurulation and the cortical tractor model for epithelial folding. J Embryol Exp Morphol 96:19-49.
Johnson KP, Klasnya R, Johnson RT (1971). Neural tube defects in chick embryos: an indirect result of influenza A infection. J Neuropath Exp Neurol 30:68-74.
Johnson RT (1982). "Viral Infections of the Nervous System." New York: Raven Press, pp 433.
Karfunkel P (1974). The mechanism of neural tube

formation. Int Rev Cytol 38:245-271.

Kreber IJ, Warr OS, Richardson C (1968). Pregnancy in a patient with a prosthetic mitral valve. J Am Med Assoc 203:223-225.

Lammer EJ, Chen DT, Hoar RM, Agnish ND, Benke PJ, Braun JT, Curry CJ, Fernhoff PM, Grix AW Jr, Lott IT, Richard JM, Sun CC (1985). Retinoic acid embryopathy: a new human teratogen and a mechanistic hypothesis. New Engl J Med 313:837-841.

Landmesser L, Pilar G (1974). Synaptic transmission and cell death during normal ganglionic development. J Physiol (Lond) 347:205-224.

Lane GA, Narhwold ML, Tait AR, Taylor-Bush M, Cohen PJ, Beaudoin AR (1980). Anesthetics as teratogens: nitrous oxide is fetotoxic, xenon is not. Science 210:899-901.

Lane GA, DuBoulay PM, Tait AR, Taylor-Bush M, Cohen PJ (1981). Nitrous oxide is teratogenic: halothane is not. Anesthesiology 55:A252.

Layde PM, Edmonds LD, Erickson JD (1980). Maternal fever and neural tube defects. Teratology 21:105-108.

Lemire RJ, Loeser JD, Leech RW, Alvord EC Jr (1975). "Normal and Abnormal Development of the Human Nervous System." Hagerstown: Harper and Row, pp 54-83.

Leung CCK (1983). Antiserum to visceral yolk sac endoderm induced abnormal embryonic development. Pediatr Res 17:313-318.

Levitt P, Rakic P (1980). Immunoperoxidase localization of glial fibrillary acidic protein in radial glial cells and astrocytes of the developing rhesus monkey brain. J Comp Neurol 193:815-840.

McLone DG, Knepper PA (1985-6). Role of complex carbohydrates and neurulation. Pediatr Neurosci 12:2-9.

Miller P, Smith DW, Shepard TH (1978). Hyperthermia as one possible etiology of anencephaly. Lancet 1:519-521.

Mottet NK (1981). Biochemical mechanisms of trace metal teratogenesis. In Juchau MR (ed): "The Biochemical Basis of Chemical Teratogenesis." New York: Elsevier, pp 201-246.

Murphy DP (1929). Outcome of 629 pregnancies in women subjected to pelvic radium or roentgen irradiation. Am J Obstet Gynecol 18:179-185.

Naeye RL, Blanc W (1965). Pathogenesis of congenital rubella. J Am Med Assoc 194:1277-1279.

Narayan O, Johnson RT (1972). Effects of viral infection on nervous system development. I. Pathogenesis of blue-tongue virus infection in mice. Am J Pathol 68:1-14.

Opitz JM (1985). The developmental field concept. Am J Med Genet 21:1-11.

O'Shea KS (1986). Gene and teratogen defects in early CNS development. Scan Electron Microsc III:1195-1213.

Ornoy A, Yanai J (1980). Central nervous system teratogenicity: experimental models and human problems. In Persaud TVN (ed): "Neural and Behavioral Teratology." Baltimore: University Park Press, pp 1-22.

Oster-Granite ML (1974). The pathogenesis of rat virus-induced cerebellar hypoplasia in the Syrian hamster, Mesocricetus auratus. A light, Golgi, and electron microscopic study. Thesis, Johns Hopkins University, Baltimore, MD pp 321.

Pass RF, Hutto C, Stagno S, Britt WJ, Alford CA (1986). Congenital Cytomegalovirus Infection: Prospects for Prevention. Ann NY Acad Sci 477:123-127.

Pass RF, Stagno S, Myers GJ, Alford CA (1980). Outcome of symptomatic congenital cytomegalovirus infection: results of long-term longitudinal follow-up. Pediatrics 66:758-762.

Press MF (1977). Neuronal development in the cerebellum of lead poisoned neonatal rats. Acta Neuropathol (Berlin) 10:259-268.

Purves D, Lichtman JW (1985). "Principles of Neural Development." Sunderland: Sinauer and Assoc, pp 433.

Rakic P (1971). Guildance of neurons migrating to the fetal monkey neocortex. Brain Res 33:471-476.

Rakic P, Sidman RL (1973a). Weaver mutant mouse cerebellum: defective neuronal migration secondary to specific abnormality of Bergmann glia. Proc Natl Acad Sci USA 70:240-244.

Rakic P, Sidman RL (1973b). Sequence of developmental abnormalities leading to granule cell deficit in cerebellar cortex of Weaver mutant mice. J Comp Neurol 152:103-132.

Ramon y Cajal S (1929). "Studies of Vertebrate Neurogenesis." (Translation of the 1929 edition by L. Guth). Springfield: Charles Thomas.

Rawls WE, Melnick JL (1966). Rubella virus carrier cultures derived from congenitally infected infants. J Exp Med 123:795-805.

Robert E, Guiband P (1982). Maternal valproic acid and congenital neural tube defects. Lancet 2:937.

Rodier PM (1986). Inhalant anesthetics as neuroteratogens. Ann NY Acad Sci 477:42-48.

Rosa FW (1983). Teratogenicity of isotretinoin. Lancet

2:513.
Roth S, MacGuire EJ, Roseman S (1971). Evidence for cell-surface glycosyltransferases. Their potential role in cellular recognition. J Cell Biol 51:536-547.
Schardein JL (1985). "Chemically Induced Birth Defects." New York: Marcel Dekker pp 879.
Schoenwolf G (1982). On the morphogenesis of the early rudiments of the developing central nervous system. Scan Electron Microsc 1982; I:289-308.
Schoenwolf G (1984). Histologic and ultrastructural studies of secondary neurulation in mouse embryos. Am J Anat 169:361-376.
Shepard TH (1986). Human teratogens: how can we sort them out? Ann NY Acad Sci 477:105-115.
Smith BE (1974). Teratology in anesthesia. Clin Obstet Gynecol 17:145-163.
South MA, Tomkins WAF, Morris CR, Rawls WE (1969). Congenital malformation of the central nervous system associated with genital (type 2) herpesvirus. J Pediatr 75:13-18.
Takeuchi T (1968). Pathology of Minamata disease. In: Katsuna M (ed). Minamata Disease. Kumamoto Univ Press, Kumamoto, Japan. pp 121-147.
Toole BP (1976). Morphogenetic role of glycosaminoglycans (acid mucopolysaccharides) in brain and other tissues. In Barondes SH (ed): "Neuronal Recognition," New York: Plenum Press pp 275-329.
Vorhees CV (1986). Fetal anticonvulsant exposure: effects on behavioral and physical development. Ann NY Acad Sci 477:49-62.
Weinbaum PJ, Cassidy SB, Vintziliess AM, Campbell WA, Ciarleglio L, Nochiman DJ (1986). Prenatal detection of a neural tube defect after fetal exposure to valproic acid. Obstet Gynecol 67 (Suppl):315-335.
Wright TL, Hoffman LH, Davis J (1967). Teratogenic effects of lithium in rats. Teratology 4:151-156.

DISCUSSION

DR. LEVY: Do you think that with bioengineering advances we will be able to observe cell migrations and many of the changes that you have demonstrated *in vivo* in animals and humans?

DR. OSTER-GRANITE: Yes. Investigators in this country are trying now to introduce retroviral agents that will be targeted to specific cell populations. Of obvious interest to mammalian developmental neurobiologists for many years has been the lineage of cells and the actual mechanisms by which their sorting is directed. Within the next few years, we should be able to target these retroviral vectors into particular parts of the central nervous system. The introduction of such vectors must take place very early in development, preceding gastrulation, in order for informative kinds of influences to be directed. Hopefully, we will be able to introduce exotic bacterial genes, coupled with appropriate promoters, for studies of their expression later in the development of particular cell populations.

DR. LEVY: Will these be able to be observed *in vivo*?

DR. OSTER-GRANITE: I think that much of what will be done will be in animal model systems. The technology for *in situ* hybridization to visualize unique proteins that would be introduced and expressed is now possible at the structural level. The current dilemma is to target such agents into specific cell populations, and it is clear that many different strategies are being employed. Whether or not they will be relevant to the actual human situation or even to primates in the near future is more doubtful.

DR. LAMMER: Could you shed any light on the controversy among clinicians about what types of caudal neural tube defects might result from an error in the process of neurulation that occurs caudal to the posterior neuropore?

DR. OSTER-GRANITE: In experimental mammalian animal models, in which the closure of the posterior neuropore is prevented even though the colonization process takes place, and the epithelialization of those mesenchymal cells occurs, an open neural tube that extends caudally from the posterior neuropore is observed. It seems that in mammals, at least, if that closure does not take place, you cannot close the rest of the neural tube. It will remain with a lumen open to the amniotic cavity. In the chick something very different occurs. The process is more autonomous among these mesenchymal elements, so that problems in discontinuity of the lumen, and in duplication of the actual caudal neural tube result in more consistent findings. It could be that we have not observed carefully enough the types of teratogenic agents that might disrupt this in mammals, but if you change the extracellular matrix in this forming caudal neural tube, you create havoc with the actual extension of that tube, and with its essential retrogression process later on.

DR. LAMMER: If the posterior neuropore closes normally, is it possible that an open neural tube defect could occur caudal to the area of closure of the neuropores?

DR. OSTER-GRANITE: Yes. I have an example of the cranial part of the neural tube that would be relevant to the posterior neural tube with a complete closure having already taken place. It is possible to demonstrate such an effect in rats administered with cyclophosphamide at 12 to 14 days of gestation, when the neural tube has closed and when major neuron populations are being generated inside the CNS--well past the closure event. One hundred percent of treated fetuses will have cranioschisis with either exencephaly or anencephaly. By simply modifying the mesenchyme around the neural tube, not only is an opening of the tube itself produced, but also a degeneration process occurs. It is quite feasible to use an agent which disrupts the proliferation of mesenchyme and condensation of mesenchyme associated with the vertebral column, in order to produce an open neural tube defect after closure has taken place. It would be most likely to occur spontaneously in the regions posterior because those events are relatively late and relatively protracted in their duration.

DR. HANSON: Some epidemiologic studies have suggested that the spinal defects in children who were exposed prenatally to valproic acid are really attributable principally to alterations in this process, and that these are actually low sacral lipomeningoceles. Can you speculate as to how that may be occurring mechanistically?

DR. OSTER-GRANITE: I am not familiar with the teratogenic processes of valproic acid but it seems that these antiepileptic agents affect cell membranes. Their primary effect is to alter the way that cell membranes respond to the environment and continue their differentiation during development. Necessary cell interaction may be arrested, affecting the proliferation of these cells, or their ability to maintain the integrity of intercellular contacts. That might be one speculative mechanism for these agents.

DR. SCARPELLI: A mechanism which is believed to be involved in differentiation is modulation of gene activitation by the methylation of DNA. Has anyone shown alterations in the CNS such as methylation of DNA in nuclei in populations, especially of children, that are continuously exposed to a protein-poor diet?

DR. OSTER-GRANITE: Not to my knowledge, but we do know that there are gene families in which methylation patterns and switching must occur during differentiation events. One good example of this is the albumin-alphafetoprotein family. You can show that certain sites are continuously methylated when the gene is on, and other sites are never methylated when the gene is off, so that the influence of methylation may be a more subtle effect.

DR. SCARPELLI: I was thinking specifically of a person subsisting on a protein-poor or essentially a methionine-deficient diet.

DR. OSTER-GRANITE: It is very clear that you will alter methylation patterns during methionine deficiency, but what effect that actually has on gene programming in the CNS of the embryo or fetus is very speculative.

Transplacental Effects on Fetal Health, pages 227–242

MATERNAL PHENYLKETONURIA

Harvey L. Levy

Department of Neurology, Harvard Medical School; Neurology Service, Massachusetts General Hospital; State Laboratory Institute, Boston, Massachusetts 02114

INTRODUCTION

Maternal phenylketonuria (PKU) is a complication of PKU. The complication consists of teratogenetic effects incurred during pregnancies of women with PKU, expressed in the offspring as any combination of mental retardation, microcephaly, congenital heart disease, and low birth weight.

Ironically, the very success of newborn screening in identifying infants with PKU and leading to early treatment has greatly increased the magnitude of the maternal PKU problem. Before routine newborn screening, early treatment was rarely possible and most individuals with PKU became mentally retarded. Thus, few women with PKU bore children. Those few who did brought maternal PKU to medical attention through the original observation of their children by Dent (1956) and the later definitive studies by Mabry and his colleagues (Denniston 1963; Mabry et al 1963; Mabry et al 1966). With the prevention of mental retardation by early treatment of PKU, a new generation of phenylketonuric girls are now coming into childbearing ages. These young women are mentally normal, have normal fertility and wish to bear children.

This review will focus on our present knowledge about maternal PKU. Before presenting this information, however, I will briefly summarize PKU for those who are not already familiar with this metabolic disorder.

PKU

This is the best known of the inborn errors of amino acid metabolism. It was discovered by Fölling in 1934 when he identified phenylpyruvic acid in the urine of several mentally retarded children (Fölling 1934). Subsequently, these children were found to have increased levels of phenylalanine in blood (Jervis 1940) and no detectable activity of phenylalanine hydroxylase, a liver-specific enzyme (Jervis 1953). Figure 1 depicts the phenylalanine metabolic pathway and the block in PKU. The clinical phenotype of untreated PKU includes mental retardation, autistic-like behavior, hyperactive behavior, muscle hypertonia, and hyperactive deep tendon reflexes.

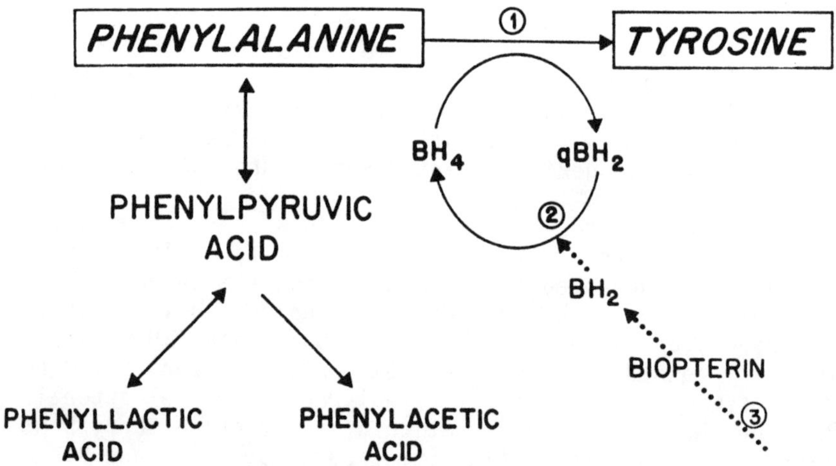

Figure 1. Pathways of phenylalanine metabolism. Tetrahydrobiopterin (BH_4) is the cofactor for phenylalanine hydroxylase (1), the defective enzyme in PKU.

Phenylalanine is an essential amino acid, i.e. not synthesized by mammals. Based on this, Bickel and coworkers developed a phenylalanine restricted diet that controlled the biochemical abnormalities and produced some clinical improvement in children with PKU (Bickel et al 1954). Mental retardation could only be prevented, however, if the diet began in early infancy before the clinical effect in PKU was expressed. Realization of this led to the development of routine newborn screening by Guthrie (1961). The success of newborn screening and early dietary therapy for PKU in virtually eliminating mental retardation from PKU has been one of the great events of modern medicine. There are now thousands of individuals with PKU the world over who are mentally normal but who would have been mentally retarded were it not for newborn screening.

MATERNAL PKU

This success has not been without a price. One of the costs is maternal PKU. As stated in the introduction, girls with PKU are at later risk for bearing children with mental retardation, microcephaly, congenital heart disease and low birth weight.

There are numerous questions about maternal PKU and its teratogenicity. The most immediate questions concern (1) the frequencies of birth defects in offspring from maternal PKU pregnancies; (2) whether teratogenic effects occur at all degrees of maternal PKU and maternal hyperphenylalaninemia; (3) whether dietary treatment during pregnancy will prevent fetal damage; and (4) the toxic agent that produces fetal damage and the mechanism of this damage.

FREQUENCIES OF OFFSPRING ABNORMALITIES

There is no doubt that classic PKU in the mother (untreated blood phenylalanine level 1200 μM or higher) presents great risk to the fetus. In an international survey of maternal PKU, we found that when the mothers had classic PKU and the pregnancies were untreated, 92% of the offspring were mentally retarded and 73% were microcephalic (Lenke, Levy 1980). These offspring quite often also had congenital heart disease and low birth weight (Table 1.)

This survey also revealed very high frequencies of abnormalities in the offspring when the mother had a high atypical degree of PKU, i.e. when her untreated blood phenylalanine concentration was 1000-1200 μM. In fact, there was little difference in the frequencies of offspring abnormalities between classic and near-classic degrees of PKU in the mother.

TABLE 1. Frequency of Abnormalities in Offspring from Untreated Pregnancies in Maternal PKU and Maternal Hyperphenylalaninemia Relative to the Maternal Blood Phenylalanine Level

Offspring Abnormalities	Maternal Blood Phenylalanine Level (μM)				
	>1200	1000-1200	600-1000	200-600	Normal
Mental Retardation (%)	92	73	22	21	3
Microcephaly (%)	73	68	35	24	5
Congenital Heart Dis. (%)	12	15	6	0	0.8
Low Birth Weight (%)	40	52	56	13	10

This could not be said for lower levels of maternal hyperphenylalaninemia. Low degrees of atypical PKU (blood phenylalanine levels 600-1000 μM) and non-PKU mild hyperphenylalaninemia (blood phenylalanine levels 200-600 μM) were associated with much lower frequencies of offspring abnormalities than when the mother had classic or near-classic PKU. Nevertheless, in that survey the prevalence of offspring abnormalities when the mother had a relatively mild degree of hyperphenylalaninemia was still higher than expected for the general population. Did this indicate that even the mildest degree of maternal hyperphenylalaninemia might damage the fetus? Or was there ascertainment bias in the survey that skewed the data in that direction? We suspected ascertainment bias, since many fewer families in which the mother had mild hyperphenylalaninemia were reported to us than families of maternal PKU despite the fact that 25-35 percent of all those with persistent hyperphenylalaninemia do not have PKU. In other words, since most of the families in the survey came to attention because of abnormalities in the offspring, could there be many families with maternal mild hyperphenylalaninemia not reported to us because the offspring were normal? If so, these normal offspring could reduce the frequency of offspring abnormalities in maternal mild hyperphenylalaninemia into the normal range.

In Massachusetts we had the opportunity to examine this question more carefully and without clinical bias in ascertainment. For a decade we routinely screened filter paper cord blood specimens for phenylalanine concentration in order to identify maternal PKU. Among 725,197 specimens representing approximately 435,000 women, we identified 22 women with persistent hyperphenylalaninemia (Levy, Waisbren 1983). Only two of these women had classic PKU. The remainder had atypical PKU or non-PKU mild hyperphenylalaninemia. Very importantly, we could examine 53 offspring from untreated pregnancies in these women. Only one offspring had congenital heart disease, a ventricular septal defect; her mother had non-PKU mild hyperphenylalaninemia. Microcephaly did not occur in offspring of mothers with non-PKU mild hyperphenylalaninemia. There was a 22 percent frequency of birth microcephaly among offspring of mothers with atypical PKU, but in only one of these offspring did the microcephaly persist. Among the four offspring from classic PKU pregnancies, however, three had birth microcephaly, and all four were microcephalic at later ages. Thus the obvious features of the maternal PKU syndrome were not seen in offspring from non-PKU mild hyperphenylalaninemic pregnancies and were less pronounced in offspring of mothers with atypical PKU than when the mother had classic PKU.

The most important question, however, is whether these offspring are mentally retarded or intellectually impaired to any degree. Figure 2 plots the IQ/DQ of the offspring against the maternal plasma phenylalanine level. There seemed to be no discernible adverse effect on offspring IQ/DQ when the maternal phenylalanine level was 600 µM (10 mg/dl) or less. The mean IQ among these offspring was 117. From a maternal phenylalanine level of approximately 700 µM continuing into the classic PKU levels greater than 1200 µM, however, there seemed to be a roughly linear reduction in offspring IQ/DQ. On the other hand, with one exception mental retardation was not observed

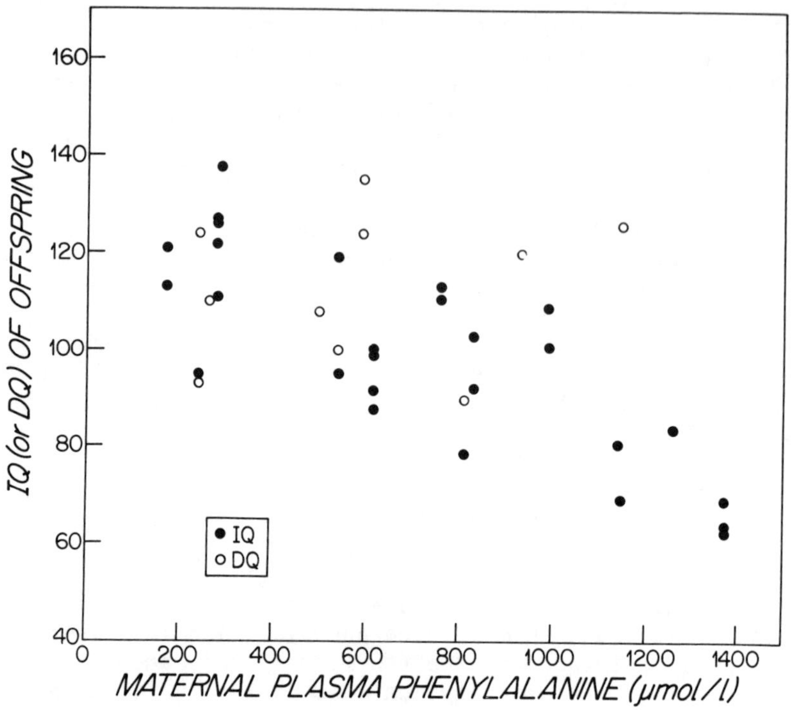

Figure 2. IQ or developmental quotient of offspring from untreated pregnancies in mothers with maternal PKU or maternal non-PKU mild hyperphenylalaninemia plotted against the maternal plasma phenylalanine level.

until the maternal phenylalanine concentration exceeded 1100 μM. In summary, it seemed that there might be no adverse effect on the fetus when the woman had nonPKU mild hyperphenylalaninemia and much less effect when the woman had atypical PKU than when she had classic PKU. Recently we reexamined many of these offspring, specifically measuring the IQ in those who had only been scored for DQ. The general impression stated above has not changed.

The question of whether non-PKU mild hyperphenylalaninemia or even atypical PKU in the pregnant woman causes fetal damage is very important and needs to be studied as carefully as possible. A substantial number of girls and young women with hyperphenylalaninemia have less than a classic degree of biochemical defect. At some centers they comprise almost 50 percent of those known to the center. The information about the risks to pregnancy that we provide to these young women and their families will have major implications for them.

TREATMENT OF MATERNAL PKU

Despite the uncertainty about risks to pregnancy when the hyperphenylalaninemic woman does not have classic PKU, there is no question about fetal damage when the woman has classic or near classic PKU. This recognition has generated an attempt to reduce or prevent the damage through dietary treatment that controls the maternal (and by extension the fetal) biochemical abnormalities. The rationale for such treatment has been the success of early dietary treatment in preventing mental retardation in individuals with PKU and the evidence that risks to the fetus are certainly less when the maternal phenylalanine level is lower.

Table 2 summarizes the experience with dietary treated maternal PKU pregnancies. Clearly the most encouraging results have been when the treatment began before conception and continued throughout the pregnancy (Rohr et al 1987). No offspring from a maternal PKU pregnancy treated in this manner has been microcephalic, has had congenital heart disease, low birth weight, or mental deficiency. Treatment begun after conception has been less beneficial. Offspring from pregnancies treated from about the middle of the first trimester have not suffered substantial intellectual loss but have often been microcephalic and have had congenital heart disease at least as often as those from untreated pregnancies. The presence of congenital heart disease in such offspring is expected, since cardiogenesis begins at about the third gestational week in the embryo and is complete by the eighth week. Treatment delayed until the second and third trimesters may be of little benefit.

TABLE 2. Results of Treated Maternal PKU Pregnancies

	Relation to Conception			
		Trimester		
	Before	1	2	3
No. Studied	13	18	18	5*
IQ or DQ	~100	~100	84	79
Microcephaly	0	27%	56%	60%
Congenital Heart Disease	0	28%	11%	0
BW <2,500 g	0	0	28%	0

*One offspring was stillborn.

Far more data about treated maternal PKU pregnancies and their outcomes need to be obtained. In recognition of this need, two large collaborative studies have begun--one combining centers in the United States and Canada and the other combining experiences in the United Kingdom and Australia. Such carefully planned studies are necessary if we are ever to know whether fetal damage from maternal PKU can be prevented by dietary therapy.

PATHOGENESIS OF THE FETAL DAMAGE

It may not be possible to adequately control the effects of maternal PKU unless we understand the origin of these effects and the mechanism that produces the fetal damage. Unfortunately, very little is currently known about pathogenesis.

One indisputable observation that may be important in our understanding of this problem is that the fetus is not only exposed to the hyperphenylalaninemia of the mother but to an even greater concentration of phenylalanine than that in the maternal circulation. This was shown by Pueschel and his coworkers through simultaneous sampling of maternal and fetal blood in hyperphenylalaninemic monkeys (Pueschel et al 1982) and by us in human maternal PKU pregnancies at term comparing phenylalanine concentrations between maternal blood and umbilical vein (Levy et al 1984). Thus the placenta concentrates phenylalanine in maternal PKU as it concentrates amino acids in normal pregnancies (Ghadimi, Pecora 1964). The placenta also concentrates tyrosine in maternal PKU, complicating the question of whether fetal tyrosine depletion is a factor in the fetal damage. We recently found that the increased phenylalanine in fetal blood is reflected in increased tissue phenylalanine in a 13-week fetus from a terminated pregnancy (Levy H: unpublished data). It is not yet known whether phenylalanine metabolites are also transferred across the placenta to the fetus. If not, current evidence would support phenylalanine per se as the toxic agent when its concentration is increased. Otherwise, any of the phenylalanine metabolites acting alone or in concert with phenylalanine might initiate the pathogenetic process. For instance, Loo et al (1983/84) believe that phenylacetate rather than phenylalanine is the culprit.

As uncertain as we are of the toxic agent, we are even more uncertain about pathogenesis in maternal PKU. Lack of a natural animal model for PKU has greatly hampered such study, as it has prevented intensive study of the nature of brain damage in individuals with PKU. In lieu of a true genetic model for PKU, a number of groups have produced "models" for maternal PKU by administering phenylalanine to pregnant rats or monkeys either alone or in combination with a phenylalanine hydroxylase inhibitor such as p-chlorophenylalanine or a-methylphenylalanine. These animals always become hyperphenylalaninemic, often more so than humans with untreated PKU, and also excrete phenylalanine metabolites, notably phenylpyruvate. Unlike human PKU, however, the animal "model" develops at least a mild-to-moderate increase in the blood tyrosine concentration.

This technique has not succeeded in reproducing the full clinical syndrome of maternal PKU. Notably, until the recent report from Japan (Suyama et al 1987), congenital heart disease had not been reported in fetuses or offspring from these hyperphenylalaninemic pregnancies. Their finding of an increased frequency of ventricular septal defects in rat fetuses exposed to hyperphenylalaninemia at 8-11 days gestation may be a breakthrough in this experimental area. Learning deficits and other signs of brain damage analogous to the mental retardation seen in maternal PKU offspring have also not been consistently noted. Kerr et al (1968) described selective learning reductions in infant monkeys exposed to maternal hyperphenylalaninemia, but Pueschel et al (1985) did not find evidence of learning impairment in monkey offspring similarly exposed to maternal hyperphenylalaninemia. Performance impairment has been observed in rat offspring from hyperphenylalaninemic pregnancies in some studies (Loo et al 1983/84; Butcher 1970). Thompson and Kano (1965) found evidence of emotional instability, but not intellectual deficits, in the rat offspring they studied; and Lewis et al (1985) described hyperactive behavior in rat offspring exposed to relatively mild maternal hyperphenylalaninemia.

Two frequently noted features of these animal fetuses and offspring, low body weight and reduced brain weight, have been consistent with what is observed in maternal PKU offspring. Body weights of rat fetuses or offspring exposed to maternal hyperphenylalaninemia have been approximately 10-20 percent below controls (Loo et al 1983/84; Brass et al 1982). This reduction is an order of magnitude similar to the reduced birth weight noted in maternal PKU offspring. Brain weights have been correspondingly reduced (Spero, Yu 1983), perhaps analogous to the microcephaly of maternal PKU. Reduced concentrations of DNA and RNA have suggested reduced numbers of cells in the brains of the experimental fetuses (Hirano et al 1985).

Beyond weight and protein content, the specific features of the brain from fetuses exposed to maternal hyperphenylalaninemia have not been extensively studied. Spero and Yu (1983) described increased packing density of cells in the cortical plate along with degenerating cells and reactive microglia, but all of these changes tended to disappear postnatally. Hirano and colleagues (1985) demonstrated reduced activity of cyclic nucleotide 3'-phosphohydrolase, a marker enzyme for myelin. Loo and coworkers (1985) described a disruption in the normal brain ganglioside pattern and reduced sialoglycoproteins. Copenhaver et al (1973) found that the polyribosomal structure in rat fetal brains was disaggregated, and Okano et al (1986) supported this in observing reduced polysomes with increased numbers of disomes and monosomes in fetal brains. Taken together, these findings would suggest an effect by maternal hyperphenylalaninemia on brain protein synthesis as well as myelin formation in the rat fetus.

A hint as to the origin of these changes has been provided by studies from Japan. Takada et al (1974) showed that hyperphenylalaninemia in the pregnant rat resulted in reduced uptake of leucine in the protein and non-protein fractions of fetal liver and brain. They interpreted this as indicating inhibition of protein synthesis by the increased phenylalanine. Recently, Okano and coworkers (1986) demonstrated a similar pattern of reduced leucine uptake in fetal plasma, liver, brain, and heart. They also found reduced concentrations of many free amino acids (other than phenylalanine) in these fetal tissues and concluded that increased maternal phenylalanine inhibited placental amino acid transport, thereby producing amino acid imbalance in fetal tissues. They related this imbalance to the polysome disaggregation observed, which they postulated resulted in reduced protein synthesis. It is not clear how an imbalance of free amino acids could produce disruption of polysomes. Nevertheless, either reduced levels of free amino acids or polysome disaggregation or both could limit protein synthesis. If applicable to human maternal PKU, this hypothesis would provide a reasonable explanation for the fetal brain effect but would leave still unanswered questions such as why the heart is not always defective and why certain other organs are not affected.

FUTURE DIRECTIONS IN MATERNAL PKU

Maternal PKU represents an unusual example of biochemical disequilibrium transmitted across the placenta and producing fetal damage. In this sense it is not unlike maternal diabetes or the fetal alcohol syndrome. Study of maternal PKU that leads to a better understanding of its pathogenesis could provide us with much information about placental function and maternal-fetal interaction. This knowledge would benefit not only young women with PKU but would have far-reaching implications for reproduction in general.

REFERENCES

Bickel H, Gerrard J, Hickmans EM (1954). The influence of phenylalanine intake on the chemistry and behavior of a phenylketonuric child. Acta Paediatr 43:64-73.

Brass C, Isaacs C, McChesney R Greengard O (1982). The effects of hyperphenylalaninemia on fetal development: a new animal model of maternal phenylketonuria. Pediatr Res 16:388-394.

Butcher R (1970). Learning impairment associated with maternal phenylketonuria in rats. Nature 226:555-556.

Copenhaver J, Vacanti J, Carver M (1973). Experimental maternal hyperphenylalaninemia: disaggregation of fetal brain ribosomes. J Neurochem 21:273-280.

Denniston JC (1963). Children of mothers with phenylketonuria. J Pediatr 63:461-462.

Dent CE (1956). Discussion of Armstrong MD: Relation of biochemical abnormalty to development of mental defect in phenylketonuria. In: "Phenylketonuria in Etiological Factors in Mental Retardation". Report of 23rd Ross Conference, Columbus: Ross, p32.

Fölling A (1934). Uber Ausscheidung von Phenylbrenztraubensäure in den Harn als Stoffwechselanomalie in Verbindung mit Imbezillität. Hoppe Seyler Z Physiol Chem 227:169-176.

Ghadimi H, Pecora P (1964). Free amino acids of cord plasma as compared with maternal plasma during pregnancy. Pediatrics 33:500-504.

Guthrie R (1961). Blood screening for phenylketonuria. J Am Med Assoc 178:863.

Hirano S, Takagi Y, Kanamatsu T, Nakai K (1985). Effects of hyperphenylalaninemia in the fetal stage on the postnatal development of fetal rat brain. Neurochem Res 10:1071-1081.

Jervis GA (1953). Phenylpyruvic oligophrenia: deficiency of phenylalanine oxidizing system. Proc Soc Exp Biol Med 82:514-515.

Jervis GA, Block RJ, Bolling D, Kanze E (1940). Chemical and metabolic studies on phenylalanine. II. The phenylalanine content of the blood and spinal fluid in phenylpyruvic oligophrenia. J Biol Chem 134:105-113.

Kerr G, Chamove A, Harlow H, Waisman H (1968). "Fetal PKU:" The effect of maternal hyperphenylalaninemia during pregnancy in the rhesus monkey (Macaca mulatta). Pediatrics 42:27-36.

Lenke RR, Levy HL (1980). Maternal phenylketonuria and hyperphenylalaninemia: an international survey of the outcome of untreated and treated pregnancies. N Engl J Med 303:1202-1208.

Levy HL, Lenke RR, Koch R (1984). Lack of fetal effect on blood phenylalanine concentration in maternal phenylketonuria. J Pediatr 104:245-247.

Levy HL, Waisbren SE (1983). Effects of untreated maternal phenylketonuria and hyperphenylalaninemia on the fetus. N Engl J Med 309:1269-1274.

Lewis S, Lyon I, Elliott R (1985). Outcome of pregnancy in the rat with mild hyperphenylalaninemia and hypertyrosinaemia: implications for the management of "human maternal PKU". J Inherited Metab Dis 8:113-117.

Loo Y, Hyde K, Lin F, Wisniewski H (1985). Cerebral biochemical abnormalities in experimental maternal phenylketonuria: gangliosides and sialoglycoproteins. Life Sci 37:2099-2109.

Loo Y, Rabe A, Potempska A, Wang P, Fersko R, Wisniewski H (1983/84). Experimental maternal phenylketonuria: an examination of two animal models. Dev Neurosci 6:227-234.

Mabry CC, Denniston JC, Coldwell JC (1966). Mental retardation in children of phenylketonuric mothers. N Engl J Med 275:1331-1336.

Mabry CC, Denniston JC, Nelson TL, Son CD (1963). Maternal phenylketonuria. A cause of mental retardation in children without the metabolic defect. N Engl J Med 269:1404-1408.

Okano Y, Chow I, Isshiki G, Inoue A, Oura T (1986). Effects of phenylalanine loading on protein synthesis in the fetal heart and brain of rat: an experimental approach to maternal phenylketonuria. J Inherited Metab Dis 9:15-24.

Pueschel S, Boylan J, Jackson B, Piasecki G (1982). A study of placental transfer mechanisms in nonhuman primates using [^{14}C] phenylalanine. Obstet Gynecol 59:182-188.

Pueschel S, Schrier A, Povar M, Boylan J (1985). Biological and behavioral assessments of young rhesus monkeys after intrauterine exposure to high phenylalanine concentrations. J Ment Defic Res 29:247-256.

Rohr F, Doherty LB, Waisbren SE, Bailey IV, Ampola M, Benacerraf B, Levy HL (1987). New England Maternal PKU Project: prospective study of untreated and treated pregnancies and their outcomes. J Pediatr 110:391-398.

Spero D, Yu M (1983). Effects of maternal hyperphenylalaninemia on fetal brain development: a morphological study. Exp Neurol 79:655-665.

Suyama I, Tani M, Isshiki G, Okano Y, Oura T, Nishimura K (1987). Fetal heart malformations following phenylalanine loading of pregnant rats. Fourth Intern Cong IEM, Sendai, p 121.

Takada G, Chow I, Tada K (1974). Maternal hyperphenylalaninemia induced experimentally: decreased incorporation of ^{14}C-leucine into protein in the brain of the fetus. Tohoku J Exp Med 113:173-179.

Thompson W, Kano K (1965). Effects on rat offspring of maternal phenylalanine diet during pregnancy. J Psychiatr Res 3:91-98.

DISCUSSION

DR. HANSON: There have been some analogies drawn between the fetal effects of maternal PKU and those of alcohol. The craniofacial abnormalities, at least in some of the children, seem to be rather similar. Certainly some of the cardiac anomalies produced in infants exposed to a large amount of alcohol prenatally are, at least, sometimes similar to this. Do you think that there are things to be learned from that analogy and whether or not this might predict the kinds of central nervous system anomalies that one might expect? In the alcohol-exposed babies, one may see migrational errors like neuroglial heterotopias and cerebellar hypoplasia. West, studying the rodent model, has suggested that there were abnormalities of arborization of dendrites in the limbic system. These findings might not be readily apparent, unless they are carefully sought for on neuropathological examination. I wonder if there is any validity in making this analogy and whether it tells us anything about mechanisms?

DR. LEVY: Yes, I certainly think there is validity in making the analogy. Whether it is telling us about mechanisms and whether they are truly analogous is a question which I certainly don't have the answer to, but you are correct. There are facial dysmorphisms reported. Bruce Beuhler and others have reported this in offspring from maternal PKU pregnancies, making one wonder whether the neural crest cell migration theory is a bit more cogent than even I had thought. There are connections or seeming connections, and I think that one of the things that we would be concentrating on in the next few years is trying to firm these up. If they exist, we should try to determine whether or not they are truly related mechanistically or pathogenetically.

DR. LAMMER: Is a suitable animal model of maternal PKU unavailable because the metabolism of phenylalanine differs among vertebrates or is the problem that we have not been able to find a mutant comparable to the human defect?

DR. LEVY: We have not been able to find a comparable mutant, but it may very well be that the reason we have not been able to find a comparable mutant is because animal metabolism of phenylalanine differs from that of the human. It is known, for instance, that murine phenylalanine hydroxylase in the liver is 10-fold higher than the specific activity of normal human phenylalanine hydroxylase in the liver. So, it may very well be that if you had the sort of mutation that produces PKU in the human it may not necessarily eradicate the phenylalanine hydroxylase activity in the animal liver, although this is pure speculation. A number of years ago we tried to produce phenylketonuric monkeys in a collaborative study with the New England Regional Primate Research Center. The macaques were injected intravenously with phenylalanine in an attempt to identify, through the phenylalanine and tyrosine responses, carriers of the PKU gene and selectively mate them. We thought we identified about 13 or 14 carriers. The best carrier was an animal named Einstein. The problem with Einstein was that while he was the best carrier, he was, also, the least interested. So, we could never get Einstein to mate with female carriers in order for us to produce the offspring that we thought might show PKU. Other investigators have also attempted to identify carriers and mate these to try to produce phenylketonuric offspring and were as unsuccessful as we were.

Screening studies at Bar Harbor, of a mouse population, have identified at least two strains of mice with mild elevations of phenylalanine and mild reductions in liver phenylalanine hydroxylase activity but not the level one associates with classical PKU. So, those attempts identifying an animal model for PKU have also been unsuccessful. I am hopeful that methods such as selective mutagenesis using recombinant DNA techniques will perhaps allow for the normal phenylalanine hydroxylase to be replaced or altered in animals. If that is true, perhaps in the future we will have an animal model of this disease.

DR. HANSON: I am almost hesitant to ask this question, but I wonder if you would care to enter into the fray regarding the effects of dietary sources of phenylalanine, such as aspartame on the human population's neurocognitive function or development?

DR. LEVY: My feeling is that the danger of aspartame has been overemphasized. In our experience, at least in one study and a limited experience in another, we have found that rather large amounts of aspartame ingested at one sitting do not raise the blood phenylalanine level of individuals who carry the gene for PKU, those who do not carry the gene, or even individuals who have mild hyperphenylalaninemia that would be considered to be biologically significant levels. Aspartame does raise the blood phenylalanine level in a statistically significant sense, but again, far below that which might be considered biologically important. The argument is that if you gave twice as much or three times as much aspartame, you would raise the level a whole lot more, but I am not sure that that is true. We and others have done some of that and found that even much larger amounts of aspartame than we gave in the study seem not to raise the blood phenylalanine into an area that we would be concerned about. The fact that aspartame does raise the phenylalanine level to some extent frightens many people, it is still a controversial point, and there is a lot more that needs to be known about it.

Transplacental Effects on Fetal Health, pages 243–263

DEVELOPMENTAL ACTIONS OF GONADAL STEROIDS

Neil J. MacLusky

Dept. of Obstetrics and Gynecology, Yale University Medical School, 333 Cedar St., New Haven CT06510

INTRODUCTION

The potential for gonadal steroids to induce developmental abnormalities in the reproductive tract and in the mechanisms controlling reproductive function was first recognized more than 40 years ago (Pfeiffer, 1936; Greene *et al*, 1940). Only within the last two decades, however, has the full significance of these effects come to be appreciated in terms of human development. Unfortunately, warning signs from studies in experimental animals were initially either disregarded, or assumed not to apply to man. This situation was dramatically altered in the early 1970's when it was reported that exposure of the human fetus to the synthetic estrogen, diethylstilbestrol (DES), resulted in developmental abnormalities of the reproductive tract. It has been estimated that more than 2 million individuals may have been affected by prenatal exposure to this drug (Newbold and McLachlan, 1985). Since the full consequences of DES exposure may not be known for many years to come, in view of the possibility that other problems may yet emerge in the affected population, this experience clearly indicates the necessity for caution in the introduction of agents which may have developmental hormonal activity into either clinical use, or the environment at large.

The developmental effects of gonadal steroids are related to the crucial role played by these hormones in sexual differentiation of the normal masculine and feminine phenotypes. In many instances, the teratogenic effects of early gonadal steroid exposure can be viewed as derangements of sexual differentiation, induced by the presence of a hormonal milieu that is inappropriate for the sex of the fetus. Not all responses to early gonadal steroid exposure can, however, be considered within this conceptual framework, since elevated levels of gonadal steroids may seriously impair developmental processes in the steroid target organs of *both* sexes - DES being a case in point. Moreover, in some instances, the actions of hormonally-active agents may represent a composite of hormonal and other biological activities, which together may be required to bring about the observed effects.

The first part of this article briefly reviews the processes involved in sexual differentiation, to provide a basis for understanding the effects of the gonadal steroids on sexually dimorphic structures. Subsequently, examples will be considered of situations in which exogenous hormonally-active agents have either been demonstrated to influence normal development during therapeutic use, or to present the potential for such effects as a result of their pharmacological properties and/or presence in the environment.

Sexual Differentiation of the Reproductive Organs

The first stage in sexual differentiation is the development of the male and female gonads. Chromosomal sex, established at the time of fertilization, directs the development of either ovaries or testes. In both sexes, the embryonic origin of the gonadal cells is similar: the primordial germ cells migrate from the yolk sac endoderm, while the somatic elements of the gonads are derived from the mesonephric ridge. In female mammals, the XX karyotype results in development of the germ cells into oocytes, while the Y chromosome of the male causes testicular differentiation.

Once the gonads have differentiated, it is their secretions that are primarily responsible for the further differentiation of the masculine or feminine phenotype. The fundamental mechanism of sexual differentiation was elucidated almost three decades ago by Alfred Jost (Reviewed in Jost, 1972), who showed that the castrated mammalian embryo develops physically as a female. These seminal experiments led to the formulation of what is now the central hypothesis of sexual differentiation: the genetic sex of the embryo determines its gonadal sex, which in turn determines its phenotypic sex. If testes are formed, their secretions organize the development of masculine reproductive organs and secondary sexual characteristics. In the absence of these secretions, anatomic development continues along feminine lines.

The nature of the two testicular hormones responsible for differentiation of the masculine phenotype was also deduced by Jost (1972). The first, Mullerian inhibitory substance, is a polypeptide of approximately 70,000 molecular weight which, as its name implies, is responsible for the degeneration of the primordium of the female reproductive tract, the Mullerian ducts. The second hormone is the principal steroidal secretion of the testes, testosterone, which is responsible for the differentiation of the precursor of the masculine reproductive tract (the Wolffian duct) and its accessory organs, as well as the male external genitalia. In addition to its effects on the developing reproductive structures, testosterone is also responsible for bringing about the masculinization of a wide range of non-reproductive tissues. Sex differences in such parameters as bone length, muscle mass and hair growth are obvious expressions of these non-reproductive effects. However, there are also more subtle testosterone effects on a large number of other tissues. For example, testosterone is responsible for sex differences in the levels of many hepatic drug and steroid metabolizing enzymes, as well as hepatic secretory proteins. Sex differences in the morphology of the kidney and in erythropoesis can also be ascribed to testosterone action (Bardin and Catterall, 1981).

Mechanisms Involved in Androgen-Induced Tissue Differentiation: the Crucial Role of Local Steroid Metabolism

The actions of testosterone on sexually-dimorphic tissues can be divided into two phases: an early "organizational" phase during embryogenesis which leads to an essentially irreversible differentiation of the tissues; and a later "activational" phase, in which the steroid may bring about transient, reversible responses in its target cells (e.g. the androgen-induced processes of irreversible differentiation of the prostatic epithelium; and subsequent reversible stimulation of prostatic growth). Although these two phases might at first sight appear to be fundamentally different, they are in fact mediated through essentially similar mechanisms. The general model for the mechanism of androgen action is summarized in Figure 1. The steroid is believed to initially enter its target tissues through passive diffusion from the bloodstream. Within the target cells, or in closely neighboring cells, it may undergo a variety of different metabolic transformations leading to biologically-active metabolites. One of the most physiologically important of these transformations is 5α reduction of the 4-5 double bond, leading to 5α dihydrotestosterone (DHT). Alternatively, the same double bond may be reduced to give the enantiomer of DHT, 5β dihydrotestosterone. The third route of metabolism entails aromatization of the androgen to estradiol. Whatever the intracellular fate of the steroid, the final step in the mechanism is the same: within the target cells, either the unchanged testosterone or the locally-synthesized metabolites bind to specific cellular receptor proteins. Interactions between the receptor-steroid complexes and acceptor sites on the chromatin result, through an as

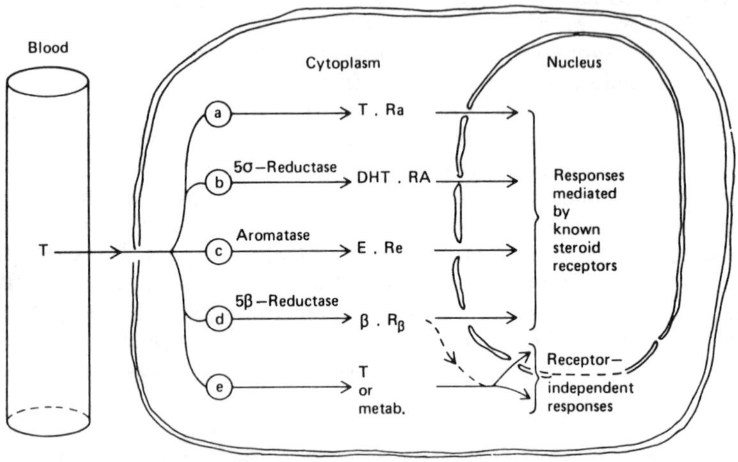

Fig. 1 Testosterone (T) metabolism and receptor binding. The known pathways of testosterone metabolism that lead to biological activities in various tissues are summarized as though they occurred in a single cell. Testosterone leaves the blood and enters the cell by diffusion. In the cytoplasm, testosterone can react in the following ways: (a) without being metabolized, in which case testosterone binds directly to the androgen receptor (Ra), and this steroid receptor complex (T.Ra) is then transferred to nuclear acceptor sites in chromatin for initiation of the steroid- specific responses; (b) testosterone is metabolized by 5α-reductase to 5α-dihydrotestosterone (DHT) which then binds to Ra and the steroid receptor complex (DHT.Ra) is bound in the nucleus; (c) testosterone is aromatized to estradiol (E) which binds to estrogen receptor (Re) which is transferred and bound in nuclei as for (a) and (b); (d) testosterone is metabolized to 5β metabolites (β) which bind to the βsteroid receptor (Rβ) and the steroid receptor complex (β.Rβ) presumably acts in the nucleus; and (e) testosterone or one of its metabolites (x.) acts in the nucleus or cytoplasm by mechanisms which are independent of known receptors (receptor-independent responses) (Reproduced from Bardin and Catterall, 1981, with permission).

yet poorly defined process, in increased messenger RNA and protein synthesis which, in turn, initiate the observed cellular response.

This system provides for considerable diversity, since the actions of the circulating hormone are dependent on the tissue concentrations of the various testosterone metabolizing enzymes as well as the cellular levels of the receptor proteins specific for each class of androgen metabolite. In many cases, the actions of testosterone appear to be dependent on conversion to 5α dihydrotestosterone, which has considerably greater androgenic potency than the parent steroid on such organs as the ventral prostate. DHT plays a particularly important role in the differentiation of the external genitalia (Wilson *et al*, 1981). Testosterone is not extensively metabolized in most muscles; but in the levator ani muscle, locally synthesized estrogen mediates the inductive effects of circulating testosterone on glucose-6-phosphate dehydrogenase activity (Knudsen and Max, 1980; Max and Knudsen, 1980). In contrast, 5β reduced androgens are more potent inducers of hemoglobin biosynthesis by erythroblasts than their 5α epimers (Granick and Kappas, 1967).

Sexual Differentiation of the Central Nervous System

Sexual differentiation of the neuroendocrine and behavioral processes involved in reproductive function can in many respects be considered to be analogous to that of the reproductive tract and of the physical secondary sexual characteristics. Like the primordium of the reproductive tract, the developing central nervous system is intrinsically bipotential with the capacity to develop along masculine or feminine lines. Which line is followed depends on a number of factors. Included among these are the gonadal steroid hormones, as well as social and environmental factors that come into play during postnatal development.

The central importance of gonadal secretions in the sexual differentiation of the central nervous system was established by Pfeiffer (1936) who showed that the transplantation of testes into the neck of the newborn female rat masculinized the development of the systems controlling pituitary function, such that the animal was no longer capable of supporting cyclical patterns of gonadotrophin release. Subsequent work demonstrated that this effect was due to an action of testosterone from the testes on the hypothalamic neurosecretory mechanisms responsible for generating cyclic surges of gonadotrophin releasing hormone (Harris and Levine, 1965). Other studies demonstrated a similar dependence of masculine behavior on early exposure to testicular androgens (Phoenix *et al*, 1968; Gorski, 1973).

Just as the effects of androgens on the reproductive tract can be divided into "organizational" and "activational" phases, so the effects of gonadal steroids on the central nervous system can also be considered in terms of whether they represent a permanent developmental change or a transient response. The effects on the CNS of androgen exposure during early development include organizational components. Thus, for example, the actions of testosterone on the developing rat brain, inducing a shift from the feminine, cyclic pattern of gonadotrophin release and sex behavior towards the male, acyclic pattern are not reversible by subsequent exposure to ovarian hormones: the effects of the early androgen are irrevocably imprinted. In contrast, the effects of gonadal steroids in adulthood are primarily activational, leading to the transient potentiation of pre-established functions and characteristics (McEwen, 1981).

The effects of androgens on the brain appear to be mediated through receptor mechanisms that are fundamentally similar to those found in non-neural androgen target organs. As in peripheral tissues, local metabolism of the androgen plays an essential role. However, in contrast to the reproductive tract, in many species it appears to be aromatization and not 5α reduction that is important for the actions of circulating testosterone on the developing central nervous system. In laboratory rodents, such as rats and mice, several lines of evidence support the concept that local estrogen biosynthesis is required for sexual differentiation of the central nervous system to take place (MacLusky and Naftolin, 1981). The question of whether androgen receptor-mediated responses also play a role in sexual differentiation of the brain remains the subject of continuing investigation. While it is clear that estrogen is of major importance in laboratory rodents such as rats and mice, there are indications that this dependence on estrogen may not extend equally well to all species. In guinea pigs and monkeys, for example, prenatal administration of 5α DHT (which cannot itself be aromatized) mimics some of the effects of testosterone on masculine behavior (Reviewed in Goy and McEwen, 1980). Even in rats, there is evidence that androgen per se is required for the normal differentiation of certain non-reproductive behaviors as well as of the spinal reflexes involved in the masculine copulatory response (Hart, 1979; MacLusky and Naftolin, 1981).

In man, hormone-dependent sex differences in the functions of the CNS appear to be rather more subtle than the essentially irreversible imprinting of masculine or feminine behavior patterns observed in sub-primate mammalian species. In contrast to rodents, the mechanisms responsible for control of reproductive function in higher primates do not appear to be "programmed" by early androgen exposure. Thus, males retain the capacity to exhibit estrogen induced surges in gonadotrophin release into adulthood (Karsch *et al*, 1973; Barbarino *et al*, 1979). The normal sex differences in the patterns of gonadotrophin release observed in man appear to be the result of activational as opposed to organizational hormonal effects, reflecting the predominance of ovarian estrogen and progesterone in the female, and testicular androgens in the male. Similarly, behavioral sex differences in human beings are not rigidly organized along masculine or feminine lines as a result of early gonadal steroid exposure. Studies of women exposed to abnormally high androgen levels prenatally as a result of genetic defects in adrenal steroid production have clearly demonstrated that gender identity and sexual orientation are not irrevocably determined by the prenatal hormone environment (Ehrhardt and Meyer-Bahlburg, 1981). Nevertheless, there is little doubt that prenatal steroid exposure does affect CNS development in man, albeit in a more subtle fashion than in experimental animals. Anatomical sex differences in the human brain (deLacoste *et al*, 1986; Swaab and Fliers, 1985) as well as sex differences in gender role behavior and the incidence of certain cognitive disorders (Ehrhardt and Meyer-Bahlburg, 1981; Geschwind and Behan, 1982) have all been suggested to reflect developmental consequences of testosterone action in the male.

An important corollary of the hypothesis that local estrogen biosynthesis is involved in sexual differentiation of the brain is that there must be some mechanism for protecting the developing brain from high levels of estrogen derived from the circulation. Paradoxically, circulating estrogen levels in neonatal rats of either sex appear to be relatively high (Weisz and Gunsalus, 1973). The great majority of this estrogen, however, is bound to a circulating estrogen binding protein, α-fetoprotein (AFP), which is synthesized by the fetal yolk sac and liver. AFP effectively sequesters the circulating estrogen in a biologically inactive form. Testosterone, in contrast, is not bound to AFP and is therefore free to enter the brain as a substrate for local estrogen biosynthesis (McEwen *et al*, 1976). This mechanism appears to be responsible for protecting the developing female fetus from circulating estrogens in several rodent species, including the rat, mouse and hamster. However, it is probably not a universal mechanism since it has now been established that in other species, including man, AFP does not bind estrogens to any appreciable extent (Uriel *et al*, 1972). It is possible that protection against high circulating estrogen levels in primates may be exerted through rapid metabolism of the steroids to inactive conjugates (Davidson *et al*, 1983), rather than binding to serum proteins.

Developmental Consequences of Postnatal Gonadal Steroid Exposure

In addition to their effects on sexual differentiation, gonadal steroids may also interfere with normal development by virtue of their roles in sexual maturation. Normally, the gonads remain relatively quiescent from shortly after birth until the time of puberty. Thus, expression of masculine and feminine secondary phenotypic characteristics is delayed until sexual maturity is reached. This entire developmental sequence can be disrupted by exposure to increased gonadal hormone levels during early life. In rats, post-natal estrogen treatment accelerates the onset of first estrus (Ramirez and Sawyer, 1965). In man, a number of cases have been documented of premature thelarche (breast enlargement) as a result of inadvertant postnatal estrogen treatment (New, 1985a).

Implications of Exposure to Exogenous Hormonally-Active Agents During Development

The critical role of the steroid hormones in the development of the reproductive system clearly indicates the necessity for careful evaluation of the potential risks associated with any disturbance of the normal hormonal milieu during pregnancy and/or the early postnatal period. Unfortunately, however, assessment of these risks is complicated by a lack of crucial information related to both the mechanisms involved, and the properties of compounds to which the mother and developing child may be exposed. As indicated above, much of our knowledge about the processes involved in sexual differentiation comes from work in sub-primate experimental animals, which may only partially be applicable to man. Simply because the principal activity of a drug is one that appears to have minimal potential risk for the embryo does not necessarily mean that such a drug will have no hormonal teratogenic activity. Moreover, it is becoming increasingly clear that there are a host of environmental agents, both natural and man-made, that have significant hormonal activity and therefore have the potential for effects on developing gonadal steroid target tissues. The remainder of this article will illustrate these problems by briefly reviewing the developmental effects of several hormonally-active therapeutic and environmental agents.

Hormonal Therapy During Pregnancy: DES and the Synthetic Progestins

The synthetic estrogen, diethylstilbestrol (DES) was used to treat pregnant women at risk for spontaneous abortion for over thirty years. In 1971, a statistical association was found between maternal ingestion of DES and the occurrence of a rare form of clear cell adenocarcinoma of the vagina (Herbst *et al*, 1971). Subsequent work established a link between prenatal DES exposure and a variety of abnormalities in the development of the reproductive tract, in both the male and female offspring, with the result that this treatment modality is no longer used. The abnormalities identified in addition to vaginal cancer included benign adenosis of the cervical and vaginal epithelium, distortion in the shape of the cervix and uterus, occasional obstruction of the fallopian tubes and paraovarian cysts in the female; and cryptorchidism, epididymal cysts and testicular lesions in the male (Newbold and McLachlan, 1985). Experimental studies suggest that these defects are at least in large part the result of DES-induced teratogenic changes in the differentiation of the Mullerian and Wolffian duct derived structures (Fig. 2). It remains to be seen whether other problems will emerge as the exposed population passes through reproductive maturity and approaches old age. For example, studies in mice and rats have demonstrated increased susceptibility to mammary tumor formation following prenatal DES exposure (Bern *et al*, 1985). It is still too early to tell whether similar effects may occur in the human population.

Prenatal DES exposure also appears to have effects on the development of the central nervous system. As indicated above, estrogens are believed to play an important role in sexual differentiation of the brain. Recent work comparing prenatally DES-exposed women with normal controls suggests that the abnormal prenatal estrogen exposure may have resulted in a subtle masculinization of certain aspects of CNS function, including the degree of cerebral lateralization (Hines and Shipley, 1984) and sexual orientation (Ehrhardt *et al*, 1985).

In addition to DES, women at risk for spontaneous abortion also were treated during pregnancy with synthetic progestins, some of which possess androgenic as well as progestational activity. The effects of this treatment varied, depending on the steroids used and the duration of therapy. In some cases of treatment with androgenic progestins, clinical masculinization of the external genitalia was observed. At the level of the central nervous system, girls exposed prenatally to such treatments exhibited significant masculinization of gender-role behavior (Ehrhardt and Money, 1967). In contrast, the offspring of women treated prenatally with estrogen-progestin combinations demonstrated subtle increases in the expression of typically feminine behavior patterns (Ehrhardt and Meyer-Bahlburg, 1981).

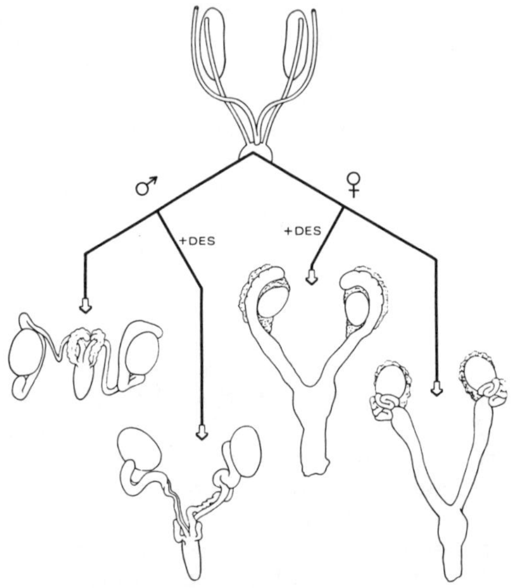

Fig. 2 Schematic representation of the early changes in the reproductive tract induced by exposure to DES (From Newbold and McLachlan, 1985, with permission)

Cimetidine: a Case of Unexpected Hormonal Activity

The H-2 histamine antagonist, cimetidine (Tagamet; Smith, Kline and French) is extremely useful in treatment of gastric hypersecretory states. Over the more than 10 years since its introduction, it has been found to be a well-tolerated and very effective agent for reduction of gastric acid secretion, which has led to its widespread use. During the early 1980s, it became apparent that reproductive side-effects occasionally occurred during long-term cimetidine treatment of adult men. In the affected patients, there was an increased frequency of infertility (Jansen *et al*, 1983), a condition which was reversed after cessation of the cimetidine therapy. Experimental studies established that the reason for this side-effect was cimetidine's significant anti-androgenic activity (Winters *et al*, 1979). Not surprisingly, given this activity, cimetidine treatment of rats during pregnancy was found to induce serious abnormalities of sexual differentiation: masculinization of the external genitalia in males was inhibited; while in adulthood masculine sexual behavior in the offspring of cimetidine-treated dams was impaired (Parker *et al*, 1984). These observations assume particular significance in view of the fact that cimetidine has been considered for use in pregnant women to treat morning sickness. Clearly, such use would constitute a hazard to developing male fetuses, in view of the potential for interference with normal androgen action. Fortunately, the development of other drugs with H-2 antagonist properties but without the unwanted antiandrogenic side-effects (notably, Ranitidine [Zantac]; Glaxo) provides excellent therapeutic alternatives.

Hormonally-Active Agents in the Environment: Estrogen Agonists, Antagonists and Inhibitors of Estrogen Biosynthesis

Recognition of the adverse effects of DES on reproductive tract development coincided with increasing concern over the occurrence of estrogenic compounds in the environment. DES itself was widely used in the farming industry to increase meat yields in cattle and poultry, with the result that contamination of meat with residual DES was occasionally observed (Jukes, 1976; Knight, 1980). Approval for this use of DES was subsequently withdrawn, although other types of hormonal therapy have been introduced to take its place (see below). Although as recently as 1977 it was estimated that almost 30,000 kg of DES were being used per annum for agricultural purposes, the available evidence suggests that it does not present an environmental hazard, since it is rapidly excreted by livestock and broken down in the soil (Knight, 1980).

In addition to synthetic estrogens, a number of other man-made chemicals that have found their way into the environment have now also been shown to exhibit significant estrogenic activity, including the polychlorinated biphenyls (PCBs) and the organochlorine insecticides methoxychlor, kepone and DDT, as well as a number of DDT metabolites (Katzenellenbogen *et al*, 1980). Although the estrogenic potencies of these agents are relatively weak, continued exposure may lead to a build-up of the compounds in the body, resulting in reproductive problems. DDT has also been shown to bind to the progesterone receptor, raising the possibility that it may exert weak progestational or anti-progestational activity (Brown and Blaustein, 1984).

Another class of compounds with significant reproductive side-effects is the imidazole antimycotics. These compounds are believed to act by inhibiting ergosterol biosynthesis. During the late 1970s, it was realized that some of these compounds also inhibit aromatase, the enzyme responsible for estrogen biosynthesis. Particularly powerful effects were noted with miconazole and ketoconazole (Mason *et al*, 1985), both of which are used clinically for treatment of fungal infections. Pharmaceutical use of these compounds is not, however, the only way in which such agents could have a biological impact, since similar preparations are also widely used as agricultural chemicals. For example, reproductive side-effects recently came to light in the toxicological evaluation of a related agricultural fungicide, fenarimol (α-(2-chlorophenyl)-α(4-chlorophenyl)-5-pyrimidine-methanol; Lilly). During reproductive trials, it was found that rats treated with high levels of this compound for prolonged periods exhibited a dose-dependent decrease in fertility, which was pronounced and irreversible in animals that were treated pre- as well as post-natally. Mating trials established that the primary reason for the loss of fertility was a failure of the males to exhibit normal copulatory behavior. This failure was subsequently demonstrated to be due to inhibition of estrogen biosynthesis in the brain, resulting in a blockade of the normal masculinizing effects of testosterone on development of the centers controlling reproductive function (Hirsch *et al*, 1987).

Naturally-Occurring Biologically-Active Compounds: the Phytoestrogens

Compared to the large body of information that has been developed with respect to the environmental concentrations of different hormonally-active xenobiotics, relatively little attention has been paid to a group of naturally-occurring compounds that are also known to exert steroid-like effects on the reproductive system. These compounds comprise a variety of substances derived from plant or fungal sources that have been found to exhibit estrogenic or antiestrogenic activity. The importance of these "phytoestrogens" lies in the fact that they are normal constituents of the diet.

Very few plants synthesize the principal mammalian estrogens, estradiol and estrone. However, a number of other plant substances have been isolated that bear a structural resemblance to either the mammalian estrogens or to DES. The major groups of phytoestrogens that are found in the human diet and their principal dietary sources are the isoflavones (soy beans, chick peas, cherries), the coumestans (alfalfa, peas, beans) and the resorcylic acid lactones (peas and a variety of grains). This last group of compounds is not intrinsic to the foodstuffs in which they are found, but is produced as a secondary metabolite of several species of the fungal genus Fusarium, which frequently accumulate on poorly stored grain.

The biological significance of the dietary phytoestrogens is a subject of continuing debate. These compounds have been shown to bind to the estrogen receptor and to exert weak estrogenic effects

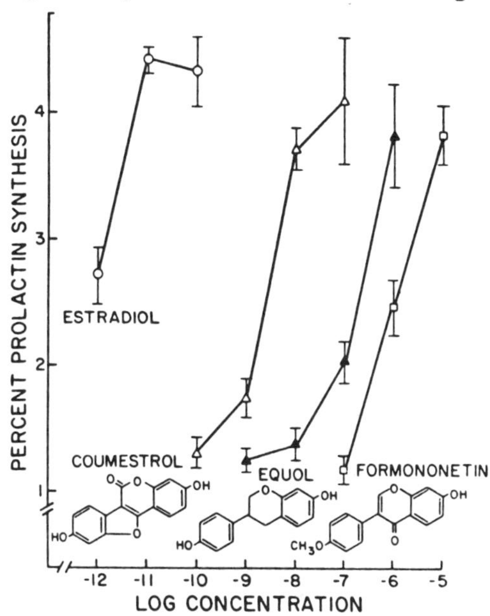

Fig. 3 Estrogenic effects of estradiol, coumestrol, equol and formonentin in primary cultures of rat pituitary cells (From Jordan *et al*, 1985, with permission).

(Shutt and Cox, 1972; Tang and Adams, 1980). Such effects may either be synergistic with those of the endogenous hormones, or antagonistic, since the complexes formed between the estrogen receptor and the phytoestrogens may not be fully active in terms of inducing the cellular responses observed with estradiol (Tang and Adams, 1980). In common with other estrogens when administered orally, the phytoestrogens appear to stimulate the synthesis of testosterone-estradiol binding globulin (TeBG), which may also serve to attenuate the actions of the endogenous hormones. Zearalenone, in addition, exhibits considerable anabolic activity, which has been exploited commercially in the use of the closely related synthetic compound, α-zearalenol as an anabolic agent in beef cattle and sheep. Finally, recent studies have shown that a number of flavonoids inhibit aromatization of androgens to estrogens (Kellis and Vickery, 1984). Phytoestrogens and their metabolites have been identified in the urine of several mammalian species (Adlercreutz *et al*, 1987); but a definitive link between the ingestion of these compounds and effects on the reproductive system has yet to be established in man. Nevertheless, the potential for such effects must clearly be considered, as a result of demonstrations in animals that dietary components can affect reproductive function. Sheep grazing on pastures rich in Trifolium subterraneum, a species of clover that is widely distributed in Australia, develop infertility ("Clover disease") as a result of the presence in this plant of the isoflavone, formonentin. Formonentin is converted to diadzein and equol by bacterial metabolism in the sheep rumen: all three of these compounds are weak estrogens (Fig. 3). Moldy feed has been repeatedly observed to cause hyperestrogenism in swine. Finally, commercially-prepared rat chow containing soy beans has been demonstrated to produce a significant uterotrophic response in laboratory rats, an effect which has been correlated with the isoflavonoid content of soy meal (Axelson *et al*, 1984).

DISCUSSION AND CONCLUSIONS

The question of the developmental risk presented by hormonally-active drugs and naturally-occurring compounds is one without a definitive answer. On the one hand, the experience with DES and the synthetic progestins clearly indicates that disturbance of the normal sex steroid milieu during pregnancy can have serious, life-long consequences for the developing fetus. On the other hand, despite a growing list of compounds with hormonal activity to which pregnant women and young children may be exposed from the environment, there is a lack of hard evidence to indicate the extent of the effects elicited by these compounds.

The picture is clearest with respect to the risks presented by man-made agents, either introduced therapeutically or derived from the environment. There is no doubt that substances with androgenic or estrogenic activity may interfere with normal sexual development. In addition to the effects of prenatal exposure to such agents cited previously, it should be noted that the risks may extend well into the postnatal period as a result of transfer of the agents to breast milk. The natural estrogens and some of the estrogen xenobiotics are excreted in the milk at sufficient quantities to induce accelerated reproductive development, at least in experimental animals (Eroschenko, 1985). The previously-mentioned effects of the fungicide, fenarimol, on sexual differentiation in rats probably result primarily from excretion into the milk, since trans-placental passage of this fungicide is limited (Hirsch *et al*, 1987)

The issue of whether low-level exposure to xenobiotics or phytoestrogens may also have reproductive consequences, however, remains unresolved. The possibility that such contamination might have contributed to unexplained instances of premature thelarche has been suggested, but not unequivocally proven (Haddock *et al*, 1985). Studies of the excretion of equol and related diphenolic compounds by human subjects have shown that a strict vegetarian diet can dramatically increase the production rates of these compounds and, as indicated previously, there seems little doubt that this raises at least the potential for reproductive effects. An area of particular concern might be the increasing use of soy protein in the human diet, especially in formula for infants, in view of the high isoflavonoid content of soy meal. However, it must be acknowledged that there have not been any documented cases of estrogenization resulting from soy-rich diets. Indeed, since the age of puberty is relatively constant in children raised on vegetarian or omnivorous diets, and infants raised from birth on soy protein formula do not appear to exhibit abnormal breast enlargement, it is difficult to argue for a major estrogen agonist role for dietary phytoestrogens in normal human development (New, 1985b).

The apparent disparity between the pharmacological estrogenic activities of the phytoestrogens and the apparent lack of effect of a diet rich in these agents on pregnancy and the developing reproductive system may perhaps be resolved by consideration of the other factors associated with such a diet. The increased fiber content of the food reduces the enterohepatic circulation of the natural estrogens, thereby increasing the excretion rates of the endogenous hormones (Adlercreutz *et al*, 1987). This would tend to counteract the effects of increased estrogen intake. The estrogenic effects of the isoflavonoids in soy meal appear to be at least partly dependent on bacterial conversion to the more estrogenic metabolite, equol. This conversion may not occur to a significant extent in nursing infants, in which the normal gut flora have not yet become established. It may be more appropriate to consider the effects of the phytoestrogens primarily in terms of their potential for interference with normal estrogen biosynthesis and action, rather than their relatively weak estrogen agonist activity. As indicated previously, dietary phytoestrogens may inhibit estrogen biosynthesis and partially antagonize the actions of the natural mammalian estrogens, as well as reducing the effective free concentrations of circulating androgens and estrogens by stimulating TeBG synthesis. These effects have been suggested to at least partially underlie the reduced risk of hormone-dependent cancer in women with primarily vegetarian diets (Setchell *et al*, 1984; Adlercreutz *et al*, 1987). It seems unlikely, however, that similar effects might play a significant role in human pregnancy as a result of the enormous changes which normally occur during gestation in both TeBG and steroid hormone biosynthesis, unless dietary phytoestrogen intake were to increase to well above normal levels.

ACKNOWLEDGEMENTS

I am indebted to Dr. Patricia Whitten for useful discussions in the preparation of this article.

REFERENCES

Adlercreutz, H, Hockerstedt, K, Bannwart, C, Bloigu, S, Hamalainen, E, Fotsis, T, Ollus, A (1987). Effect of dietary components, including lignans and phytoestrogens, on enterohepatic circulation and liver metabolism of estrogens and on sex hormone binding globulin (SHBG) J Steroid Biochem 27:1135-1144.

Axelson M, Sjovall J, Gustaffson B, Setchell K (1984). Soya - a dietary source of the non-steroidal oestrogen equol in humans and animals. J Endocrinol 102:49-56.

Barbarino A, De Marinis L, Lafuenti G, Muscatello P, Matteucci B (1979). Presence of positive feedback between oestrogen and LH in patients with Klinefelter's syndrome, and Sertoli-cell-only syndrome. Clin Endocrinol (Oxf). 10:235-242.

Bardin C, Catterall J (1981). Testosterone: a major determinant of extragenital sexual dimorphism. Science 211:1285-1294.

Bern H, Mills K, Edery M (1985). Estrogen-associated defects in rodent mammary gland development. In McLachlan JA (ed): "Estrogens in the Environment II: Influences on Development" New York: Elsevier, pp 319-326.

Brown T, Blaustein J (1984). 1-(o-chlorophenyl).-1-(p-chlorophenyl).2,2,2-trichloroethane induces functional progestin receptors in the rat hypothalamus and pituitary gland. Endocrinology 115:2052-2058.

Davidson I, Stott J, Longstaff, A, Abramovich D, Pearson C (1983). Oestrogen concentration in mid-trimester human fetal brain: a possible role in its sexual differentiation. J Steroid Biochem 18:525-529.

De Lacoste M, Holloway R, Woodward D (1986). Sex differences in the fetal human corpus callosum. Hum Neurobiol 5:93-96.

Ehrhardt AA, Meyer-Bahlburg H (1981). Effects of prenatal sex hormones on gender-related behavior. Science 211:1312-1318.

Ehrhardt A, Meyer-Bahlburg H, Rosen L, Feldman J, Veridiano N, Zimmerman I, McEwen BS (1985). Sexual orientation after prenatal exposure to exogenous estrogen. Arch Sex Behav 14:57-77.

Ehrhardt A, Money J (1967). Progestin-induced hermaphroditism: I.Q. and psychosexual identity in a study of ten girls. J Sex Res 3:83-100.

Eroschenko V (1985). Morphological analysis of chlordecone (kepone). action in different mouse organs: choroid plexus in adult males and vaginal epithelium in suckling neonates. In McLachlan JA (ed): "Estrogens in the Environment II: Influences on Development" New York: Elsevier, pp 86-103.

Geschwind N, Behan P (1982). Left-handedness: association with immune disease, migraine, and developmental learning disorder. Proc Natl Acad Sci USA 79:5097-5100.

Gorski R (1973). Perinatal effects of sex steroids on brain development and function. Prog Brain Res 39:149-163.

Goy R, McEwen BS (1980). Sexual Differentiation of the Brain. MIT Press, Cambridge, Mass.

Granick S, Kappas A (1967). Steroid control of porphyrin and heme biosynthesis: a new biological function of steroid hormone metabolites. Proc Natl Acad Sci USA 57:1463-1467.

Greene R, Burrill M, Ivy A (1940). Experimental intersexuality. Am J Anat 67:305-343.

Haddock L, Lebron G, Martinez R, Cordero J, Freni-Titulaer L, Carrion F, Cintron C, Gonzalez L (1985). Premature sexual development in Puerto Rico: background and current status. In McLachlan JA (ed): "Estrogens in the Environment II: Influences on Development" New York: Elsevier, pp 86-103.

Harris G, Levine S (1965). Sexual differentiation of the brain and its experimental control. J Physiol 181:379-400.

Hart B (1979) Activation of sexual reflexes of male rats by dihydrotestosterone but not estrogen. Physiol Behav 23:107-109

Herbst A, Ulfelder H, Poskanzer D (1971). Adenocarcinoma of the vagina: association of maternal stilbestrol therapy with tumor appearance in young women. N Engl J Med 284:878-881.

Hines M, Shipley C (1984). Prenatal exposure to diethylstilbestrol (DES) and the development of sexually dimorphic cognitive abilities and cerebral lateralization. Dev Psychobiol 20:81-94.

Hirsch K, Weaver D, Black L, Falcone J, Maclusky NJ (1987). Inhibition of central nervous system aromatase activity: a mechanism for fenarimol-induced infertility in the male rat. Tox Appl Pharmacol 91:235-245.

Jansen R, Collen M, Pandol S, Allende H, Raufman J-P, Bissonette B, Duncan W, Durgan P, Gillin J, Gardner J (1983). Cimetidine-induced impotence and breast changes in patients with gastric hypersecretory states. N Engl J Med 308:883-888.

Jordan, VC, Koch, R, Bain, RR (1985). Prolactin synthesis in cultured rat pituitary cells: an assay to study estrogens, antiestrogens and their metabolites in vitro In McLachlan JA (ed): "Estrogens in the Environment II: Influences on Development" New York: Elsevier, pp 221-237

Jost A (1972). A new look at the mechanisms controlling sex differentiation in mammals. Johns Hopkins Med J 130:38-53.

Jukes T (1976). Diethylstilbestrol in beef production: what is the risk to consumers? Ann NY Acad Sci 111:665-670.

Karsch F, Dierschke D, Knobil E (1973). Sexual differentiation of pituitary function: apparent difference bewteen primates and rodents. Science 179:484-486.

Katzenellenbogen J, Katzenellenbogen B, Tatee T, Robertson D, Landvatter S (1980). The chemistry of estrogens and antiestrogens: relationship between structure, receptor binding and biological activity. In McLachlan JA (ed): "Estrogens in the Environment" New York: Elsevier, pp 33-51.

Kellis JJ, Vickery L (1984). Inhibition of human estrogen synthetase (aromatase). by flavones. Science 225:1032-1034.

Knight W (1980). Estrogens administered to food-producing animals: environmental considerations. In McLachlan JA (ed): "Estrogens in the Environment" New York: Elsevier, pp 391-401.

Knudsen J, Max S (1980). Aromatization of androgens to estrogens mediates increased activity of glucose-6-phosphate dehydrogenase in rat levator ani muscle. Endocrinology 106:440-443.

MacLusky N, Naftolin F (1981). Sexual differentiation of the central nervous system. Science 211:1294-1303.

Mason J, Murry B, Olcott M, Sheets J (1985). Imidazole antimycotics: inhibitors of steroid aromatase. Biochem Pharmacol 34:1087-1092.

Max S, Knudsen J (1980). Effect of sex hormones on glucose-6-phosphate dehydrogenase in rat levator ani muscle. Mol Cell Endocrinol 17:111-118.

McEwen BS (1981). Neural gonadal steroid interactions. Science 211:1303-1311.

McEwen BS, Lieberburg I, MacLusky NJ, Plapinger L (1976). Interactions of testosterone and oestradiol with the neonatal rat brain; protection mechanisms and possible relationship to sexual differentiation. Ann Biologie 16:471-478.

New M (1985a). Premature thelarche and estrogen intoxication. In McLachlan JA (ed): "Estrogens in the Environment II: Influences on Development" New York: Elsevier, pp 349-357.

New M (1985b). Discussion Comment. In McLachlan JA (ed): "Estrogens in the Environment II: Influences on Development" New York: Elsevier, p 84.

Newbold R, McLachlan J (1985). Diethylstilbestrol associated defects in murine genital tract development. In McLachlan JA (ed): "Estrogens in the Environment II: Influences on Development" New York: Elsevier, pp 288-318.

Parker S, Schade R, Pohl C, Gavaler J, Van Thiel D (1984). Prenatal and neonatal exposure of male rat pups to cimetidine but not ranitidine adversely affects subsequent adult sexual functioning. Gastroenterology 86:675-680.

Pfeiffer C (1936). Sexual differences of the hypophyses and their determination by the gonads. Am J Anat 58:195-210.

Phoenix C, Goy R, Resko J (1968). Psychosexual differentiation as a function of androgenic stimulation. In Diamond M (ed): Reproduction and Sexual Behavior, Bloomington, Indiana: Indiana University Press, pp 33-49.

Ramirez V, Sawyer C (1965). Advancement of puberty in the female rat by estrogen. Endocrinology 76:1158-1168.

Setchell K, Borriello S, Hulme P, Kirk D, Axelson M (1984). Non-steroidal estrogens of dietary origin: possible roles in hormone-dependent disease. Am J Clin Nutr 40:569-578.

Shutt D, Cox R (1972). Steroid and phytoestrogen binding to sheep uterine receptor in vitro. J Endocrinol 52:299-310.

Swaab D, Fliers E (1985). A sexually dimorphic nucleus in the human brain. Science 228:1112-1115.

Tang B, Adams N (1980). The effect of equol on oestrogen receptors and on synthesis of DNA and protein in the immature rat uterus. J Endocrinol 85:291-297.

Uriel J, DeNechaud B, Dupiers M (1972). Estrogen binding properties of rat, mouse, man fetospecific serum proteins. Demonstration by immuno-autoradiographic methods. Biochem Biophys Res Commun 46:1175-1180.

Weisz J, Gunsalus G (1973). Estrogen levels in immature rats: true or spurious - ovarian or adrenal? Endocrinology 93:1059-1065.

Wilson J, George F, Griffin J (1981). The hormonal control of sexual development. Science 211:1278-1284.

Winters S, Banks J, Loriaux D (1979). Cimetidine is an antiandrogen in the rat. Gastroenterology 76:504-508.

DISCUSSION

DR. KELLOGG: I just recalled that Dick Swaab recently presented some data indicating that the sexual differentiation of the sexually dimorphic nucleus in human males actually may be taking place 2 to 5 years postnatally. This puts a whole different perspective on considering the effects of exposure to compounds that you were discussing.

DR. MACLUSKY: In my presentation there was of necessity a good deal of oversimplification. In most species, the critical period for sexual differentiation has been defined on the basis of the period in which you can see effects on reproductive behavior or the control of reproductive cyclicity. If androgen exposure occurs, you get a shift towards masculine patterns of behavior and gonadotropin release. That is, however, not necessarily the only time at which androgen can have a developmental effect.

In the case of the sexually dimorphic nucleus of the preoptic area, it seems clear from animal studies that this doesn't have a major role to play in the control of reproductive behavior. One can functionally remove this nucleus by experimentally producing a lesion in it, and reproductive behavior remains intact. At present the function of the sexually dimorphic nucleus is not known.

In animal studies, the differentiation of aggression, which is very much influenced by testosterone, goes on well into the postnatal period. Morphological differentiation of the hippocampus can be affected up to puberty in mice. Again, with respect to aromatase activity in the prefrontal cortex in primates, testosterone can effect the maturation of the association cortex well into postnatal life, in just those regions which retain aromatase activity. So, I don't mean to exclude the possibility of androgen effects at other time intervals.

DR. MUELLER: Maybe an indication for this postnatal influence of aromatase inhibitors is the fact that some aromatase inhibitors (i.e. antifungal agents) are now being used to modify sexual behavior in male children.

DR. MACLUSKY: Yes, that is right. In those cases, there are questions about whether these drugs, which have a fairly wide specificity in terms of P450 inhibition, may produce their effects through a general inhibition of steroidogenesis. The question is at which point do the drugs exert their effects, is it at the level of steroid production, or in the action of the steroids. The fungicide miconazole is a very good aromatase inhibitor.

DR. MUELLER: I was thinking of ketoconazole.

DR. MACLUSKY: Yes, but that also produces a fairly good inhibition of steroidogenesis in the adrenal. So, again there would be the question of whether aromatase inhibition was responsible for the effects. The question of the role of aromatase and effects of androgen on behavior in people is a controversial one. I would certainly like to believe that there is a role for aromatase and that inhibitors of aromatase, therefore, produce their effects in this way; but in this case I am not sure that is so.

DR. QUINN: In light of the observations on cimetidine and Accutane, how were the negative side effects managed before release of these drugs? I believe that Accutane was known to be a teratogen before being released for marketing. What kind of guidelines are given regarding its use?

DR. MACLUSKY: Cimetidine was a real problem because they did not know about the antiandrogenic effects before they marketed it. These came out later; but I don't think anyone had any idea how popular cimetidine was going to be, or how much it was going to be prescribed, and particularly how many people were going to take it at high doses for extended periods of time. The side effects became apparent more or less simultaneously from research in animals and from clinical studies of infertility. The initial animal studies indicated that it did not significantly inhibit androgen receptor binding. In the case of cimetidine, the problem is that it remains at high levels for a long time. It is a relatively simple problem to deal with by changing an infertile male's prescription of cimetidine to ranitidine. The suggestion that cimetidine might be used in pregnant women to control excessive gastric acid secretion has stimulated a number of studies, particularly from Dr. Van Thiel's group.

Transplacental Effects on Fetal Health, pages 265–277

DEVELOPMENTAL EFFECTS OF NEUROACTIVE DRUGS

Carol K. Kellogg and Ronnie Guillet

Department of Psychology,
University of Rochester,
Rochester, New York 14627

INTRODUCTION

That drugs elicit their effects on organisms through combination with specific receptors has been a well accepted concept since its introduction by Langley (1906). And in recent years, neural receptors that mediate the pharmacologic effects of many neuroactive drugs (such as antipsychotic, antidepressant and anxiolytic agents) have been identified. If occupancy of specific neural receptors mediates the actions of neuroactive drugs in adult organisms, it would seem likely that the existence of specific receptors in developing brains could render the developing brain vulnerable to the presence of specific exogenous compounds. Vulnerability could of course simply mean that the developing brain was sensitive to the compounds, but that once a response was elicited, there would be no lasting effect. On the other hand, because there is a high degree of plasticity in the central nervous system, vulnerability could imply that generation of a response in the developing brain could influence the continued course of neural development, with functional consequences that might be expressed throughout the lifespan of the organism.

Precisely how a drug will influence developing nervous systems cannot be predicted, however, based simply on the presence of recognition sites for the drug. Receptor function depends not only on the presence of a specific, high affinity recognition site but also on the existence of effector mechanisms that translate the interaction of a drug with its binding site into a response in the receptive cell. Studies on the development of transmitter receptors in the brain indicate that some early appearing sites are linked to active effector mechanisms while other early appearing receptors are unable to mediate appropriate effector responses (see Miller, Kellogg and Saltzman, 1987 for review). Additionally, effector mechanisms present during development may differ from those present in the adult.

The full expression of drug interaction with neural receptors during development will also depend upon the neural interactions that receptive cells make with other neurons and upon the maturational state of specific neural circuitry. Because neuroactive drugs can influence chemical neurotransmission, the developmental profile of specific neurotransmitters may be an important determinant of the effect of early developmental drug exposure. The processes underlying chemical transmission in specific neural populations, such as the catecholamine-containing neurons, are known to appear early in fetal rat brain (Coyle, 1977), and these early developing transmitter systems respond in a predictable manner to many neuroactive drugs (Coyle and Henry, 1973). An involvement in regulation of cell proliferation, in differentiation, and in organization of specific neural circuitry has been proposed for these early appearing systems (Lauder and Krebs, 1986). Thus, interference with specific transmitter function during development could have profound consequences on brain function.

Experimental studies have indicated that early drug exposure can indeed elicit a lasting imprint on neural function (see below). Some of these drugs may have altered transmitter availability, while others may have acted directly on receptors mediating communication between neurons. Some neuroactive drugs that may be utilized during pregnancy and their respective sites of interaction in the nervous system are listed in Table 1.

This paper will present some of the reported transplacental effects on the offspring of *in utero* exposure of experimental animals to selected neuroactive agents. Since the ultimate goal of these studies is to provide relevant information that may be extrapolated to

Table 1. Some Agents Utilized During Pregnancy and Their Actions in the Central or Peripheral Nervous System[a]

Drug	Effect
Antipsychotic agents	
Halperidol (Haldol)	DA receptor antagonists; some action at 5-HT
Phenothiazines (e.g., Thorazine)	and NE receptors.
Antidepressant agents	
Imipramine (Tofranil)	Block reuptake of released transmitter into
Amitriptyline (Elavil)	5-HT and NE neurons; induce down regulation of β receptors.
Ataractic drugs	
Chlordiazepoxide (Librium)	Agonists at specific benzodiazepine binding
Diazepam (Valium)	site; may influence GABA neurotransmission via GABA receptor.
Anticonvulsant agents	
Diazepam (Valium)	See above.
Phenobarbital	May bind to particular domain of GABA–receptor complex and influence GABA transmission.
Phenytoin (Dilantin)	May bind to GABA–receptor complex.
Valproic acid	
Antihypertensive agents	
Methyldopa (Aldomet)	Amine metabolite may act directly on adrenergic receptors in CNS.
Clonidine (Catapres)	Agonist at α_2 receptors.
Sympathomimetic agents	
Selective β_2 agonists	
Salbutamol (Albuterol)	Stimulate β_2 receptors
Terbutaline (Bricanyl)	
Amphetamine (Benzadrine)	Promote release of catecholamines; may block reuptake and MAO.
Methylxanthines (caffeine)	Precise action unclear; may act at adenosine sites, benzodiazepine binding sites.
Cold medications containing ephedrine, phenylephrine	Act like NE on adrenergic receptors; may release CA.
Analgesic agents	
Morphine	Agonists to opiate receptors.
Hydromorphine (Dilaudid)	
Methadone (Dolophine)	
Meperidine (Demerol)	
Codeine	

[a]Abbreviations: DA, dopamine; NE, norepinephrine; 5-HT, 5-hydroxytryptamine (serotonin); CA, catecholamine; MAO, monoamine oxidase.

humans, important considerations that must be taken into account in the design and interpretation of experimental studies will be discussed. Lastly, neural mechanisms that may translate the effect of *in utero* drug exposure into lasting functional consequences will be addressed, as the significance to humans of information obtained from experimental studies rests in the understanding of mechanisms whereby exogenous substances may influence the developing brain.

INTERPRETING EXPERIMENTAL STUDIES

When interpreting the consequences induced by *in utero* exposure of experimental animals to neuroactive drugs, specific information is essential. If one wishes to interpret the effects in terms of the significance for humans, one needs to understand species differences in comparable phases of brain development. In terms of selected biochemical indices, the rat brain at birth, *e.g.*, has been compared to a human brain around 20 weeks of gestation, whereas maturational events during late gestation in humans (*i.e.*, the third trimester) may be comparable to those events taking place during the first postnatal week in rats (Dobbing, 1974). Therefore, the developmental events taking place in the brain of a rat during the third week of pregnancy are not the same as those taking place in the human brain during the third trimester (see Miller, Kellogg, and Saltzman, 1987 for a discussion of brain development). What is most important to bear in mind is that the sequencing of specific neural events is similar during rodent (*e.g.*) and human brain development. That is, specific transmitter-identified neural populations undergo chemical differentiation prior to the appearance of certain drug receptors in both species. Thus, the appropriate substrates for specific drug-CNS interactions are present developmentally in both species. Figure 1 demonstrates the comparable period of development for selected systems in human and rodent brain.

For cross-study as well as cross-species extrapolation of observations, it is important to establish a reference of drug exposure level. Simply giving the dosage in terms of mg/kg body weight can be misleading. Expressed in these terms, dosages of the anxiolytic compound diazepam (DZ), for example, that

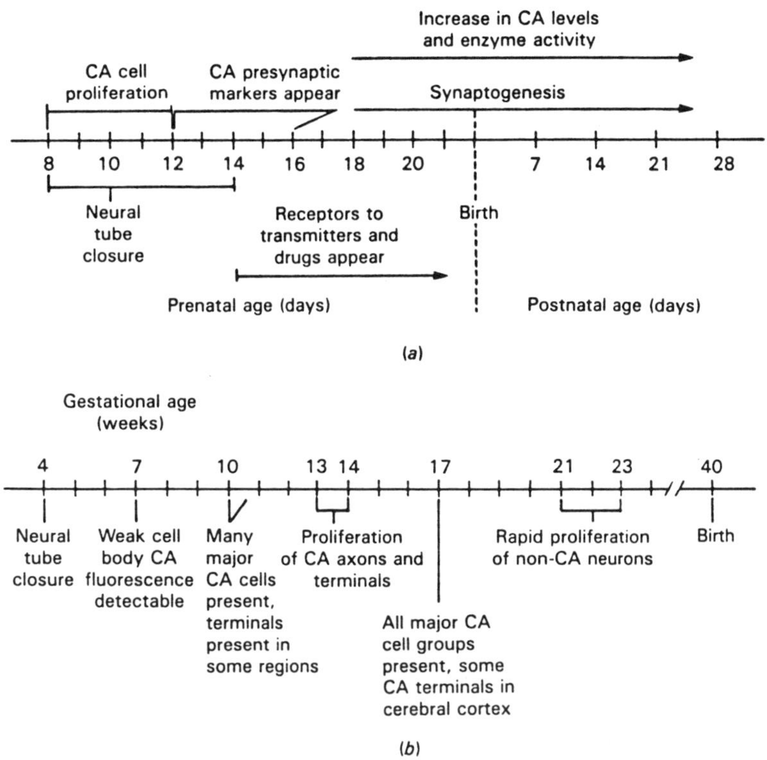

Figure 1. (a) Development of catecholamine neurons in the rat. (b) Development of catecholamine neurons in the human. CA, catecholamine. From Miller, Kellogg, and Saltzman (1987).

induce lasting effects in the rat offspring (see Kellogg, 1988) seem high when compared to clinical doses. However, the maximum plasma levels reached in the pregnant rat dam following subcutaneous administration of DZ at 2.5 mg/kg are in the range of 0.26 ug/ml, which is comparable to levels reached in clinical reports of DZ administration during labor. One must keep in mind that the clearance rate of compounds differs between species. Likewise, the route of administration used in experimental studies can influence the plasma levels reached.

Finally, in any work considering the consequences of prenatal drug exposure on the offspring, it is essential to determine whether alterations in the offspring resulted from a direct action of the drug in the fetal brain. The consequences in the offspring may reflect an action that was secondary to a direct effect of the drug in the dam. The drug must be shown to be present in the fetal brain following administration to the dam, to interact at its relevant binding site in the fetal brain, and to initiate a response in the fetal brain. Availability of such information should markedly assist in the interpretation of experimental studies.

FUNCTIONAL ALTERATIONS INDUCED BY *IN UTERO* EXPOSURE TO NEUROACTIVE DRUGS

Functional defects have been reported in offspring following *in utero* exposure to many neuroactive agents, including neuroleptic, antidepressant, anxiolytic, and antihypertensive compounds (see Brown and Fishman, 1984; Mirmiran *et al*., 1985; and Boer *et al*., 1988). Some general principles appear to govern the outcome of these early developmental exposures. Observations made in experimental animals following such exposures have indicated that the induced effects are dependent upon the timing of the exposure, are dependent upon the age of the offspring at testing, and are most obvious in the offspring when the offspring are challenged either behaviorally or pharmacologically.

With respect to the timing of drug exposure, exposure to the neuroleptic drug haloperidol (which is an antagonist at specific dopamine (DA) receptors) during late gestation in rats induces specific effects on the neural receptors for the nigral striatal DA projection. Late gestational exposure induces a decrease in the density of DA receptors in the striatum that is associated with a decreased functional response in the offspring when administered apomorphine, a DA receptor agonist. On the other hand, early postnatal exposure to haloperidol produces an increase in DA receptor density in the striatum (Friedhoff and Miller, 1983). Also, early postnatal exposure of rats to penfluridol, another neuroleptic drug, induces biochemical changes in DA projections to limbic structures rather than to the neostriatum. Similarly exposed offspring also demonstrate an impairment in the acquisition of a conditioned avoidance response (Lundborg and Engel, 1978). Therefore, the timing of early developmental exposure to neuroleptic compounds determines the specific DA projections that will be most influenced, which will in turn be an important determinant of any consequent functional alteration. The timing of exposure has also been a factor in determining the consequences of exposure to other neuroactive drugs.

As indicated above, the age of the offspring at examination also appears to be an important factor in determining any neural or functional alterations. Late gestational exposure of rats to the anxiolytic compound diazepam induces effects on the noradrenergic projection to the hypothalamus (Kellogg, 1988). This effect is not evident, though, until the offspring reach young adulthood. If the neurons are examined in prepubertal pups, little effect is evident. There is, however, a dramatic dose-related effect on these neurons in young adult offspring. Functionally, these neuronal changes can also be correlated with altered responses to a stressor in the adult offspring.

In utero exposure to diazepam also induces effects on cellular metabolism in the brain that are modified as the organism ages from young adulthood (3 months of age) to around two years of age (Kellogg, 1988). These observations indicate that the plasticity of the central nervous system can be a determinant not only of the initial response to *in utero* drug exposure but also of the expression of that initial insult throughout the lifespan of the organism. That is to say, the effects of *in utero* drug exposure are related to and altered by developmental and aging processes. This is a critical observation to consider when designing any clinical study to evaluate the effects of early developmental drug exposure.

A third observation made from experimental studies is that the functional alterations induced by *in utero* exposure to neuroactive compounds (particularly exposures after the embryonic period of organogenesis) may require a specific, but often common, environmental cue for full expression. For example, the functional effects of prenatal exposure to diazepam reflect interference with arousal-attention and stress-related functions (see

Kellogg, 1988 for review). As indicated in Table 2, changes in these types of functions can be observed at many ages. That the environment must contain cues necessary to engage these functions in order for the impairment to be detected appears critical.

Table 2. Functional Alterations in Rat Offspring Following Exposure to Diazepam During the Last Week of Gestation.

Dose (mg)	Postnatal Age At testing	Functional Changes	Implications	Investigator(s)[1]
2.5-10	days 11-20	decrement in age-specific locomotor hyperactivity	Interference in age-specific arousal mechanisms	Kellogg et al.
2.5-10	days 12-22	decrease in basal acoustic startle response (ASR) to a 110 dB stimulus	ASR may represent a response to an environmental stressor	Kellogg et al.
		absence of noise potentiation of the ASR	Interference with development of arousal mechanisms	
1-10	days 90-100	dose-specific alteration in the ASR	altered processing of specific environmental information	Kellogg et al.
1-10	days 90-100	altered neural and hormonal responses to restraint stress	may reflect alterations in neural circuitry responsible for organized responses to stressors	Simmons et al.
2.5-10	days 21-70	delayed development and altered mature performance of auditory temporal resolution	function relates to speech perception and language and learning abilities, in humans	Kellogg et al.
5.7-7.5	Adult	impaired sleep EEG patterns suggestive of impaired synchronization	interference with arousal processes	Livezey et al.
10	Adult	deficits in complex simultaneous discrimination maze; no impairment in simple maze performance or motor learning	could reflect changes in processing of environmental information or in specific memory functions	Gai and Grimm

[1] A complete discussion of the results outlined above and complete references can be found in Kellogg (1988).

Early developmental exposure of experimental animals to antihypertensive and antidepressant compounds has led to altered sleep patterns (Mirmiran _et al._, 1981; Mirmiran *et al.*, 1985). A recent report also implicates prenatal exposure in humans to the antihypertensive compound clonidine in excessive sleep disturbances in the offspring (Huisjes *et al.*, 1986). This type of functional alteration in an organism may very well be a factor in precipitating other disruptions in neuronal function. Sleep states are indeed often utilized as a biologic marker for affective disorders, for example.

Thus, it is of primary importance to realize that the initial effects induced by prenatal exposure to neuroactive compounds may, by altering the organism's response to environmental interactions, precipitate secondary effects. Not only can specific compounds given at specific developmental ages have direct consequences for the developing organism, but they may also have indirect effects. Furthermore, these effects may not be readily apparent unless specific environmental conditions are met.

POSSIBLE NEURAL MECHANISMS UNDERLYING THE FUNCTIONAL DEFICITS

While neural mechanisms that may translate the effect of prenatal occupancy of specific receptor sites into lasting and changing functional alterations are not in any way precisely understood, several possibilities exist. A likely consequence of early receptor occupancy is a change in the characteristics of the receptor itself. Hence *in utero* exposure to specific neuroactive drugs, such as neuroleptic compounds, may induce a change in receptor density in the offspring (see above), while exposure to other drugs, such as anxiolytic compounds, may not readily elicit such a change (Kellogg, 1988). However, an influence on receptor function can also be expressed as a change in effector mechanisms and responsiveness. The implication of a change in receptor function of any type is that responses to endogenous ligands or even exogenous compounds will be altered.

To more fully understand how such a change may account for altered responses to specific environmental cues, one must remember that neuroactive compounds interact with high affinity binding sites that, in general, have a specific, non-uniform distribution pattern in the brain and reside upon specific receptive cells. Hence, if certain cues activate specific neural circuitry, the neural response could be altered if the function of selective receptors in the circuitry has been influenced by early developmental drug exposure. In addition, early receptor occupancy may influence the organization of specific neural circuits such that environmental cues do not activate appropriate neural systems following early drug exposure. The plasticity that may involve changes in neural circuits during development and aging may account in part for the dynamic aspect of functional changes observed following early drug exposure.

The possibility must also be considered that early developmental exposure to exogenous neuroactive substances could influence the neurotransmitter profile of specific neurons. Neuropeptides, the most recently identified group of neurotransmitter substances, often coexist in the same neuron with other transmitters. Recent evidence has demonstrated that developmental exposure to neuropeptides can influence brain development and induce physiologic and behavioral effects in adulthood (Handelmann, 1985). Additionally, recent studies have indicated that specific neuropeptides may reside in a neuron only at certain developmental stages and that the expression of a particular neuropeptide in a given neuron may be dependent upon the environment of that neuron (Schultzberg et al., 1986). Hence, the presence of exogenous substances, such as drugs, may alter the environment of the developing brain in a manner that could influence the neuropeptide profile of selective neuronal populations.

CONCLUSIONS

The consequences of early developmental exposure to exogenous compounds may be subtle or profound. The effects are dependent on timing of exposure, timing of examination, and specific challenges. The ultimate effect may also be species-specific. Although basic neurotransmitter systems are similar and develop in the same sequence across species, the complexity of neural interactions in whole brain varies depending on the experimental subject. The implications of this increasing complexity of organization from rodent to human, for example, are unclear. On one hand, increasing complexity may allow for greater plasticity and alternative pathways and thus minimalize functional deficits following *in utero* drug exposure. On the other hand, increasing complexity may compound the effects of early developmental alterations in neural transmission. It would be impossible, therefore, to extrapolate *a priori* from differences in timing of brain development and drug metabolism.

What animal experimentation has allowed, however, is the focussing of investigations in humans. The results of studies in rodents given neuroactive drugs, for example, has suggested the most appropriate indices of function to be examined clinically. Although specific cause and effect relationships for any particular drug and any particular behavior cannot be extrapolated directly from animal studies to humans, general principles will apply. The experience thus far with neuroactive drugs, neural receptors, and resultant functional/behavior alterations in animals suggests that early developmental exposure to exogenous compounds in humans will have significant long-term effects.

REFERENCES

Boer GJ, Feenstra MGP, Mirmiran M, Swaab DF, VanHaanen F, Chen-Pelt W, Eikelboom T (1988). Neurochemistry of functional neuroteratology. Prog Brain Res (In Press).

Brown RM, Fishman HB (1984). An overview and summary of the behavioral and neural consequences of perinatal exposure to psychotropic drugs. In Yanai J (ed): "Neurobehavioral Teratology," Amsterdam: Elsevier, pp 3-54.

Coyle JT (1977). Biochemical aspects of neurotransmission in the developing brain. Int Rev Neurobiol 20:65-103.

Coyle JT, Henry D (1973). Catecholamines in fetal and newborn rat brain. J Neurochem 18:2061-2075.

Dobbing T (1974). Prenatal nutrition and neurologic development. In Crovido J, Hambraeus L, Vahlquist B (eds): "Early Malnutrition and Mental Development," Stockholm: Almquist and Wiksel, pp 96-110.

Friedhoff AJ, Miller JC (1983). Prenatal psychotropic drug exposure and the development of central dopaminergic and cholinergic neurotransmitter systems. Monogr Neural Sci 9:91-98.

Handelmann GE (1985). Neuropeptide effects on brain development. J Physiol 80:268-274.
Huisjes M, Hadders-Algra M, Touwen BCL (1986). Is clonidine a behaviorial teratogen in the human? Early Hum Dev 14:43-48.
Kellogg CK (1988). Benzodiazepines: Influence on the developing brain. Prog Brain Res (In Press).
Langley JN (1906). On nerve-endings and on special excitable substances in cells. Proc R Soc Lond [Biol] 78:170-194.
Lauder JM, Krebs H (1986). Do neurotransmitters, neurohumors, and hormones specify critical periods? In Greenough WT, Junaska JM (eds): "Developmental Neuropsychobiology," New York: Academic Press, pp 119-174.
Lundborg P, Engel J (1978). Neurochemical brain changes associated with behavioral disturbances after early treatment with psychotropic drugs. In Vernadakis A, Giacobini E, Filogamo G (eds): "Maturation of Neurotransmission," Basel: Karger, pp 226-235.
Miller RK, Kellogg CK, Saltzman RA (1987). Reproductive and perinatal toxicology. In Berndt WO, Haley W (eds): "Fundamentals of Toxicology," Washington DC: Hemisphere Pub Corp, pp 159-309.
Mirmiran M, Brenner E, Van Der Gugten J, Swaab DF (1985). Neurochemical and electrophysiological disturbances mediate developmental behavioral alterations produced by medicines. Neurobehav Toxicol Teratol 7:677-683.
Mirmiran M, Van de Poll NE, Corner MA, Van Oyen HG, Bour HL (1981). Suppression of active sleep by chronic treatment with chlorimipramine during early postnatal development: Effects upon adult sleep and behavior in the rat. Brain Res 204:129-146.
Schultzberg M, Foster GA, Gage FH, Bjorklund A, Hokfelt T (1986). Coexistence during ontogeny and transplantation. Prog Brain Res 68:129-145.

DISCUSSION

DR. HOLMES: Are there any data on the effects of diazepam on the behavior of human children who had been exposed *in utero*?

DR. KELLOGG: No not to my knowledge. We would need to study individuals from early into late adolescence, around 18 to 20. To find that population and to determine precisely its early developmental exposure would be very difficult. I wouldn't want to start a prospective study now and finish it 20 years later. That, I think is the real problem posed with neuroactive drugs; the effects of early exposure become more pronounced as the organism grows older. As we look more carefully at the data gathered in experimental animals, we may find that some early observations are good predictors for later functional impairment.

DR. LAMMER: This is a comment rather than a question. I am struck by the Lamarckian nature of some of your findings in the sense that maternal exposures during pregnancy alter reproductive and other behavior of the offspring. While xenobiotic drugs are unlikely to have influenced evolutionary processes, the behavior of offspring may be affected by substances that mothers may ingest from their environment during their pregnancies. In the same way that prenatal exposure to diazepam may induce long-term changes in offspring behavior, ingesting certain plants may alter the behavior of the offspring of some animals. It suggests that there may be a possible mechanism for one of Lamarck's hypotheses about how certain behavioral traits are transmitted in a non-genetic fashion.

DR. KELLOGG: Since the effects noted on the organism occur only in the exposed offspring, and do not cross generations, this data would not appear to support Larmarck's ideas. One can hypothesize reasonable biologic mechanisms that can mediate lasting effects of early drug exposure on an individual.

Transplacental Effects on Fetal Health, pages 279–287

THE NEUROTOXIC, TERATOGENIC, AND BEHAVIORAL TERATOGENIC EFFECTS OF LEAD AT LOW DOSE: A PARADIGM FOR TRANSPLACENTAL TOXICANTS

Herbert L. Needleman, M.D.

Professor of Psychiatry, School of Medicine, University of Pittsburgh, 3811 O'Hara Street, Pittsburgh, PA 15213

In this paper I review briefly some data from the growing field of pollutant effects on fetal development. I focus particular attention on the behavioral effects of doses of lead below those which produce clinical states. The study of lead provides a full curriculum in the methodological, epistemological and political issues encountered by investigators who would study environmental pollutants in developing humans. I first examine the neurotoxicology of lead at low dose, then the teratogenic properties of lead, and finally the behavioral teratogenic effects of lead in humans. Implications for the study of other fetotoxic agents are mentioned in conclusion.

NEUROTOXICOLOGY OF LEAD AT LOW DOSE

The neurotoxic properties of lead have been known since antiquity. Childhood lead poisoning was first described in Australia at the end of the 19th century. In the United States, the disease was recognized in the early 20th century, and described as solely an affliction of the poor. The conventional wisdom was that children who were not killed by the disease were left without residue. Byers and Lord (1943) followed up on 20 children who had recovered from severe lead intoxication, and found that 19 had severe intellectual, perceptual, or behavioral difficulty. In the 1960's, the blood lead level accepted as safe for children was 59 ug/dl. Children with levels at 68 or greater were considered intoxicated and treated; those with lower levels were followed. When screening studies showed that in some populations, as many as 20% of children had blood lead levels in the range of 40 ug/dl, the question of low level toxicity was raised. Three studies in the early 1970's showed a relationship between lesser blood lead levels and IQ scores (de la Burde and Choate, 1975; Landrigan et al., 1975; Perino and Ernhart, 1974). Some studies failed to find an association (Baloh et al., 1975; Lansdown et al., 1974; McNeil et al., 1975).

A review of the methodological issues that contributed to the dissonant conclusions revealed that four problems weakened the confidence with which assertions could be drawn. They were: (1) Weak markers of exposure. Most studies relied on blood lead levels as the exposure measure. Since the blood is a short term storage system, blood levels could decline after exposure, and subjects could be misclassified. (2) Insensitive measures of outcome. Use of screening measures, or group tests, could miss effects that were present. (3) Inadequate control of confounders. Lead is correlated with other factors which can affect brain function, and these could confound lead's effect. (4) Selection bias. Subjects who refused participation may have differed from participants in some systematic fashion related to the outcome of interest.

We designed a study to overcome these difficulties (Needleman et al., 1979). We used the shed deciduous tooth to measure body lead levels, and administered a group of standardized psychological tests which tapped functions known to be perturbed in clinical lead poisoning. We controlled for 39 non-lead covariates, and compared included and excluded subjects on two dimensions: distribution of tooth lead levels, and classroom behavior.

After controlling for 39 covariates, asymptomatic children with elevated tooth lead levels were found to score significantly lower on IQ scales, three measures of language functioning, reaction time under varying intervals of delay, and on teachers' ratings of classroom performance (TABLE I). Similar data has been reported by others from the United Kingdom, Germany, and Greece (Hatzakis et al., 1987; Winneke et al., 1982; Yule et al., 1984).

We conclude that lead at doses below those which produce symptoms severe enough to bring children to medical attention is associated with disturbances in brain function, and that these are expressed in poor test and classroom performance.

Table I

PSYCHOMETRIC TEST SCORES IN HIGH AND LOW LEAD SUBJECTS
AFTER ADJUSTMENT FOR COVARIATES (ANACOVA)

WISC-R	LOW LEAD X	HIGH LEAD X	P VALUE (2 tail)
Full Scale I.Q.	106.6	102.1	.03
Verbal I.Q.	103.9	99.3	.03
Performance I.Q.	108.7	104.9	.08
Seashore Rhythm Test			
Subtest A	8.2	7.1	.002
Subtest B	7.5	6.8	.03
Subtest C	6.0	5.4	.07
Sum	21.6	19.4	.002
Token Test			
Block 1	2.9	2.8	.37
Block 2	3.7	3.7	.90
Block 3	4.1	4.0	.42
Block 4	14.1	13.1	.05
Sum	24.8	23.6	.09
Sentence Repetition Test	12.6	11.3	.04
Reaction Time Under Varying Intervals of Delay	(X±S.D.)	(X±S.D.)	
Block 1 (3 sec.)	.35±.08 sec.	.37±.09 sec.	.32
Block 2 (12 sec.)	.41±.09	.47±.12	.001
Block 3 (12 sec.)	.41±.09	.48±.11	.001
Block 4 (3 sec.)	.38±.10	.41±.12	.01

MUTAGENIC AND TERATOGENIC PROPERTIES OF LEAD

The fetotoxic properties of lead at high dose have long been known. British factory inspectors at the turn of the century recorded the extraordinary fetal and neonatal death rate of infants born to mothers in the pottery industry. The high rate of sterility and fetal loss also were well known (Nogaki, 1957). Lead is a possible mutagen. It affects the fidelity of DNA synthesis in vitro (Sirover and Loeb, 1976), and perturbs DNA synthesis in vivo (Choie and Richter, 1979). A slight increase in dicentric chromosomes in lead cultured lymphocytes has been reported (Beek and Obe, 1974).

Wibberly et al (1977) examined the lead content of placentae of normal and malformed human births and stillbirths. A significant increase in placental lead levels was found in samples from stillbirths and malformed fetuses.

We collected umbilical cord blood samples from 4354 consecutive deliveries at the Boston Hospital for Women (Needleman et al., 1984). We then examined the relationship between umbilical cord blood lead level and birth outcome (birth weight, major and minor malformations) controlling for race, socioeconomic status, smoking, alcohol, coffee, and marijuana use. Lead was found to be significantly related to the risk of minor malformations (Table II). The

TABLE II

COVARIATE ADJUSTED RISK OF MALFORMATION AT SELECTED BLOOD LEAD LEVELS

Blood Lead (ug/dl)	Relative Risk*	% of Neonates at Greater Lead Levels
0.7	1.0	98.7
6.3	1.87(1.44-2.42)	50.0
15.0	2.39(1.66-3.43)	1.7
24.0	2.73(1.80-4.16)	0.2

*mean - 95% confidence limits

mean blood lead level in this study, it should be noted, was 6.7 ug/dl. We conclude that lead during pregnancy is a minor teratogen. The association between minor malformations and undisclosed malformations and later behaviorial aberration is well known.

BEHAVIORAL TERATOLOGY

Many toxic compounds have as their early, if not their first, effects, CNS changes, and corresponding behavioral alterations. It also is increasingly clear that many of those agents that possess psychoactive properties also produce enduring changes in the developing CNS. The converse of this observation also is true enough to be considered a rule: agents which are CNS teratogens at one dose, are likely to perturb behavior at a lesser dose. They are, to use a term proposed by Vorhees and Butcher (1982) "psychoteratogens." Among the agents which have led to the development of the nascent field of behavioral teratology are mercury, alcohol, opiates, the major tranquilizers, and the polyhalogenated hydrocarbons.

Lead qualifies as a suspected behavioral teratogen. It has demonstrated effects on the brain at high dose, is an animal CNS teratogen, and alters neurochemistry and neuropharmacology at doses not very much higher than those experienced by a large proportion of fetuses.

We set out to evaluate the relationship of lead exposure in the human fetus upon later cognitive, social and emotional behavior (Bellinger et al., 1987). From the same population of 12,000 births from which we drew the sample of 4385 infants to study birth outcome, we selected 249 newborns to study their neuropsychological development. These were almost evenly divided into three groups according to umbilical cord blood lead level (low=<3 ug/dl; mid=6-7 ug/dl; high=>10ug/dl). These infants were seen at 1, 6, 12, 18, 24 and 48 months of age to measure their psychological development. A large panel of demographic, medical, and experiential variables were scaled in order to evaluate and control for confounding. Blood lead levels were measured at these epochs to allow us to separate out the variance due to postnatal lead exposure. Environmental lead sampling was done to partition out the various sources of lead for human exposure.

The unadjusted difference between mean IQ scores at 6, 12, and 24 months was 3.1, 4.4, and 5.3 points respectively. We then entered into the regression model those covariates which differed between high and low lead groups and were potential confounders. The mean differences between groups increased (4.3, 5.8 and 7.8 points respectively). (Table III). This increase in effect after covariate control was due to unique properties of the sample. Because of the demographics of the patient population, an elevated blood lead level was associated with favored socioeconomic indicators. In this sample, higher status was linked with urban residence. Adjusting for covariates increased the lead effect.

TABLE III

INFANTS' MENTAL DEVELOPMENTAL INDEX SCORE ACCORDING TO CORD-BLOOD GROUP

Cord lead group	Mental Developmental Index Score		
	6 mo	12 mo	24 mo
Crude score			
low	109.2±12.9	113.1±12.5	115.9±17.2
medium	108.6±12.0	115.4±12.9	119.9±16.5
high	106.1±11.1	108.7±12.8	110.6±16.5
		(mean±sd)	
Covariate adjusted score			
low	110.2±1.3	114.7±1.6	118.9±1.8
medium	108.9±1.3	114.4±1.9	117.8±1.7
high	105.9±1.4	108.9±1.6	111.1±1.8
		(mean±sd)	

We conclude that lead exposure during pregnancy is associated with decreased IQ scores until at least 24 months of age.

Similar data has been reported by Dietrich et al (1987) in a sample of primarily black children of lower socio-economic status from Cincinnati. Prenatal exposure of nonhuman primates to lead at comparable doses has produced similar deficits in learning (Bushell and Bowman, 1979; Rice and Willes, 1979).

The implications of these data for studies of behavioral effects of other environmental pollutants are self evident. The same logic applies: if large doses of a toxicant produce clinical effects, lesser deficits can be expected at lesser doses. The internal dose at which an effect can be expected will depend upon the sensitivity of the outcome measures employed, the rigor of the epidemiologic design, and the size of the sample utilized. Appropriate candidates for investigation include, but are not limited to, the following classes of toxicants: methylmercury, cadmium, pesticides, and common household solvents. All of these agents listed above, and many others are candidates for study of behavioral alterations secondary to intrauterine exposure. Badly needed are forward studies of large cohorts in which real time measures of exposure are made, and follow-up for substantial periods of time are conducted with panels of sensitive, appropriate outcome measures.

REFERENCES

Baloh R, Sturm R, Green G, Gleser G (1975). Neuropsychological effects of chronic asymptomatic increased lead absorbtion: a controlled study. Arch Neurol 32:326-330.

Beek B, Obe G (1974). Effect of lead acetate on human leucocyte chromosomes in vitro. Experientia 30:1006-1007.

Bellinger D, Leviton A, Waternaux, Needleman H, Rabinowitz M (1987). Longitudinal analyses of prenatal and postnatal lead exposure and early cognitive development. N Engl J Med 316:1037-1043.

Bushnell PJ, Bowman RE (1979). Reversal learning deficits in young monkeys exposed to lead. Pharmacol Biochem Behav 10:733-42.

Byers RK, Lord E (1943). Late effects of lead poisoning on mental development. Am J Dis Child 66:471-494.

Choie D, Richter G (1979). Cell proliferation in the rat kidney produced by lead. I. Synthesis of desoxyribonucleic acid. Lab Invest 30:647-651.

de la Burde B, Choate MS (1975). Early asymptomatic lead exposure and development at school age. J Pediatr 87:638-664.

Dietrich K, Krafft K, Bier M, Bornschein R, Naraine S, Succop P (1987). Early effects of fetal lead exposure developmental findings at 6 months. Proc Int Conf Heavy

Metals in the Environ. CEP Associates Edinburgh, pp 63-65.
Hatzakis A, Kokkevi A, Katsouyanni K, Maravalias K, Salainios F, Kalandidi A, Koutselinis A, Stefanis K, Trichopoulis D (1987). Psychometric intelligence and attentional performance deficits in lead-exposed children. Proc Int Conf Heavy Metals in the Environ. CEP Associates Edinburgh, pp 204-209.
Landrigan P, Baloh R, Whitworth R, Staehling N, Rosenblum B (1975). Neuropsychological dysfunction in children with chronic low level lead absorbtion. Lancet 1:708.
Lansdown RG, Shepherd J, Clayton BE, Delves HT, Graham PJ, Turner WC (1974). Blood lead levels, behaviour, and intelligence: a population study. Lancet 1:538-541.
McNeil J, Ptasnik J, Croft D (1975). Evaluation of long-term effects of elevated blood lead concentrations in asymptomatic children. Arch Industrial Hyg Toxicol 26:97-118.
Needleman H, Gunnoe C, Leviton A, Reed RR, Peresie H, Maher C, Barrett P (1979). Deficits in psychologic and classroom performance in children with elevated dentine lead levels. N Engl J Med 300:584-695.
Needleman HL, Rabinowitz M, Leviton A, Linn S, Schoenbaum S (1984). The relationship between prenatal exposure to lead and congenital anomalies. J Am Med Assoc 251:2956-2959.
Nogaki K (1957). On action of lead on body of lead refinery workers: particularly on the conception, pregnancy and parturition in the case of females and on vitality of their newborn. Igaku Kenkyu 27:1314-1338.
Perino J, Ernhart C (1974). The relation of subclinical lead level to cognitive and sensory impairment in black preschoolers. J Learn Disorders. 7:26-30.
Rice DC, Willes RF, (1979). Neonatal low level lead exposure in monkeys Macaca fascicularis: effect on two-choice non-spatial form discrimination. Environ Pathol Toxicol 2:1195-1203.
Sirover MA, Loeb LA (1976). Infidelity of DNA synthesis in vitro: screening for potential metal mutagens or carcinogens. Science 194:1434-1436.
Vorhees C, Butcher R (1982). Behavioral teratogenicity. In Snell K (ed): "Developmental Toxicology", London: Croom Helm Press, pp 247-298.
Wibberly D, Khera A, Edwards J, Rushton D (1977). Lead levels in human placentae from normal and malformed births. J Med Genet 14:339-345.

Winneke G, Hrdina K, Brockhaus A (1982). Neuropsychological studies in children with elevated tooth lead concentrations. Part I: Pilot study using a matched pair approach. Int Arch Occup Environ Health, 51:169.
Yule W, Urbanowitz MA, Lansdown R, Millar IB (1984). Teachers' ratings of children's behavior in relation to blood lead levels. Brit J Develop Psychol 2:295-305.

DISCUSSION

DR. LAMMER: Lead levels are continuously distributed. I do not understand why lead levels were grouped into these quintiles or quartiles instead of using lead levels as a continuous variable in the data analyses.

DR. NEEDLEMAN: One could do that. This is an approximation. It employs Cox's rule for dividing samples into classes to give symmetry around the median.

DR. LAMMER: I think that your statistical power would be greater if lead levels were treated as a continuous variable.

DR. NEEDLEMAN: It would be a little stronger, but we did calculate the probability that this occurred by chance, and it was vanishingly small.

DR. MILLS: If I understood correctly, you said that you found a relationship between the rate of minor malformations but not major malformations.

DR. NEEDLEMAN: That is correct.

DR. MILLS: Could you speculate on why you might find something like that?

DR. NEEDLEMAN: I think our sample size of 4000 children wasn't large enough to detect an effect of low incidence such as a major malformation. If there was an effect on the rate of major malformations, one would need more than 4000 children to detect it.

Transplacental Effects on Fetal Health, pages 289–300

ESTIMATING FETAL MORBIDITY AND MORTALITY RESULTING FROM CIGARETTE SMOKE EXPOSURE BY MEASURING COTININE LEVELS IN MATERNAL SERUM

James E. Haddow, George J. Knight, Glenn E. Palomaki, Paula K. Haddow

Research Center for Perinatal and Child Health
Foundation for Blood Research, Scarborough, Maine 04074

BACKGROUND INFORMATION ABOUT BIOCHEMICAL MARKERS OF CIGARETTE SMOKE

In recent years, considerable effort has been directed at developing biochemical tests that can reliably measure cigarette smoke exposure, both in cigarette smokers themselves and in nonsmokers exposed to other people's smoke. Markers such as carboxyhemoglobin and thiocyanate have provided some useful information about smoking, but both these markers are influenced not only by cigarette smoke but by other environmental agents as well. This shortcoming interferes with both the sensitivity and the specificity of these two tests, especially in relation to passive smoke exposure. Nicotine is specific to tobacco smoke and also has been measured with some success, but it has two major shortcomings: it has a short circulating half-life in the body (about 30 minutes), and it is so ubiquitous on fingers and clothing of smokers that it can contaminate a laboratory and render the test system useless. The most promising marker to date is cotinine, a metabolic product of nicotine produced in the liver. Cotinine has a circulating half-life of about a day, making it very reliable to measure average exposure to smoke, and it can be measured accurately in passively exposed as well as actively exposed individuals in serum, urine, or saliva. Preliminary studies have demonstrated cotinine measurements to be more reliable than smoking history when assessing both exposure and health consequences. In the future, biochemical markers are likely to be applied more and more frequently both to study smoking and to help people modify smoking behavior, and this type of testing will be very helpful in assisting the community both to explain environmental cigarette smoke exposure and to monitor progress in reducing exposure. In this paper, we describe studies involving serum cotinine measurements in a population of pregnant women in Maine, aimed at learning more about how the fetus is affected when the mother is either actively or passively exposed to cigarette smoke products.

BACKGROUND INFORMATION ABOUT HOW MATERNAL SMOKING AFFECTS THE FETUS

It has been well established that maternal smoking has an adverse effect on fetal growth and development. Low and depressed Apgar scores at one and five minutes after birth are found almost four times as often in infants of women who smoke 41-60 cigarettes per day during pregnancy as in infants of nonsmokers. Furthermore, women who smoke cigarettes during pregnancy deliver infants whose birthweight is, on average, 150-200 grams lower than that of infants born to nonsmoking women (Stein, Kline 1983). This appears to be a dose-response effect, with 10-20 cigarettes per day throughout pregnancy producing a birthweight reduction of approximately 200 gm (Meyer et al 1976). The relationship between decreased birthweight and smoking remains after correcting for such confounding factors as maternal age, parity, weight gain, weight and/or height, socioeconomic status, race, and sex of offspring (Frazier et al 1961; Lowe 1959; Meyer et al 1976; Underwood et al 1967; USDHEW 1973). Women who stop smoking during the first half of their pregnancy deliver infants whose birthweights average close to those of nonsmokers (Sexton, Hebel 1984).

Placental blood flow, fetal activity, and fetal breathing movements all decrease when a pregnant woman smokes cigarettes, and fetal adrenergic activity increases (Hill, Kleinberg 1984). Placental vascular histologic changes also have been documented. Prostacyclin synthesis is severely depressed in the neonate's umbilical artery when the mother smokes, and it has been suggested that this may be responsible for decreased placental perfusion and umbilical artery flow (Dadak et al 1982). SP_1, a pregnancy protein produced by the placenta, has been found to be significantly reduced in smokers in both the second and the third trimesters (Lee et al 1981).

Perinatal mortality is usually defined as a reproductive loss after the twentieth week of gestation and before the seventh day of life. Although studies on the relationship between smoking and perinatal mortality have shown conflicting results, some associations have emerged (Meyer et al 1976; Rantakallio 1978). For example, smoking seems to affect the fetus of a mother in a low socioeconomic status group more than the fetus of a mother in a high socioeconomic status group; and women who are at increased risk for perinatal mortality because of low social class, advanced maternal age, and history of a previous loss are at an even greater risk if they smoke (Comstock et al 1971). In a large sample of women from all social classes, those women who decreased or stopped smoking during pregnancy had infants with lower rates of perinatal mortality than women who did not reduce their cigarette consumption (Butler et al 1972).

Vaginal bleeding during pregnancy, abruptio placentae, placenta previa, prematurity alone, pneumonia, and premature or prolonged rupture of membranes have been found to be the cause of perinatal mortality in a greater proportion of the offspring of smokers than nonsmokers (Andrews, McGarry 1972; Meyer, Tonascia 1977; Naeye 1980). Cessation of smoking during pregnancy was found to result in a decreased risk for abruptio placentae and placenta previa (Naeye et al 1979).

The spontaneous abortion rate is higher in women who smoke during pregnancy than in nonsmokers (Butler et al 1972; Comstock et al 1971; Rantakallio 1969; Yerushalmy 1972). Data from the Ontario Perinatal Mortality Study, taking into account a number of possible confounding variables such as maternal age, parity, history of previous abortions, alcohol use, and exposure to waste anesthetic gases, show an overall 27 percent higher spontaneous abortion rate among women who smoke during pregnancy. Again, a dose-response relationship has been reported, with a 20 percent higher risk associated with fewer than 20 cigarettes per day and a 35 percent higher risk with more than 30 cigarettes per day throughout pregnancy (Harlap, Shiono 1980; Himmelberger et al 1978).

By and large, abortuses of women who smoke during pregnancy are chromosomally normal, indicating an increased rate of abortions among otherwise viable products of conception, due to smoking (Werler et al 1985). Kline et al (1983) found that women smokers under the age of 30 are less likely to have a chromosomally abnormal abortus than nonsmokers, while, conversely, those women over 30 who smoke are more likely to have a chromosomally abnormal abortus than nonsmokers. Whether this indicates that smoking affects meiosis or that it affects the survivability of an embryo/-fetus in utero or whether if affects both is unclear (Werler et al 1985).

Until now, there has been no information relating cotinine or other biochemical measurements to fetal morbidity and mortality. We now report such an experience, using a cotinine assay developed by our laboratory (Knight et al 1985), and compare the strength of its birthweight association with the traditional method of assessing cigarette smoke exposure: self-reporting.

RESULTS

The present study group includes 8,063 second trimester pregnant women enrolling in a maternal serum alpha-fetoprotein (MSAFP) screening program in Maine between 1979 and 1983 who were routinely asked about their smoking habits, including how many cigarettes they smoked per day. Sera from these women were coded and frozen, and cotinine measurements were subsequently performed. After the pregnancies had gone to term, outcome information was sought on all of the pregnancies, including fetal viability and birthweight. The initial analysis was directed at comparing the yes/no answer about cigarette smoking with serum cotinine levels. A serum cotinine level of ≤10 ng/mL was used as a demarcation line between smoking and nonsmoking, based on information available from other laboratories. Table 1 presents a two way analysis of self-reporting versus serum cotinine, expressed as percentages of the total population studied. Among the women who declared themselves to be nonsmokers, cotinine levels were in agreement in 95 percent, while for self-declared smokers, cotinine levels agreed 93 percent of the time. Good agreement was thus found between the two methods, indicating that either could be used reliably to assess whether or not the population of pregnant women smoked. The proportion of self-declared smokers with cotinine values ≤10 ng/mL was somewhat higher than expected, probably due to some of the women stopping smoking between the time of answering the question and having the serum sample drawn. Next, the self-reported number of cigarettes smoked per day was compared with serum cotinine levels (Fig. 1). Considerable variability was identified between these two methods of assessing the actual dose exposure to cigarette smoke products. It might be assumed that such discrepancy might arise from women underestimating the number of cigarettes smoked, but the data in Fig. 1 are only partially consistent with this hypothesis. In fact, a number of women who reported smoking 20 or more cigarettes per day actually had relatively low serum cotinine levels. Much of the variability in serum cotinine levels throughout the range of cigarettes smoked might be explained by individual differences in the metabolic handling of the absorbed products (in this case, nicotine) or by differences in smoking technique or brand of cigarette smoked.

These preliminary study results led to the conclusion that self-reporting and serum cotinine levels both were reliable for studying whether or not our pregnancy population smoked, but further analysis was necessary to determine whether self-reported numbers of cigarettes smoked or the serum cotinine level correlated more closely with fetal morbidity.

Because smoking during pregnancy is known to be associated with lower birthweight, an analysis was performed comparing tertiles of serum cotinine at fixed numbers of cigarettes smoked to discover which was more closely associated with birthweight (Figure 2). There was a significant association between serum cotinine and birthweight, given a constant number of cigarettes smoked per day, and this pattern was evident at both the 10 and 20 cigarette/day level. When the analysis was reversed (not shown) holding cotinine constant, the tertiles of cigarettes smoked per day showed no association with birthweight. A further two-way analysis, using the complete data set is reported elsewhere (Haddow et al 1987), again demonstrating a significantly better association between cotinine and birthweight.

A preliminary study was carried out in the study population to examine the relationship between serum cotinine levels and fetal deaths occurring between the second trimester and term. This analysis was considered preliminary because there were relatively few events (fetal death) available to study trends. Table 2 demonstrates that

TABLE 1

The Percent of Serum Cotinine Values Above or Below 10 ng/mL in Pregnant Women. According to Whether They Answered No or Yes to the Smoking Question.

		Cotinine (ng/mL)	
		≤10	>10
Self Reported Smoking	NO	95	5
	YES	7	93

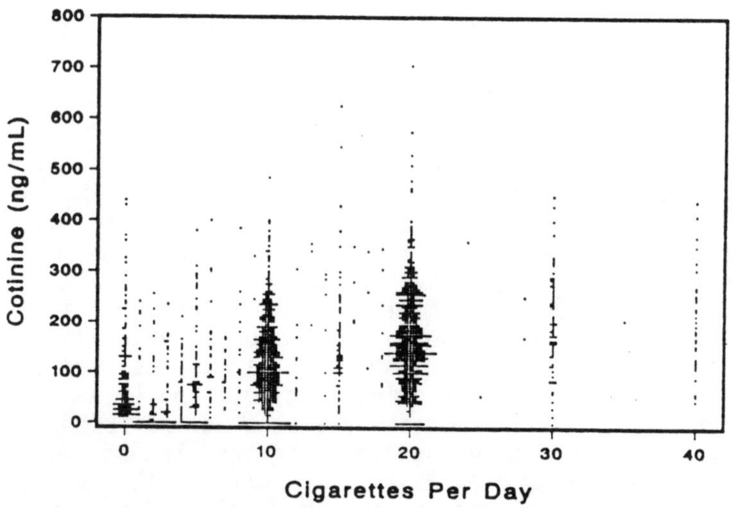

FIGURE 1. The scatter plot indicates serum cotinine levels in relation to numbers of cigarettes smoked per day. Digit preference is clearly visible for self reporting, and cotinine levels vary widely among both light and heavy smokers. Represented by a single dot at (0.0) are 3.174 cotinine measurements from women who reported nonsmoking and whose cotinine levels were ≤10 ng/mL.

maternal smoking was associated with a greater risk for fetal death as classified according to serum cotinine level. A dose response trend was clearly seen with cotinine, and the major increase in risk occurred in the upper two cotinine categories. This analysis does not take into account other variables associated with maternal smoking that might contribute to risk for fetal death.

Recently, we have employed serum cotinine measurements to study the extent to which nonsmoking pregnant women are exposed to environmental tobacco smoke products and to evaluate whether passive exposure might be associated with lower birthweight. Our study group included pregnant women who declared themselves to be nonsmokers and who also had serum cotinine levels ≤ 10 ng/mL. Approximately one-third of the nonsmoking pregnant women were being exposed passively to tobacco smoke (serum cotinine level 1 ng/mL) (Figure 3), and the average birthweight in this exposed group of women was 107 gm lower than in those women who were not exposed. This birthweight difference remained after multivariate analysis, taking into account maternal weight and height, infant's sex, maternal age, gravidity, and years of education.

Our studies support serum cotinine measurement as a reliable method for establishing the presence or absence of smoking and as a superior method for measuring the dose of cigarette smoke products absorbed into the circulation. We find a strong association between serum cotinine and birthweight, the difference in mean birthweight between the lowest and highest exposure groups being 441 gm, and we have identified an association between the nonsmoking mother's passive exposure to tobacco smoke and low birthweight, as well. There also is evidence by serum cotinine level for a dose-response relationship between serum cotinine and fetal death. Serum cotinine measurements appear well suited for biochemical epidemiologic studies involving cigarette smoking.

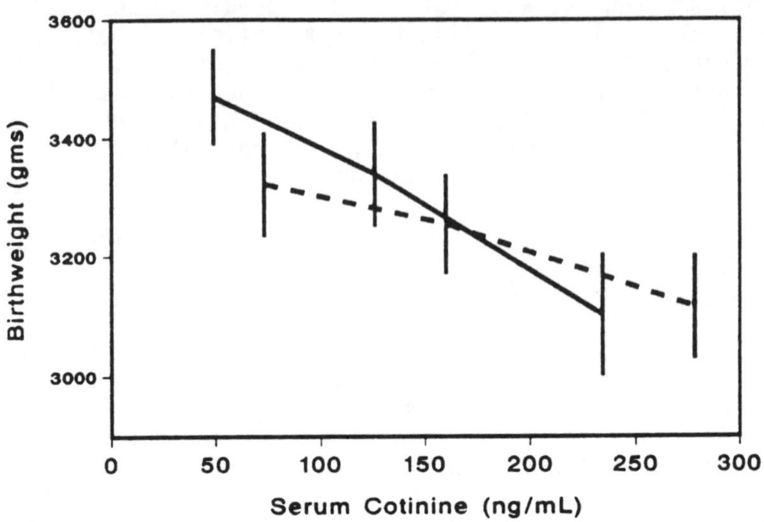

FIGURE 2. The line graph plots mean birthweights (with 95% confidence intervals) by tertile of serum cotinine for 378 women reporting 10 cigarettes/day (solid line) and the 468 women reporting 20 cigarettes/day (dashed line). At both levels of self-reported smoking, the mean birthweight goes down as serum cotinine levels go up.

TABLE 2
Serum Cotinine Levels in Relation to Fetal Death

	Cotinine (ng/ml)			
	≤10	11-100	101-175	>175
Observation	5.997	767	630	669
Deaths/1,000	11.8	10.4	17.5	28.4
Relative Risk*	1.0	0.9	1.5	2.4

* P=0.003 Chi square test for trend.

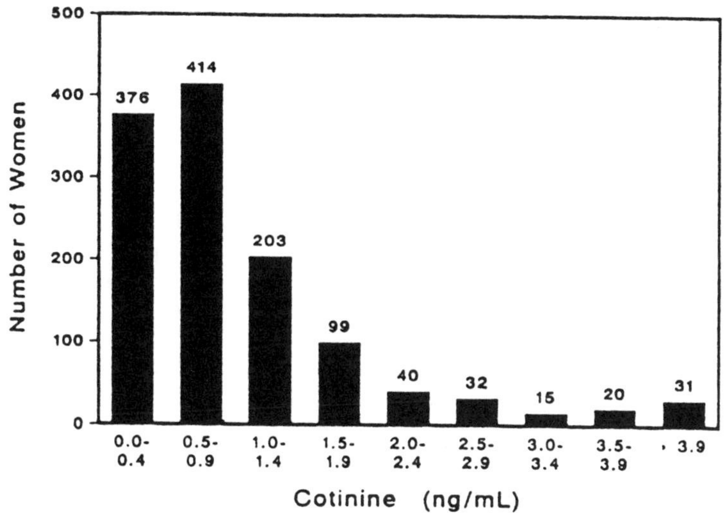

Figure 3. The bar chart shows the distribution of serum cotinine in 1,230 nonsmoking pregnant women by self-reporting who also had serum cotinine levels under 10 ng/mL. Approximately one-third of these women are passively exposed to cigarette smoke, as defined by a serum cotinine level >1.0 ng/mL.

REFERENCES

Andrews J, McGarry J (1972). A community study of smoking in pregnancy. J Obstet Gynecol Br Commonwlth 79:1057-1073.

Butler NR, Goldstein H, Ross EM (1972). Cigarette smoking in pregnancy: Its influence on birthweight and perinatal mortality. Br Med J 2:127-130.

Comstock GW, Shah FK, Meyer MB, Abby H (1971). Low birthweight and neonatal mortality rate related to maternal smoking and socioeconomic status. Am J Obstet Gynecol 111:53-59.

Dadak C, Kefalides A, Sinzinger H, Weber F (1982). Reduced umbilical artery prostacyclin formation in complicated pregnancies. Am J Obstet Gynecol 144:792-795.

Frazier TM, Davis GH, Goldstein H, Goldberg ID (1961). Cigarette smoking and prematurity: A prospective study.

Am J Obstet Gynecol 81:988-996.
Haddow JE, Knight GJ, Palomaki G, Kloza EM, Wald NJ (1987). Cigarette consumption and serum cotinine in relation to birthweight. Br J Obstet Gynecol 94:678.
Harlap S, Shiono P (1980). Alcohol, smoking and incidence of spontaneous abortion in first and second trimester. Lancet ii:173-176.
Hill LM, Kleinberg F (1984). Effects of drugs and chemicals on the fetus and the newborn. Mayo Clin Proc 59:755-756.
Himmelberger D, Brown B, Cohen E (1978). Cigarette smoking during pregnancy and the occurrence of spontaneous abortion and congenital abnormality. Am J Epidemiol 108:470-479.
Kline J, Levin B, Shrout P, Stein Z, Susser M, Warburton D (1983). Maternal smoking and trisomy among spontaneously aborted conceptions. Am J Hum Genet 35:421-431.
Knight GJ, Wiley P, Holman M, Haddow JE (1985). Improved 125-I radioimmunoassay for cotinine by selective removal of bridge antibodies. Clin Chem 31(1):118-121.
Lee JN, Grudzinskas JG, Chard T (1981). Effect of smoking on blood SP1 levels in late pregnancy. Obstet Gynecol 57:220-223.
Lowe CR (1959). Effect of mothers' smoking habits on birthweight of their children. Br Med J 4:673-676.
Meyer M, Jonas B, Tonascia J (1976). Perinatal events associated with maternal smoking. Am J Epidemiol 103:464-476.
Meyer MB, Tonascia JA (1977). Maternal smoking, pregnancy complications, and perinatal mortality. Am J Obstet Gynecol 128:494-502.
Naeye R, Harkness W, Utts J (1979). The duration of maternal cigarette smoking, fetal and placental disorders. Early Hum Dev 3:229-237.
Naeye RL (1980). Abruptio placentae and placenta praevia: Frequency, perinatal mortality, and cigarette smoking. Obstet Gynecol 55:701-704.
Rantakallio P (1969). Groups at risk. In: Low Birthweight Infants and Perinatal Mortality. Acta Pediatr Scand [Suppl] 193:1-71.
Rantakallio P (1978). Relationship of maternal smoking to morbidity and mortality of the child up to the age of five. Acta Paediatr Scand 67:621-631.
Sexton M, Hebel JR (1984). A clinical trial of change in maternal smoking and its effect on birth weight. J Am Med Assoc 251:911-915.
Stein Z, Kline J (1983). Smoking, alcohol, and reproduction. Am J Public Health 73:1154-1156.

Underwood PB, Kesler KF, O'Lane JM, Callagan DA (1967). Parental smoking empirically related to pregnancy outcome. Obstet Gynecol 29:1-8.

U.S. Department of Health, Education, and Welfare (1973). The women and their pregnancies. The Collaborative Perinatal Study of the National Institute of Neurological Diseases and Stroke. DHEW Publication No. (NIH) 73-379:72-80.

Werler MM, Pober B, Holmes LB (1985). Smoking and pregnancy. Teratology 32:473-481.

Yerushalmy S (1972). The relationship of parents' cigarette smoking to outcome of pregnancy: Implications as to the problem of inferring causation from observed associations. Am J Epidemiol 93:443-456.

DISCUSSION

DR. LAMMER: Among your group of nonsmokers who had very low levels of cotinine, is it possible that the cotinine is coming from a source other than cigarette smoke? You mentioned earlier that cotinine was a specific marker for cigarette smoke. This may not be true, however, when cotinine levels are that low. My second question is, could the nonsmokers with detectable cotinine levels be smoking something other than tobacco?

DR. HADDOW: On the first question, we have just completed a related study in men and nonpregnant women, involving a questionnaire survey of hours of passive tobacco smoke exposure over the few days preceding the time of blood and urine sampling to determine the extent of correlation between self-reported passive exposure and blood and urinary cotinine levels in the passive exposure range. Also, we wanted to determine how closely urine cotinine levels correlated with blood cotinine levels. There is good correlation between passive tobacco smoke exposure as reported by self and blood and urine cotinine levels, and the urine levels are about 10-fold higher than the sera, so that if you had 3 ng/mL in the serum, you might get about 30 ng/mL in the urine. These data support that we are, in fact, measuring cotinine, even at low concentrations.

Concerning cotinine as a measure of people's smoking products other than tobacco, anything that contained nicotine and was absorbed into the blood stream would be converted to cotinine in the liver. Otherwise, cotinine would not be detected.

IV. GENETIC ENGINEERING

Transplacental Effects on Fetal Health, pages 303–323

MOLECULAR BIOLOGIC APPROACHES TO PRENATAL DEFECTS

George H. Sack, Jr.

Departments of Medicine, Biological Chemistry and Pediatrics, The Johns Hopkins University School of Medicine and the John F. Kennedy Institute, Baltimore, Maryland, 21205

The principles and techniques of molecular biology provide new approaches for the delineation and correction of genetic defects in many organisms. While not all prenatal defects are inherited, an attempt at molecular characterization is warranted in order to put them into perspective and permit further study. In practice, it is rational to seek molecular definition of the spectrum of changes which require correction prior to developing therapy.

Due to the overwhelming amount of study of human genetic disorders, this review will inevitably include many examples from human biology. However, most approaches are applicable to the majority of animals and specific principles and non-human data will be presented whenever possible. Non-human systems are particularly appropriate for embryo manipulation techniques as described below.

GENETIC LESIONS

The simplest genetic change is the point mutation - alteration of a single nucleotide in the genome of the organism. Point mutations have a remarkable spectrum of consequences from none at all ("silent" when the base change does not cause an amino acid change) through trivial protein changes ("conservative" where the amino acid substitution is of minimal consequence to function) to significant changes in protein structure and/or function such as sickle cell anemia and other problems including the prevention or termination of protein synthesis. Point mutations are widespread and contribute to the spectrum of genetic diversity in all organisms without causing gross genomic reorganization.

More complicated than point mutations, but also becoming recognized as important contributors to genetic change, are chromosomal deletions. Varying from a small number of nucleotides to extensive stretches of nucleic acid losses, deletions are becoming recognized more frequently as the sensitivity of diagnostic technology improves. Deletions are almost always consequential to the organism but their consequences may vary depending on their position and extent. Some are visible at the light microscopic level, but many are too short for such detection. Gene deletions have been recognized more frequently with the use of molecular probes (for example, in X-chromosomal genes: Youssoufian et al., 1987; Kunkel et al., 1987).

Chromosomal translocations and other reorganizations are the most prominent lesions detectable by light microscopy. Classically, these have been studied as consequences of radiation but in recent years other etiologies have been recognized including errors in recombination and replication as well as mobile chromosomal elements. Mobile elements are particularly important in such organisms as Drosophila where "P elements" can cause striking genetic instability (O'Hare and Rubin, 1983). Some visible chromosomal translocations may be without immediate consequence to the organism if there is no loss of genetic material. However, these still may create serious difficulties with chromosome alignment during meiosis resulting in substantial deletions and providing another source of prenatal and developmental defects.

The combination of the rich history of developmental biology and the more recent techniques of molecular genetics has begun to reveal a series of programs for the changes of normal development. Altering these programs can cause long-term and grave consequences to the host. The organism in which these have been studied best is Drosophila where such genetic changes as bithorax and antennapedia have been recognized (Bender et al., 1983;

Scott, 1985). These genetic developmental changes have been shown to reflect altered regulation of a series of genes and are frequently mediated through the "homeo box" system (Gehring, 1985). Homeo boxes are short nucleotide sequences which are remarkably conserved in vertebrates (Hart et al., 1985) and which serve as markers and control signals at the 5' (or upstream) ends of some developmentally regulated genes. Changes in homeo boxes or homeotic genes, their organization and their temporal and spatial expression may have great and varied consequences which may appear unconnected when first encountered. However, molecular analysis has revealed that the various changes encountered by the clinician or biologist ultimately reflect embryonic gene expression patterns which have been altered by regulatory changes.

More complex familial biologic changes have been recognized by both human and animal biologists for many years. However, such phenomena as size, weight, and general health are probably determined by the interaction of multiple genetic and environmental components; none of these "multifactorial" conditions has successfully been dissected into individual, manipulatable determinants.

MOLECULAR BIOLOGIC TECHNIQUES

The molecular biologic techniques applicable to genetic defects have increased in complexity, specificity and precision in recent years. However, it is important to recall that certain simpler approaches have made and continue to make significant contributions to genetic understanding. These older methods will be considered briefly both because of their historic value and since they are still useful for specific problems.

The formation of hybrid cells (heterokaryons) between cells of different organisms has had a productive history with many contributions to understanding genetic interactions. Heterokaryons frequently are unstable since some parental chromosomes usually are lost. Nevertheless, some traits derived from each parent frequently are retained by the heterokaryons.

Heterokaryons have been used in studies of the control of virus production (Payne et al., 1969; Baccara and

Kelly, 1978), in the formation of hybrid products such as muscle proteins and structures (Quinn et al., 1981), in the analysis of control factors (Baron and Maniatis, 1986) and as reagents useful for gene assignment and chromosomal mapping (Ruddle, 1981). Nevertheless, the inherent instability of such lines has, over the long term, precluded their usefulness in prevention or treatment of genetic defects. Furthermore, the large number of genetic changes introduced by heterokaryon production generally complicates interpretation of the experiment.

Chromosome-mediated gene transfer (CMGT) is somewhat less complicated than heterokaryon formation and also has been useful in somatic cell genetics. The transfer of an entire chromosome or a chromosome fragment to a foreign cell has been used to help establish linkage between chromosomal markers (Weiss et al., 1984; Porteous, 1987). CMGT also can verify the presence of functional genetic information within a given chromosomal fragment and thus confirm a map position. However, the long-term stability of such constructs is questionable. While there have been rare mouse cell lines in which autonomous genetic elements have been reasonably stable (Rassoulzadegan et al., 1986), this technique cannot be the major basis of therapeutic genetic alterations.

The goal of therapeutic corrections has become based on manipulation of single genes. The initial applications of genetic technology have used methods for isolating specific genes and gene fragments - the process of cloning. Once clones become available, by whatever technique they have been derived, molecular genetics permits determining precise details of the structure of the cloned material. Clone characterization includes determining the nucleotide sequence, the structural elements of the gene(s) involved and, ultimately, the chromosomal assignment of the genes or fragments in the growing gene map.

Such efforts result in genes which have been mapped, which have been related to one another (in what frequently are gene families of similar function and structure) and which can be detected in both their normal structures and as variants. Many examples exist but our own laboratory has been interested in the small serum protein gene family of serum amyloid A (SAA). Study of recombinant clones of members of this gene family has yielded detailed structural information regarding the internal organization of the genes as well as their control sequences (Sack, 1983; Sack and Lease, 1986). Clones of DNA (excluding repeated sequences or those present in multiple sites) can be assigned to specific chromsomal sites and used to detect normal and pathologic variations within the population; this is useful for mapping and studies of pathophysiology (e.g. Aubourg et al., 1987). Thousands of cloned fragments from human and other genomes are being related to one another to generate long- and short-range linkage groups. Groups of linked markers are evolving more slowly into an organized picture of sites throughout vertebrate chromosomes.

MOLECULAR DIAGNOSIS

The accumulating data relating chromosomal linkage groups and molecular markers serve as the basis for the most important current application of molecular genetics to genetic disorders - the detection of abnormalities. The methods and problems of prenatal diagnosis have been discussed widely elsewhere and will not be reviewed here (for example, see Donis-Keller et al., 1986a, b; Latt et al., 1986; Wallace et al., 1986). Nevertheless, it is important to emphasize that the detection of genetic disorders either by precise abnormalities of known genes, for example globin (Geever et al., 1981; Chang and Kan, 1982), or by linkage to known markers as seen with Huntington chorea (Gusella et al., 1983), cystic fibrosis (White et al., 1985) and adrenoleukodystrophy (Aubourg et al., 1987) has been prominent in genetic analysis.

Detection of genetic abnormalities has been aided by the growing recognition of gene conservation between organisms. Despite well recognized interspecies differences, there frequently is sufficient similarity between gene systems to aid the interpretation of structural relationships. This has been particularly useful in relating human and mouse genes and in evaluating homologous gene clusters in other organisms. Examples include the globin (Koop et al., 1986), histocompatibility (Geliebter and Nathenson, 1987) and immunoglobulin (Hinds and Litman, 1986) genes and our own studies of SAA genes noted above (Sack, 1983, Sack and Lease, 1986, Lowell et al., 1986).

Many single gene disorders now can be detected in the early prenatal period but this has been limited largely to human biology despite their potential applicability in other animal systems. Nevertheless, it is in the detection of genetic changes that genetic technology has made its first and most prominent therapeutic appearance.

INTRODUCTION OF GENES

The cloning of individual genes and the increasing understanding of gene structure and cell- and tissue-specific controlling factors have set the stage for direct gene manipulation including introducing specific genes into cells and providing appropriate gene expression in specific cells and tissues. Although these techniques are only evolving, their potential application underlies the practice and planning for correction and control of genetic defects. The approaches will be considered in turn but it is important at this point to introduce the term "transgenic" to refer to an organism with an altered genotype reflecting the introduction of genes from another individual or species by _in vitro_ techniques.

The goal of molecular intervention already has been achieved in yeast where it is generally possible to produce homologous replacement of a resident chromosomal region. As shown in Figure 1, the exchange is usually precise and results in the insertion of a new sequence. This can be either the "correct" gene (in effect "gene therapy" for an identified lesion) or an altered gene (a new, known mutation whose consequences are to be studied).

Unfortunately, there is no reliable method of producing such site-specific replacements in more complex organisms but the appeal of this possibility drives many current efforts. Precise replacement at a single site should, in theory, place the new genetic information under control of the appropriate temporal and physical regulatory machinery of the locus and assure normal biologic function of the exogenous gene.

In order to introduce new genes into mammalian cells it is necessary to overcome the basic difficulty of actually getting the gene into the cell of interest. (See Table 1)

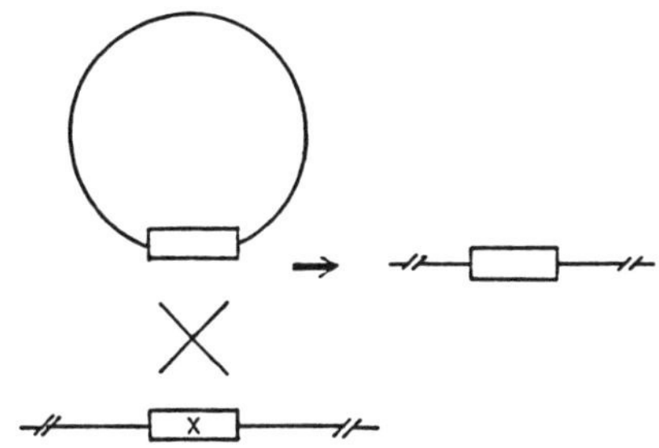

Figure 1: Schematic diagram of recombination of introduced DNA clone containing a sequence (open rectangle) homologous to resident (chromosomal) sequence (below). In yeast, such events frequently lead to replacement of the endogenous sequence by the new sequence, as shown.

TABLE 1 - TECHNIQUES FOR MAKING TRANSGENIC CELLS

Cell Fusion
Chromosome-mediated gene transfer
Calcium-mediated precipitation
Electroporation
Microinjection
Retroviral constructs

Cell fusion and chromosome transfer have been discussed above. More recently developed techniques are applicable to the transfer of smaller DNA fragments and include precipitation of DNA over tissue culture cells and electroporation whereby a transient electric shock actually opens spaces in the cell membrane permitting DNA to enter the cell (Pellicer et al., 1980). Physically injecting DNA into the pronucleus of a fertilized egg using a micropipette also has been useful in the creation of transgenic animals (e.g. Brinster et al., 1982).

Small RNA tumor viruses (or "retroviruses") have several features which have led to their use as vectors for introducing new genetic information into cells. They are small, but capable of carrying a reasonable amount of cloned material (see Figure 2). Their structure is well known and the information responsible for neoplastic changes can be eliminated by appropriate in vitro recombinations. They are bounded by long terminal repeats (LTR's) which also contain strong promoters for transcription of cloned genes. The retroviral genome is single-stranded RNA but is converted into double-stranded DNA within the recipient cell. A normal part of the retroviral life cycle is the integration of a double-stranded DNA copy into the DNA of the host cell.

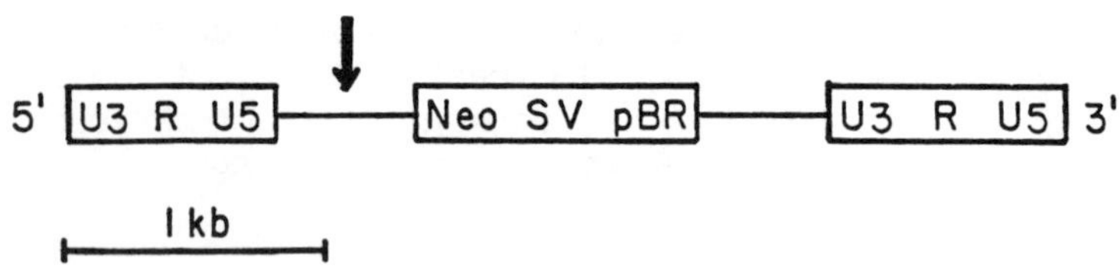

Figure 2: Diagram of basic structure of a retrovirus modified to be suitable for introducing an exogenous gene by deleting the sequences responsible for neoplasia. The tripartite long terminal repeats (LTRs) are shown in the flanking boxes; these serve replication and promoter functions. A gene permitting selection (e.g. Neomycin resistance) may be included to assist recovery of transfected host cells. The new gene or sequence can be introduced at the position of the arrow where it will be under control of the 5' LTR promoter.

Constructs derived from retroviruses can be transfected into recipient cells with relative ease using precipitation or electroporation. It also is possible to package the constructs into authentic retroviral particles using other proteins supplied by a defective "helper" virus (Mann et al., 1983); such viruses then can infect the target cell directly. The genes contained in these constructs are expressed frequently and, although the site(s) of integration are not yet well controlled in mammalian cells, phenotypic changes can be obtained. A selected group of references for results in transgenic animals is included in Table 2.

RESULTS OF GENE INTRODUCTION

Introducing exogenous DNA into eukaryotic cells has both predictable and unpredictable consequences depending, in part, on the number, location and control of the introduced genes. Table 2 presents a representative summary of studies of this problem which will be discussed in more detail below.

TABLE 2 - PHENOTYPIC CHANGES IN TRANSGENIC ANIMALS

Hormone production	
supermouse	Palmiter et al., 1982a,b
growth factor	Rosenthal et al., 1986
Neoplasia - tissue-specific	
lymphatic	Adams et al., 1985
mammary, testicular	Leder et al., 1986
Cell-specific protein production	
murine beta lactoglobulin in sheep milk	Simons et al., 1987
phenylalanine hydroxylase	Ledley et al., 1985
alpha-1-antitrypsin	Krumlauf et al., 1986
globins	Chada et al., 1986 Kollias et al., 1986
alcohol dehydrogenase	Goldberg et al., 1983
diphtheria toxin	Palmiter et al., 1987
Widespread protein production	
neomycin resistance	Eglitis et al., 1985 Keller et al., 1985
globin	Lacy et al., 1983
Defect correction	
HPRT	Willis et al., 1984
adenosine deaminase	Belmont et al., 1986
glucocorticoid receptor	Miesfeld et al., 1986
thalassemia (murine)	Constantini et al.,1986
Insertional mutation	
HPRT (murine)	Kuehn et al., 1987
actin (yeast)	Shortle et al., 1982
limb deformity (murine)	Woychik et al., 1985

An important determinate of the physiologic consequences of gene introduction is the appropriate expression of the introduced material, made possible by specific replacement of resident genetic material with exogenous sequences. As described above, direct replacement is not yet possible at high frequency in mammalian cells. However, recent improvements in vector systems, mostly based on retroviruses (see Figure 2, above), have improved the prospects for this approach.

Particular progress on this problem has involved the construction of precisely defined molecules to permit detection and quantitation of the events following the introduction of the exogenous DNA. Several systems have now provided data for an initial assessment of the events. Thomas and Capecchi (1986) observed the results of introducing marked neomycin resistance genes into cells where another neo gene already resided. They found 3 types of interaction between the incoming and the resident genes: 1) the resident gene was replaced, 2) the introduced gene was modified by the resident, 3) there were various types of changes in the resident gene which could be explained by recombination with the new DNA.

An estimate of the frequency of gene replacement events was provided by studies of the beta globin locus. Having a double-stranded DNA break in the region of interest increased the frequency of recombination between the exogenous and endogenous sequences (Kucherlapati et al., 1984). When appropriately marked globin genes were used Smithies et al (1985) obtained stable recombinants into the globin gene of the host human cell at a frequency of about 10^{-3}. After some more recent refinements; this occurred a bit more frequently permitting several conclusions: 1) the notion of gene replacement may be considered in mammalian cells, 2) the event is of low but detectable frequency, 3) obtaining the desired recombinant will require some type of screening or in vitro selection, and 4) the product of such replacement could be used in conjunction with bone marrow transplantation or embryo (e.g. blastocyst) implantation (see below).

Refinements of these approaches hold the best promise for making unique gene changes in animal cells. They offer a reasonable way of obtaining the highly specific changes which will be necessary in, for example, the human genome where the target may be as small as a single nucleotide in $3X10^9$.

The difficulties inherent in current approaches to site-specific gene replacement have led to experiments with less precise methods. One approach to circumventing the technical problems of inserting genes into their ideal positions has been to develop gene control systems which, following introduction, can be regulated either by exogenous factors or by gene control sequences incorporated into the recombinant molecule. Both approaches have had some success and considerable notoriety.

One approach has exploited the sensitivity of the gene for metallothionein (MT) to transcriptional regulation by divalent cations (particularly cadmium and manganese). Since the MT gene was cloned it was possible to connect its upstream control region to another gene thus placing the new gene under MT (and divalent cation) control. The entire construct, in a recombinant plasmid, was microinjected into fertilized mouse eggs which were reimplanted and permitted to develop. The result of such experiments using growth hormone recombinants was the production of transgenic mice which grew to a large size when their diet contained a divalent cation supplement. Such "supermice" represent the consequence of exogenously controlled expression of growth hormone production. (Brinster et al., 1982; Mayo et al., 1982; Palmiter et al., 1982a, b; Palmiter et al., 1983).

In another group of useful and informative constructs the oncogene "myc" has been introduced into cells leading to various tumors in the resulting transgenic animals depending on the enhancing and control region to which the gene was connected. For example, when connected to immunoglobulin gene control regions, myc leads to lymphoid malignancies (Adams et al., 1985). Alternatively, connecting myc to a mouse mammary tumor virus construct led to testicular, breast, lymphocytic and mast cell tumors (Leder et al., 1986).

It is occasionally possible to depend on features connecting the control region of the construct and the physiology of the recipient cell to result in appropriate gene expression. Such effects have been seen with phenylalanine hydroxylase (Ledley et al., 1985), alpha-1-antitrypsin (Ciliberto et al., 1985), alpha-fetoprotein, (Krumlauf et al., 1986), fetal and other globins (Chada et al., 1986; Kollias et al., 1986) and alcohol dehydrogenase (Goldberg et al., 1983). There is no common structural feature to these individual expression systems except that the newly-introduced and differentially expressed genes also were subject to regulation in the host from which they were derived. Unfortunately, there also is precedent, using similar gene introduction methods, for having variable or non-specific expression of foreign genes: generalized neomycin resistance in marrow-derived cells (Eglitis et al., 1985; Keller et al., 1985) and globin in non-hematologic tissues (Lacy et al., 1983).

A new technique for gene expression which has particular biological consequence and may prove useful for domestic animal genetics and protein production has been the attachment of genes to control regions which are specific for a given tissue. A recent example has been provided by the work of Simons et al (1987) where sheep beta lactoglobulin was introduced into mice. The transgenic mice resulting from this experiment produced significant amounts of the sheep protein in their milk. Not only does this show tissue specific protein production, (and, hence, the reliability of the control signals in the recombinant) but it also offers a potentially useful approach to producing valuable animal proteins through their expression in a renewable fluid such as milk.

Other experiments have led to the correction of specific biochemical and developmental defects by introducing an appropriate enzyme or protein. These have included amelioration of the changes of the Lesch-Nyhan syndrome with HPRT gene correction (Willis et al., 1984), correction of adenosine deaminase deficiency (Belmont et al., 1986) and correction of a glucocorticoid receptor deficiency (Miesfeld, 1986). Murine thalassemia also has been corrected by transfer of globin genes into the germ line (Constantini et al., 1986). Palmiter et al (1987) have used developmental stage-specific control sequences attached to the gene for diphtheria toxin A. When expressed in accord with its built-in developmental signals, this construct causes the death of the cell in which it resides and the consequent loss of potential progeny - thus providing an approach to developmental analysis.

The intrinsic difficulty with DNA mediated gene transfer is the random and potentially mutagenic insertion of the introduced DNA into multiple sites in the host genome. Many of these events seem to be without great consequence to the host; however, it has been possible to cause insertional mutations by these techniques. For example HPRT deficiency has been introduced in the mouse (Kuehn et al., 1987), the actin gene in yeast has been disrupted by the integration of DNA (Shortle et al., 1982) and a developmental limb deformity has been created in a transgenic mouse by insertional mutagenesis (Woychik et al., 1985). Such insertional mutations are generally negative factors from the perspective of using these techniques for therapy. On the other hand, some may prove useful by providing molecular markers for gene cloning as the P element mutants have done for Drosophila (O'Hare and Rubin, 1983). This also has been done for the limb deformities referred to above.

While DNA may be introduced into embryos and thus enter all (or most) cells of the recipient, this is not always necessary for therapeutic effects. A useful adjunct to these methods is bone marrow transplantation (BMT). Although the extensive possibilities of BMT cannot be explored here in detail, they have been reviewed elsewhere (Barranger, 1984; Parkman, 1986). As BMT becomes more reliable (it is still used largely for neoplastic disorders), the possibility of producing in vitro alteration of the cells prior to their introduction (or reintroduction in the case of autologous BMT) becomes important (Dick et al., 1985; Gruber et al., 1985; Hock and Miller, 1986). Using retrovirus-derivatives with selectable markers (e.g. neomycin resistance as discussed above) or a selection system based on the function of the newly-introduced gene in initially defective cells (e.g. HPRT replacement) it should be possible to prepare a group of transplantable cells which contain the specific change desired. Therapeutic effects in the nervous system have been produced using BMT in Twitcher mice (Yeager et al., 1984); this serves as a useful test system for perfecting details of the procedure as an approach to correcting genetic disorders.

EMBRYO MANIPULATION

The possibilities presented by recombinant DNA manipulation using specific gene promoters and various introduction methods are multiplied when combined with embryo manipulation techniques. The use of both of these approaches promises even more useful methods for diagnosis and treatment of prenatal and developmental defects in man and other animals.

The techniques of embryo manipulation have been developed over several decades. Much has been derived from animal husbandry studies including such methods as embryo transfer, embryo splitting and fusion, and *in vitro* fertilization. Only the latter has reached any prominence in human developmental biology. By contrast, the reintroduction of transgenic cells of early embryos or teratocarcinomas into pregnant female mice has led to chimeric progeny (Wagner et al., 1985; Lovell-Badge et al., 1985).

The basic technique involves the *in vitro* introduction of recombinant molecules into various embryo preparations. The results of such interventions (see Figure 3) include transgenic animals, genetically identical animals, sex-selected animals and a wide spectrum of progeny - the products of various cloning and embryonic techniques (Church, 1987; Womack, 1987). This combination of techniques has extremely broad applicability for animal breeding and developing desired characteristics in domestic animals and other organisms. It also opens possibilities for using animals as sources of production for important medical and biological compounds including hormones, drugs and unique proteins. The possibility of using milk as a renewable source of these proteins has been noted above and has potential application to making proteins specific for individual genetic disorders and other therapeutic purposes (Simons et al., 1987; Clark et al., 1987; Cartwright, 1987).

Since it now is possible to produce virtually any desired recombinant molecule, the growing knowledge of gene expression control as well as the improving methods for introducing specific genes into specific chromosomal regions provide an opportunity for applying these molecular techniques to a wide variety of problems in therapy and diagnosis as well as the production of pharmaceutical and other molecules.

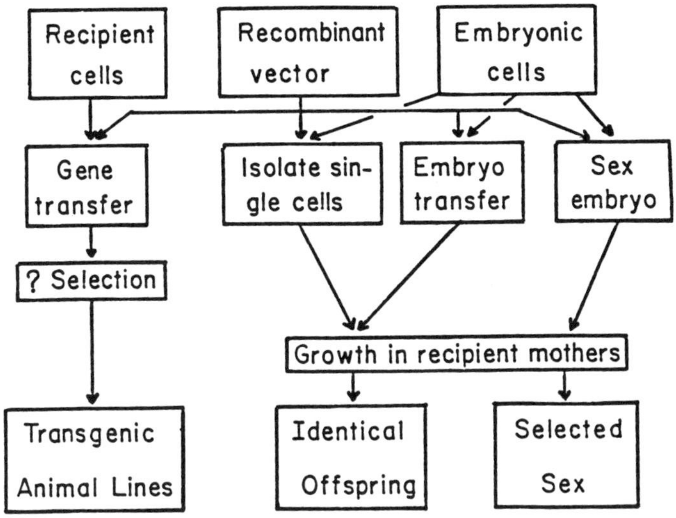

Figure 3: A schematic view of possible combinations of molecular genetic and embryonic manipulation methods as described in text.

This rapidly evolving field offers hope for definitive management of genetic defects first by their detailed characterization and then by specialized intervention. Long term possibilities for the applications of these approaches have only begun to be appreciated.

ACKNOWLEDGEMENTS

The author gratefully recognizes support from USPHS grants AM 31745 and HD 10981 as well as gifts from Mr. Daniel M. Kelly and Mr. and Mrs. William M. Griffin. Mrs. Mary A. Mix provided careful manuscript preparation and Mr. C. Conover Talbot, Jr. added thoughtful comments.

REFERENCES

Adams JM, Harris AW, Pinkert CA, Corcoran LM, Alexander WS, Cory S, Palmiter RD, Brinster RL (1985). The c-myc oncogene driven by immunoglobulin enhancers induces lymphoid malignancy in transgenic mice. Nature 318:533.

Aubourg PR, Sack GHJr, Meyers DA, Lease JJ, Moser HW (1987). Linkage of adrenoleukodystrophy to a polymorphic DNA probe. Ann Neurol 21:349.

Baccara M, Kelly F (1978). Expression of polyoma virus in heterokaryons between embryonal carcinoma cells and differentiated cells. Virology 90:147.

Baron MH, Maniatis T (1986). Rapid reprogramming of globin gene expression in transient heterokaryons. Cell 46:591.

Barranger, JA (1984). Marrow transplantation in genetic diseases. New Engl J Med 311:1629.

Belmont JW, Henkel-Tigges J, Chang SMW, Wager-Smith K, Kellems RE, Dick JE, Magli MC, Phillips RA, Bernstein A, Caskey CT (1986). Expression of human adenosine deaminase in murine haematopoietic progenitor cells following retroviral transfer. Nature 322:385.

Bender W, Akam M, Karch F, Beachy PA, Peifer M, Spierer P, Lewis EB, Hodness DS (1983). Molecular genetics of the bithorax complex in Drosophila melanogaster. Science 221:23.

Brinster RL, Chen HY, Warren R, Sarthy A, Palmiter RD (1982). Regulation of metallothionein - thymidine kinase fusion plasmids injected into mouse eggs. Nature 296:39.

Cartwright T (1987). Isolation and purification of products from animal cells. Trends in Biotechnol 5:25.

Chada K, Magram J, Costantini F (1986). An embryonic pattern of expression of a human fetal globin gene in transgenic mice. Nature 319:685.

Chang JC, Kan YW (1982). A sensitive new prenatal test for sickle cell anemia. New Engl J Med 307:30.

Church RB (1987). Embryo manipulation and gene transfer in domestic animals. Trends in Biotechnol 5:13.

Ciliberto G, Denter L, Cortese R (1985). Cell-specific expression of a transfected human alpha-1-antitrypsin gene. Cell 41:531.

Clark AJ, Simons P, Wilmut I, Lathe R (1987). Pharmaceuticals from transgenic livestock. Trends in Biotechnol 5:20.

Constantini F, Chada K, Magram J (1986). Correction of murine β-Thalassemia by gene transfer into the germ line. Science 233:1192.

Dick JE, Magli MC, Huszar D, Phillips RA, Bernstein A (1985). Introduction of a selectable gene into primitive stem cells capable of long-term reconstitution of the hemopoietic system of w/wv mice. Cell 42:71.

Donis-Keller H, Barker D, Knowlton R, Schumm J, Braman J (1986 a). Applications of RFLP probes to genetic mapping and clinical diagnosis in humans. In Lerman LS (ed): "DNA Probes," New York: Cold Spring Harbor, p 73.

Donis-Keller H, Barker DF, Knowlton RG, Schumm JW, Braman JC, Green P (1986 b). Highly polymorphic RFLP probes as diagnostic tools. Cold Spring Harbor Symp Quant Biol 51:317.

Eglitis MA, Kantoff P, Gilboa E, Anderson WF (1985). Gene expression in mice after high efficiency retroviral-mediated gene transfer. Science 230:1395.

Geever RF, Wilson LB, Nallaseth FS, Milner PF, Bittner M, Wilson JT (1981). Direct identification of sickle cell anemia by blot hybridization. Proc Natl Acad Sci USA 78:5081.

Gehring WJ (1985). The homeo box: a key to the understanding of development. Cell 40:3.

Geliebter J, Nathenson SG (1987). Recombination and the concerted evolution of the murine MHC. Trends in Genet 3:107.

Goldberg DA, Posakony JW, Maniatis T (1983). Correct developmental expression of a cloned alcohol dehydrogenase gene transduced into the Drosophila germ line. Cell 34:59.

Gruber HE, Finley KD, Hershberg RM, Katzman SS, Laikind PK, Seegmiller JE, Friedmann T, Yee J-K, Jolly DJ (1985). Retroviral vector-mediated gene transfer into human hematopoietic progenitor cells. Science 230:1057.

Gusella JF, Wexler NS, Conneally PM, Naylor SL, Anderson MA, Tanzi RE, Watkins PC, Ottina K, Wallace MR, Sakaguchi AY, Young AB, Shoulson I, Bonilla E, Martin JB (1983). A polymorphic DNA marker genetically linked to Huntington's disease. Nature 306:234.

Hart CP, Awgulewitsch A, Fainsod A, McGinnis W, Ruddle FH (1985). Homeo box gene complex on mouse chromosome 11: molecular cloning, expression in embryogenesis, and homology to a human homeo box locus. Cell 43:9.

Hinds KR, Litman GW (1986). Major reorganization of immunoglobulin VH segmental elements during vertebrate evolution. Nature 320:546.

Hock RA, Miller AD (1986). Retrovirus-mediated transfer and expression of drug resistance genes in human haematopoietic progenitor cells. Nature 320:275.

Keller G, Paige C, Gilboa E, Wagner EF (1985). Expression of a foreign gene in myeloid and lymphoid cells derived from multipotent haematopoietic precursors. Nature 318:149.

Kollias G, Wrighton N, Hurst J, Grosveld F (1986). Regulated expression of human a γ-, β-, and hybrid $\gamma\beta$-globin genes in transgenic mice: manipulation of the developmental expression patterns. Cell 46:89.

Koop BF, Goodman M, Xu P, Chan K, Slighton JL (1986). Primate globin DNA sequences and man's place among the great apes. Nature 319:234.

Krumlauf R, Chapman VM, Hammer RE, Brinster R, Tilghman SM (1986). Differential expression of α-fetoprotein genes on the inactive X-chromosome in extraembryonic and somatic tissues of a transgenic mouse line. Nature 319:224.

Kucherlapati RS, Eves EM, Song K-Y, Morse BS, Smithies O (1984). Homologous recombination between plasmids in mammalian cells can be enhanced by treatment of input DNA. Proc Natl Acad Sci USA 81:3153.

Kuehn MR, Bradley A, Robertson EJ, Evans MJ (1987). A potential animal model for Lesch-Nyhan syndrome through introduction of HPRT mutations into mice. Nature 326:295.

Kunkel LM and coauthors (1987). Analysis of deletions in DNA from patients with Becker and Duchenne muscular dystrophy. Nature 322:73.

Lacy E, Roberts S, Evans EP, Burtenshaw MK, Constantini FD (1983). A foreign β-globin gene in transgenic mice: integration at abnormal chromosomal positions and expression in inappropriate tissues. Cell 34:343.

Latt SA, Lalande M, Donlon T, Wyman A, Rose E, Shiloh Y, Korf B, Muller U, Sakai K, Kanda N, Kang J, Stroh H, Harris P, Bruns G, Wharton R, Kaplan L (1986). DNA-based detection of chromosome deletion and amplification: Diagnostic and mechanistic significance. Cold Spring Harbor Symp Quant Biol 51:299.

Leder A, Pattengale PK, Kuo A, Stewart TA, Leder P (1986). Consequences of widespread deregulation of the c-myc gene in transgenic mice: multiple neoplasms and normal development. Cell 45:485.

Ledley FD, Grenett HE, DiLella AG, Kwok SCM, Woo SLC (1985). Gene transfer and expression of human phenylalanine hydroxylase. Science 228:77.

Lovell-Badge RH, Bygrave AE, Bradley A, Robertson E, Evans MJ, Cheah KSE (1985). Transformation of embryonic stem cells with the human Type-II collagen gene and its expression in chimeric mice. Cold Spring Harbor Symp Quant Biol 50:707.

Lowell CA, Potter DA, Stearman RS, Morrow JF (1986). Structure of the murine serum amyloid A gene family - Gene conversion. J Biol Chem 261:8442.

Mann R, Mulligan RC, Baltimore D (1983). Construction of a retrovirus packaging mutant and its use to produce helper-free defective retrovirus. Cell 33:153.

Mayo KE, Warren R, Palmiter RD (1982). The mouse metallothionein-1 gene is transcriptionally regulated by cadmium following transfection into human or mouse cells. Cell 29:99.

Miesfeld R, Rusconi S, Godowski PJ, Maler BA, Okret S, Wikstrom A-C, Gustafsson J-A, Yamamoto KR (1986). Genetic complementation of a glucocorticoid receptor deficiency by expression of cloned receptor cDNA. Cell 46:389.

O'Hare K, Rubin GM (1983). Structures of p transposable elements and their sites of insertion and excision in the drosophila melanogaster genome. Cell 34:25.

Palmiter RD, Behringer RR, Quaife CJ, Maxwell F, Maxwell IH, Brinster RL (1987). Cell lineage ablation in transgenic mice by cell-specific expression of a toxin gene. Cell 50:435.

Palmiter RD, Brinster RL, Hammer RE, Trumbauer ME, Rosenfeld MG, Birnberg NC, Evans RM (1982 a). Dramatic growth of mice that develop from eggs microinjected with metallothionein-growth hormone fusion genes. Nature 300:611.

Palmiter RD, Chen HY, Brinster RL (1982 b). Differential regulation of metallothionein - thymidine kinase fusion genes in transgenic mice and their offspring. Cell 29:701.

Palmiter RD, Norstedt G, Gelinas RE, Hammer RE, Brinster RL (1983). Metallothionein-Human gH fusion genes stimulate growth of mice. Science 222:809.

Parkman, R (1986). Application of bone marrow transplantation to treatment of genetic diseases. Science 232:1373.

Payne FE, Baublis JV, Itabashi HH (1969). Isolation of measles virus from cell cultures of brain from a patient with subacute sclerosing panencephalitis. New Engl J Med 281:585.

Pellicer A, Robins D, Wold B, Sweet R, Jackson J, Lowy I, Roberts JM, Sim GK, Silverstein S, Axel R (1980).

Altering genotype and phenotype by DNA-mediated gene transfer. Science 209:1414.

Porteous DJ (1987). Chromosome mediated gene transfer: a functional assay for complex loci and an aid to human genome mapping. Trends in Genet 3:177.

Quinn CA, Goodfellow PN, Povey S, Walsh FS (1981). Human-rat muscle somatic cell hybrids form myotubes and express human muscle gene products. Proc Natl Acad Sci USA 78:5031.

Rassoulzadegan M, Leopold P, Vailly J, Cuzin F (1986). Germ line transmission of autonomous genetic elements in transgenic mouse strains. Cell 46:513.

Rosenthal A, Lindquist PB, Bringham TS, Goeddel DV, Derynck R (1986). Expression in rat fibroblasts of a human transforming growth factor-α cDNA results in transformation. Cell 46:301.

Ruddle FH (1981). A new era in mammalian gene mapping: Somatic cell genetics and recombinant DNA methodologies. Nature 294:115.

Sack GHJr (1983). Molecular cloning of human genes for serum amyloid A. Gene 21:19.

Sack GHJr, Lease JJ (1986). Human serum amyloid A genes - molecular characterization. In Glenner GG, Osserman EF, Benditt EP, Calkins E, Cohen AS, Zucker-Franklin D (eds): "Amyloidosis," New York: Plenum Publishing Company, p 61.

Scott MP (1985). Molecules and puzzles from the antennapedia homoeotic gene complex of Drosophila. Trends in Genet 1:74.

Shortle D, Haber JE, Botstein D (1982). Lethal disruption by the yeast actin gene by integrative DNA transformation. Science 217:371.

Simons, JP, McClenaghan M, Clark, AJ (1987). Alteration of the quality of milk by expression of sheep beta lactoglobulin in transgenic mice. Nature 328:530.

Smithies O, Gregg RG, Boggs SS, Koralewski MA, Kucherlapati RS (1985). Insertion of DNA sequences into the human chromosomal β-globin locus by homologous recombination. Nature 317:230.

Thomas KR, Folger KR, Capecchi MR (1986). High frequency targeting of genes to specific sites in the mammalian genome. Cell 44:419.

Wagner EF, Keller G, Gilboa E, Ruther U, Stewart C (1985). Gene transfer into murine stem cells and mice using retroviral vectors. Cold Spring Harbor Symp Quant Biol 50:691.

Wallace RB, Petz LD, Yam PY (1986). Application of synthetic DNA probes to the analysis of DNA sequence variants in man. Cold Spring Harbor Symp Quant Biol 51:257.

Weiss JH, Nelson DL, Pryzborski MJ, Chaplin DD, Mulligan RC, Housman DE, Seidman JG (1984). Eukaryotic chromosome transfer: linkage of the murine major histocompatibility complex to an inserted dominant selectable marker. Proc Natl Acad Sci USA 81:4879.

White R, Woodward S, Leppert M, O'Connell P, Hoff M, Herbst J, Lalouel J-M, Dean M, Vande Woude G (1985). A closely linked genetic marker for cystic fibrosis. Nature 318:382.

Willis RC, Jolly DJ, Miller AD, Plent MM, Esty AC, Anderson PJ, Chang H-C, Jones OW, Seegmiller JE, Friedmann T (1984). Partial phenotypic correction of human Lesch-Nyhan (hypoxanthine-guanine phosphoribosyltransferase-deficient) lymphoblasts with a transmissible retroviral vector. J Biol Chem 259:7842.

Womack JE (1987). Genetic engineering in agriculture: animal genetics and development. Trends in Genet 3:65.

Woychik RP, Stewart TA, Davis LG, D'Eustachio P, Leder P (1985). An inherited limb deformity created by insertional mutagenesis in a transgenic mouse. Nature 318:36.

Yeager AM, Brennan S, Tiffany C, Moser HW, Santos GW (1984). Prolonged survival and remyelination after hematopoietic cell transplantation in the twitching mouse. Science 225:1052.

Youssoufian H, Antonarakis SE, Aronis S, Tsiftis G, Phillips DG, Kazazian HHJr (1987). Characterization of five partial deletions of the factor VIII gene. Proc Natl Acad Sci USA 84:3772.

V. REASSESSMENT OF TRANSPLACENTAL HAZARDS

Transplacental Effects on Fetal Health, pages 327–335

CLINICAL ASPECTS RISK ASSESSMENT AND MANAGEMENT OF TRANSPLACENTAL HAZARDS FOR THE FETUS: CONSIDERATIONS FOR PUBLIC POLICY

James W. Hanson and Elizabeth J. Thomson

Department of Pediatrics, University of Iowa, Iowa City, Iowa 52242

The participants in this conference have addressed mechanisms of action of transplacental hazards. The occurrence of such a conference reflects not only the increased emphasis on this important research area among medical scientists but also the immense and growing public concern regarding these issues. The twin tragedies of thalidomide and rubella epidemics in the early 1960s stimulated this concern. Subsequent episodes such as exposure of human populations to Agent Orange in Viet Nam, the banning of spray adhesives after anecdotal reports from Oklahoma City, dioxin contamination in Times Beach, Missouri, real and potential release of radioactive materials at 3 Mile Island and Chernobyl, and clusters of leukemia associated with contamination of water supplies in Woburn, Massachusetts, as well as the highly publicized legal events involving such drugs as Bendectin and various contraceptive agents, have further galvanized these fears. Unfortunately, public concern has outstripped scientific knowledge and the ability of health care providers to provide meaningful consultation and care.

Concurrently, there has been an increasing recognition of the significance of transplacental hazards to fetal growth and development as a major public health problem. The U.S. Centers for Disease Control and other agencies provide eloquent data which reveal that 3-4% of babies have birth defects recognized within the first year of life. Such defects are a principal cause of mortality among full-term neonates in developed areas of the world and are the fifth leading cause of years of potential life lost in the

United States at the present time. Furthermore, developmental disabilities and birth defects are the largest single category for expenditure of dollars for chronic health care purposes in most state budgets. Clearly, these disorders consume a disproportionate share of our health care resources. This is a group of conditions for which care is often difficult and inaccessible, for which most care providers have relatively little preparation and/or knowledge, and for which care is poorly reimbursed.

It is now recognized that a significant proportion of all birth defects have a major environmental (transplacental) contribution to their cause, many of which may be subject to prevention strategies. Of course, birth defects are only one category of adverse reproductive outcomes which can stem from transplacental effects on the fetus. Other outcomes include infertility, sterility, fetal loss, stillbirth, low birth weight, developmental disabilities, behavioral effects, and cancer.

Though the past 25 years have seen a substantial growth in our scientific knowledge of the types of potentially hazardous agents (Table 1), their mechanisms of action, other potentially contributing risk factors, and approaches to their control and treatment, there remain substantial barriers to the widespread effective implementation of this information at the clinical level.

Partially in response to the continued need for access to information regarding these agents, various governmental agencies, such as the National Institutes of Health and the National Library of Medicine, have collaborated in developing information resources. Examples of existing services include: 1) Environmental Teratology Information Center File, a subfile of TOXLINE which is a part of MEDLARS, the National Library of Medicine's computerized information system, 2) the Chemical Carcinogenesis Research Information System (CCRIS), a joint program of the National Cancer Institute and the National Library of Medicine, 3) the Information Retrieval and Analysis Section of the National Institute of Occupational Safety and Health, 4) the National Toxicology Program, and 5) the National Pesticide Telecommunications Network at the Texas Tech Health Science Center School of Medicine. Other sources of information include the U.S. Centers for Disease Control, the Agency for Toxic Substances and Disease Registries (ATSDR) and the

Food and Drug Administration. Whereas these agencies and programs have access to an immense amount of information, until relatively recently even knowledgeable scientists and public health officials had serious problems appropriately accessing this information and obtaining comprehensive and authoritative information upon which to base public policy decisions, to say nothing of interpreting the information in clinical management settings. For the average health practitioner or consumer, the vast array of available information was both inaccessible and incomprehensible.

TABLE 1. Categories of Teratogenic Agents

I. Infectious Agents
1. viruses
2. bacteria
3. parasites
examples: rubella, cytomegaloviruses, syphilis, toxoplasmosis

II. Physical Agents
1. ionizing radiation
2. hyperthermia
3. mechanical factors
examples: therapeutic radiation, fever, oligohydramnios, amniotic bands

III. Drug and Chemical Agents
1. environmental chemicals
2. nonprescription drugs
3. prescription drugs
examples: organic mercurials, alcohol, warfarin, valproic acid, isotretinoin

IV. Maternal Factors
1. metabolic conditions
2. genetic disorders
3. nutritional factors
examples: diabetes mellitus, PKU, myotonic dystrophy, vitamin deficiency

In the 1970's the health care community began to focus attention (in part because of medical tort liability actions) on ways of providing information to potentially pregnant couples and their health care providers (Brent and Jackson, 1985). In 1979 the first such program was developed at the University of California, San Diego, by Dr. Kenneth Jones (Jones et al., 1986). The California Teratogen Registry had, as an early objective, the identification of a cohort of individuals whose exposure to given environmental agents could be identified so that reproductive outcome could be prospectively assessed. However, the subsequent response of the public suggested more interest in the service aspects of this project than in the research aspects. Subsequently over 25 other such systems or programs have developed throughout the United States and Canada, most of which emphasize the service components (Vogt, 1985). These systems are extremely heterogeneous in terms of their organizational base, operational methods, type and quality of personnel, information retrieval and interpretation, target audience, sponsorship and program of services (O'Brien et al., 1986; Vogt and Librizzi, 1986; Manchester et al., 1986; Quirk et al., 1986; Biesecker et al., 1986; Shepard et al., 1986; Shulman et al., 1986; Martinez et al., 1986; Allen and Hoyme, 1986; Peters and Garbis, 1986).

Relatively recently more organized programs with a national perspective have evolved. The two principal such programs include REPROTOX (Brown and Scialli, 1986), a computerized information service of the Reproductive Toxicology Center of the Research Foundation of the Columbia Hospital for Women in Washington, D.C. developed by Dr. Sergio Fabro and the Teratogen Information System (TERIS) under development by Drs. Jan Friedman and Thomas Shepard at the University of Washington through a grant from the Federal Office of Maternal and Child Health.

The development and operation of these service programs has resulted in the identification of a number of problems which have been the basis for extensive discussion in recent years at national meetings of the Teratology Society (Public Affairs Forum, 1986), the American Society of Human Genetics and meetings sponsored by the March of Dimes Birth Defects Foundation.

The central question concerning exposure to a potentially teratogenic agent is: "Has the risk to the baby been increased?" However, various parties to the communication process resulting from this question have somewhat different areas of emphasis in this risk assessment. To the degree that a teratogen information service meets these needs it may be judged effective.

From a consumer perspective, the patient who requests information in general is asking: "Is my baby well?" Families wish reassurance that nothing has gone wrong and are likely to be equally distressed by the presence of birth defects unrelated to a given exposure. Hence such information needs to be given in the context of other pregnancy risk assessment data. Reproductive decisions are based on complex value systems in which alternatives are considered, each having its own risks and uncertainties (Pern, 1979). If the information to be given is to be beneficial it must be desired, understood, believed, remembered, and accepted as having personal relevance. There are many factors which influence reproductive decision making. Some such as risk assessment and risk communication are almost entirely influenced by health care providers, while others are solely influenced by family understanding, interpretation and values. Figure 1 shows several factors which are important in reproductive decision making.

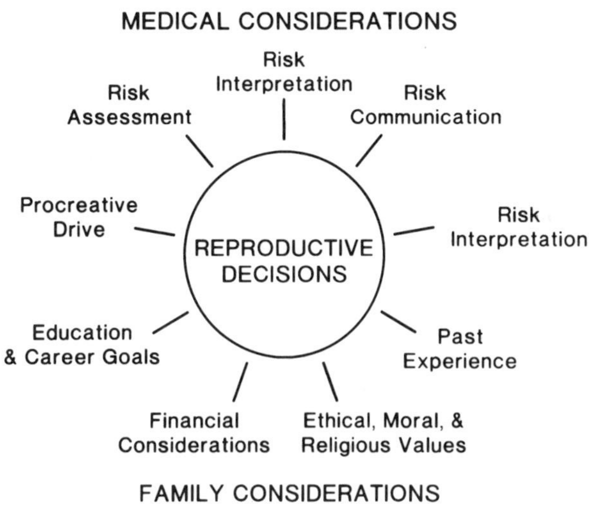

Figure 1. Factors influencing reproductive decision-making.

Furthermore, it should be understood that attitudes regarding the desirability of pregnancy and acceptable risks vary widely. In addition, patients may, when told of possible increases in risk, infer that they (or someone) is guilty of some misconduct.

From the physician or other health care provider perspective a different question arises: "What should be done?" Thus the physician's risk assessment must evaluate the interplay of many factors and must allow negotiation of a complex interpersonal communication process resulting in appropriate management steps. In this process the physician must confront often inadequate, incomplete or even contradictory information. Furthermore, the physician inevitably becomes aware that he/she may be held responsible for the outcome. In view of questions in the minds of many obstetricians as to whom (mother or baby) is his/her patient, potentially serious conflicts of interest often arise.

Finally, from the standpoint of scientists, public health officials and regulatory agencies, the risk assessment questions of interest are substantially different: What is the nature and magnitude of reproductive risks associated with exposure? How should these be reflected in public health policy? What regulatory actions are necessary to protect the public? Can teratogen information services be effectively used to collect scientific information to be utilized in risk assessment or risk management?

It should also be noted that teratogen information services are asked to respond to a wide array of concerns. Agents of concern include not only drugs (prescription and non-prescription) and chemicals (environmental and in the home and work place) but also a host of infectious agents, physical factors and maternal factors such as health conditions, genetic disorders and nutritional status. Questions about agent interactions and genetic susceptibility as well as dosage and exposure timing often arise. Thus the information is often complex, raising a host of psychological, educational, and communication problems which cannot be resolved inexpensively or briefly.

Any consideration of the problems such concerns engender identifies a wide range of issues to be addressed. A few observations are in order:

1) Integration of this information into the existing health care system seems highly desirable. The alternative would be unacceptably inefficient and expensive.

2) Follow-up on identified exposed pregnancies is essential to any proposed scientific utilization of information collected. Furthermore, without appropriate follow-up activities there can be no satisfactory quality assurance or evaluation of program effectiveness.

3) A unified authoritative information resource is highly desirable and could be effectively shared by many programs. This would reduce costs, duplication of efforts and improve the quality and accessibility of information.

4) Appropriate administrative mechanisms are needed at state and/or national levels. This could help to assure the development of adequate public policy, sufficient financing, and a rational process for the resolution of legal and ethical concerns.

5) Finally, it must be noted that education of both health care providers and the public is essential to the success of any such program. This must lead to a basic understanding of the health risk/benefit comparison process and should be sufficient to assure appropriate and timely access to information for decision-making.

CONCLUSIONS AND RECOMMENDATIONS

From the foregoing considerations it is obvious that there is clear indication of a need for and interest in improved access to reliable information on potentially teratogenic exposures. This need is currently unmet and developing systems are not yet adequate to this task. An orderly consideration of numerous issues will be necessary if this situation is to be remedied. Adequate program development will include consideration of several areas of public policy. These are summarized in Table 2.

TABLE 2. Areas of Public Policy for Consideration

1. Research Policy
   a. animal
   b. human

2. Health Services Policy
   a. public
   b. private

3. Education Policy
   a. public
   b. provider

4. Development of Comprehensive Strategy
   a. federal vs. state vs. private
   b. interagency coordination

Furthermore, a planned evaluation system is essential to assure that existing or new programs attain their objectives and meet the needs of health care providers, governmental officials, scientists and the general public.

Lastly, there is a clear need for national level interagency commitment and planning if these needs are to be met. A variety of agencies and groups including FDA, NIH, CDC and EPA as well as private and voluntary groups such as the pharmaceutical and chemical industries and the March of Dimes Birth Defects Foundation have a vested interest in assuring that such information is economically, reliably and comprehensively collected, analyzed and made accessible to those who need it.

REFERENCES

Allen EF, Hoyme HE (1986). The Vermont teratogen information network. Teratology 33:55c,

Biesecker BB, Feldman P, Weik L (1986). Clinical teratology programs in Wisconsin. Teratology 33:52c.

Brent RL, Jackson L (1985). The development of teratology hotline or teratology referral services: Their place in the medical care system. Teratology 31:40a.

Brown NA, Scialli AR (1986). REPROTOX: A computerized information system in reproductive toxicology. Teratology 33:50c.

Jones KL, Johnson KA, Aylor AR, Dick LM (1986). The California teratogen registry. Teratology 33:54c.

Manchester D, Pettersen B, Sujansky E, Capra J, Davis A, Golightly L, Wruk K, Rumack B (1986). Teratogen information system: Use of existing resources to contain costs. Teratology 33:51c.

Martinez LP, Gunderson SA, Carey JC, Kocherour NK, Emery MG, Stock C, McCormick M, Well T, Van Dyke PC (1986). Pregnancy risk line: Teratology information service for the state of Utah. Teratology 33:53c.

O'Brien J, Rosenwasser S, Feingold M (1986). Teratology information services: Preliminary analysis of data. Teratology 33:51c.

Pern J (1979). Decision-Making and Reproductive Choices. In Hsia YE, Hirschorn K, Silverberg RL, Goodmilow L (eds): "Counseling in Genetics," New York: Alan R. Liss, p. 223.

Peters, TWJ, Garbis JM (1986). The operation of the Dutch information center. Teratology 33:55c.

Public Affairs Forum of Teratogen Information Services in honor of Sergio Fabro (1986). Teratology 33:27c.

Quirk JG, Hill D, Kepper L, Char F, Brewster M, Butler B, Hawks F, Hale M, Mattison DR (1986). Teratology information and counseling in a rural state. Teratology 33:52c.

Shepard TH, Fantel AG, Mirkes PE, Nelson D (1986). Teratogen information service: 25 years of experience by the Central Laboratory for Human Embryology. Teratology 33:53c.

Shulman SA, Quinn DL, Cassidy SB (1986). Connecticut pregnancy exposure information service. Teratology 33:53c.

Vogt BL (1985). Coordination of clinical teratogen information programs. Teratology 31:40a.

Vogt BL, Librizzi RJ (1986). The pregnancy health line: Characteristics of callers, exposures and utilization. Teratology 33:51c.

VI. SUMMATION

Transplacental Effects on Fetal Health, pages 339–347

SUMMATION

Hugo W. Moser, M.D.

Kennedy Institute

707 N. Broadway, Baltimore, Maryland 21205

This symposium has brought together veterinary pathologists, virologists, geneticists, pediatricians and neuroscientists in order to examine transplacental effects on fetal health. The topic was selected because of its clinical and societal importance, awareness of recent strides in knowledge, and the need and potential for additional research in this field. The organizers of the symposium also recognized that advances have been achieved in a variety of separate disciplines, but that knowledge of these advances may not have crossed disciplinary barriers. The presentations and interchanges that took place at the symposium confirmed all these suppositions and indicate that they apply with even greater force than had been anticipated. In this summation I will begin with an overview of the individual presentations and will then highlight the major findings.

CONGENITAL VIRAL INFECTIONS IN MAN

Dr. John Sever lists 11 viral agents that cross the placenta and affect the fetus. The HIV virus of AIDS is transmitted to the child in 30 to 50% of pregnancies of infected mothers. Primary cytomegalovirus infections occur in about 2% of pregnant women, and 10% of congenitally infected children have reduced hearing and/or mental retardation. These two infectious agents alone highlight the importance of transplacentally transmitted viral agents as causes of handicapping conditions in children and adults. For most of the 11 viral infections transmission occurs across the placenta by the hematogenous route; however in some cases the infection ascends from the infected vagina, or the child is exposed at time of delivery. The most effective approach is to prevent the infection in the mother. For rubella this has been enormously effective: while in 1964-65 there were 20,000 children damaged by congenital rubella, in recent years there have been less than 10 cases a year.

CONGENITAL VIRAL INFECTION IN DOMESTIC ANIMALS

The next 4 presentations deal with viral infections in domestic animals and also examine important biological phenomena.

Dr. Bennie Osburn examines the factors which contribute to the large number of congenital infections in domestic animals. These include the lack of transplacental transfer of maternal immunoglobulins and the "leisurely" maturation of the immune system in the fetus, with several immune responses remaining underdeveloped until a short time before birth or even after birth. As also noted by other speakers, undifferentiated cells are favored sites for viral infection and replications, and this leads to malformations in the nervous, skeletal, urogenital and endocrine systems. "Immune tolerance" is another consequence of the late maturation of the immune system. When pestiviruses or bovine virus diarrhea viruses infect fetal calves before they develop immune competence to these viruses, the newborns remain persistently viremic and fail to develop immune responses to the virus. In contrast, fetuses infected after immune competence to the virus comes about develop an immune response that clears the infection.

James MacLachlan and Bennie Osburn examine the mechanism of the severe cavitating encephalopathy that accompanies congenital bluetongue virus infection in ruminants and mice. The severe malformation develops only in animals inoculated during the first half of gestation, and is dependent upon the presence of susceptible cell populations, that is, stem cell populations, within the ventricular and subventricular zones. The effect is the result of direct virus-mediated destruction of susceptible populations, and not secondary to vascular endothelial changes or interferon production.

Dr. Pohlenz and associates review the complex problems associated with congenital pestivirus disease (bovine virus diarrhea). Similar to congenital bluetongue virus, cerebral teratogenic effects in the fetus occur only when infection takes place at the time of organogenesis (100-150 days of gestation). Other important factors are the existence of cytopathogenic and noncytopathogenic strains and the previously cited phenomenon of immune tolerance. It is proposed that the sporadic severe disease, which may fatally affect 3 to 5% of a herd of cattle at 6 months to 2 years of age, takes place mainly in animals who became immunologically tolerant because of exposure to the non-cytopathogenic virus early in fetal life and then become unable to resist postnatal infection with the cytopathogenic strain.

Charles A. Anderson and associates examine the mechanism of hypomyelination that occurs in sheep congenitally infected with the border disease virus. They found hypomyelination even when virus was present only minimally in the nervous system. In contrast, they demonstrated extensive non-inflammatory non-cytolytic infection of the thyroid gland and a depression in circulating thyroid hormone levels. Since myelination is known to be retarded in hypothyroid states, these findings suggest that the nervous system effects of congenital border disease virus infection may be mediated through its effects on the thyroid gland.

CONGENITAL BACTERIAL AND OTHER INFECTIONS

Dr. Richard L. Naeye presents data which point to the importance of acute chorioamnionitis in respect to perinatal mortality and morbidity. Acute chorioamnionitis starts as an ascending infection that reaches the placental membranes through the cervical os. Bacteria and mycoplasma can be recovered in 70% of the cases and most often are single organisms with fastidious growth characteristics. A smear to search for the presence of polymorphonuclear leukocytes between the amnion and chorion is the most reliable diagnostic procedure. Acute chorioamnionitis frequently initiates labor, presumably secondary to release of phospholipase from leukocytes. This in turn leads to release of arachidonic acid with formation of prostaglandins that initiate labor. Through this mechanism acute chorioamnionitis causes premature labor with its consequent perinatal mortality and morbidity. Predisposing factors to chorioamnionitis include impaired maternal antimicrobial activity due to malnutrition and zinc deficiency. This factor is thought to be of great significance in developing countries. Coitus during pregnancy also appears to be a predisposing factor.

Dr. Patricia Quinn's studies emphasize the importance of mycoplasma infections in the fetus and newborn. Using sensitive culture techniques she demonstrated genital mycoplasma infections in 15-30% of newborns and in 38% of adult women who had had one sexual partner, and in 75% of those with 3 or more sexual partners. Mycoplasma infection was demonstrated in 60% of placentas that showed signs of inflammation. Dr. Quinn presented evidence for a role of mycoplasma in the causation of chorioamnionitis, premature labor and fetal lung disease. The antibiotics erythromycin and clindomycin have been shown to be effective against mycoplasma organisms. The provocative findings presented by Drs. Naeye and Quinn provide important new leads for the prevention of fetal mortality and morbidity.

Dr. David M. Judge provides a needed update on the pathogenesis of congenital syphilis. He notes that the frequency of this disease has increased again since 1983. Congenital syphilis is <u>not</u> a first trimester disease; its major manifestations occur during the third trimester. The appearance of the disease concomitant with the maturation of the immune system suggests that its pathogenesis is related to that response. Dr. Judge also notes that there is the likelihood that an increasing number of pregnant women will have combined infections with syphilis and the HIV virus. Because of the apparently central role of the immune response in the pathogenesis of congenital syphilis, it will be important to determine how the decreased immunocompetence of HIV infected mothers and fetuses alters the manifestations of congenital syphilis.

Drs. Fayer and Dubey review the complex series of events by which infection with protozoan parasite genus *Sarcocystis* causes abortion and fetal death. For the intensely studied sheep model it has been proposed that the initial event is at the level of the fetal hypothalamus, which eventually triggers release of steroids and prostaglandins from the placenta. While endocrine studies available so far do not provide support for such a mechanism, Fayer's recent *in vitro* studies suggest that

Sarcocystis lysates release tumor necrosis factor from macrophages. This is a significant observation since tumor necrosis factor can trigger the arachidonic acid cascade leading to prostaglandin release.

Antenatal malarial infections, an issue of prime importance in many parts of the world, are reviewed by Dr. Richard L. Naeye. A sharp distinction must be made between their occurrence in settings where the disease is endemic, and in those where they are not. In endemic settings most newborns have antibodies that passed the placenta from their mothers with the result that they are partially immune from birth and their first postnatal malarial attacks are mild. These findings stand in sharp contrast to epidemic malaria, i.e., situations where a poorly immune or non-immune population is suddenly exposed to the parasite. Poor pregnancy outcomes are associated particularly with epidemics of *P. falciparum*. The density of plasmodial parasites is usually greater in placental than maternal peripheral blood. The pathogenesis of fetal damage is in need of investigation. Rapid hemolysis, metabolic acidosis and a drop in placental blood flow may all be important contributory factors. Antimalarial treatment of non-immune mothers can protect the fetus, but the universal use of these medications is difficult to achieve. In addition, there is concern that maternal HIV infection may alter the degree to which maternal antibodies can protect the fetus in the previously protected populations in which malaria is endemic.

METABOLIC DRUG AND CHEMICAL TERATOGENS

Dr. Lewis B. Holmes presents a list of known human teratogens. These include 16 drugs, 2 heavy metals and 6 maternal conditions. He noted that this list is surprisingly small, and that this may well reflect methodological difficulties. He cited several important considerations which highlight these difficulties and presented several strategies that will help to overcome them.

The spectrum of potential effects of intrauterine exposure to teratogens is wide, and it is important to include surveillance for late effects, such as the increased frequency of insulin-dependent diabetes among individuals with congenital rubella syndrome.

A point of great importance is his admonition that epidemiological surveys must be targeted as specifically as is possible. For instance, a retrospective survey of the thalidomide epidemic in Sweden indicated that this would not have been detected if the survey had tabulated only the general category of "limb reduction deficits", but detection was achieved when the tabulation included more specific features. Detection of relatively low incidence teratogenic effects presents a difficult challenge. It requires long-term follow-up, maximum specification of the teratogenic abnormalities under suspicion, and whenever possible, observers who are blind to the exposure-status of the infants being examined.

Dr. Edward Lammer presents important data about a newly described human teratogen isotretinoin (13-cis-retinoic acid). He cites preliminary data on a prospectively identified cohort of 57 exposed pregnancies. There were 9 spontaneous abortions and 10 malformed live births. Characteristic facial, brain and cardiopulmonary malformations are traceable to adverse effects on cranial neural crest cells. Provocative preliminary studies about the biochemical mechanisms of these adverse effects are also presented.

Dr. Mary Lou Oster-Granite provides an overview of three critical periods of brain and nervous system development, namely neurulation; cell proliferation and migration; and cell differentiation and survival. She then examines effects of teratogenic agents within this context. For example, the _in utero_ effects of radiation are traced to the particular sensitivity of exponentially dividing cell populations; those of rubella virus due to depression of mitotic activity in chronically infected cells leading to organ hypocellularity; those of anticonvulsants to effects on folate metabolism through reduction of polyamine levels; and those of organic mercury and cadmium to limitation of energy metabolism as a result of their action on sulfhydryl groups of enzymes.

Dr. Harvey Levy provides an up-date on the problem of maternal phenylketonuria (PKU), i.e., intrauterine damage to the child of a phenylketonuric woman. It had been shown previously that 92% of children born to untreated "classic" PKU patients are mentally retarded. Levy reports encouraging new data which indicate that children born to mothers with milder forms of PKU (blood levels less than 600 micromolar) appear to escape brain damage, and that this is also true for children of "classic" PKU mothers who were placed on dietary therapy prior to conception. Levy also presents important new data on the pathogenesis of brain damage in maternal PKU. These data suggest that the brain damage is attributable to impaired brain protein synthesis secondary to reduced levels of free amino acids other than phenylalanine, and to polysome disaggregation.

Dr. Neil J. MacLusky provides insights about the far-reaching effects of intrauterine exposure to gonadal steroids. He reminds us that 2 million individuals were exposed prenatally to diethylstilbesterol (DES). This exposure resulted not only in an increased incidence of clear-cell adenocarcinoma of the vagina but also in subtle masculinization of certain aspects of central nervous system function. The existence of prenatal central nervous system effects of gonadal steroids is now firmly established. MacLusky emphasizes that they are subtle and complex and that studies in rodents and lower animals do not adequately reflect those that occur in human beings. An additional important observation is that gonadal activity and reproductive side-effects are produced by a variety of pharmacological agents and naturally occurring compounds. These include cimetidine, certain insecticides, antimycotic agents and phytoestrogens.

Drs. Carol K. Kellog and Ronnie Guillet summarize the large and evolving literature relating to developmental aspects of neural receptors for neuroactive drugs. These developmental profiles must be evaluated in terms of the stage of fetal development, nervous system region, and species. While the maturity of the fetus at birth varies among species, the developmental patterns show points of commonality, so that studies in animals do have relevance for man. Data available so far suggest that early developmental exposure to neuroactive drugs may have significant long-term effects and mandate great caution in the use of such medications during pregnancy.

Dr. Needleman's contribution provides carefully developed and evaluated evidence that relatively low level fetal lead exposure has a small but statistically significant effect on IQ scores at 12 and 24 months of age.

Dr. Needleman makes the generally applicable point that teratogens that cause clearly evident malformations at high dosage, at a lower dosage may be associated with effects that are discernible only in the behavioral sphere. Study of these behavioral effects requires precise measurements, long-term follow-up and elimination of confounding factors.

Dr. James E. Haddow and associates present data on an important new epidemiological tool - namely the use of plasma continine levels to provide quantitative data about the extent of nicotine exposure. With this biochemical marker they demonstrate a clear relationship between level of smoking and fetal death, and the birth weight of live-born children. While these relationships had been known to exist before, this new biochemical marker permits more precise epidemiological studies, and the evaluation of controversial issues, such as the role of passive smoking and low-level exposure.

The Conference closed with Dr. George Sack's discussion of the role of molecular biologic approaches to the diagnosis, therapy and study of prenatal defects. Molecular biology approaches, including the use of recently developed amplification techniques, will improve, and in some instances, revolutionize techniques of prenatal diagnosis. Molecular biology techniques are already being used to develop transgenic lines and valuable animal models of human genetic disease. Dr. Sack closed with a discussion of the potential and limitations of gene therapy, a topic of intense interest as a possible means of treating genetic disorders prenatally and postnatally.

CONCLUDING REMARKS

This meeting highlighted the overwhelming importance of transplacental influence for the health and well-being of man and animal species. The influences are wide-ranging and complex: ranging from infectious agents, to natural and man-made teratogens, and genetic disorders. Virtually all of these factors interact with cultural and socio-economic issues, particularly in developing countries. Transplacental influences are more widespread and pervasive than has been realized. There is need for more precise diagnostic techniques, and more widespread application of those that are presently available. Follow-up periods need to be extended to school age and even to adulthood, with greater emphasis on behavioral assessments. Finally, as noted so incisively by Drs. James Hanson and Elizabeth Thomson, there needs to be a reassessment of public policy in respect to risk assessment and management of transplacental hazards for the fetus. The authors note that if risk assessment information is to be of benefit, it must be "desired, understood, believed, remembered and accepted as having personal relevance". They also emphasize the need for improved access to reliable information on potentially teratogenic exposures. Fulfillment of this goal requires strengthening and improvement of interagency planning and cooperation. It is my fervent hope that this symposium represents a step toward the accomplishment of this goal.

Index